Feeding Challenges in Young Children

Feeding Challenges in Young Children
Strategies and Specialized Interventions for Success

by

Deborah A. Bruns, Ph.D.
Southern Illinois University, Carbondale

and

Stacy D. Thompson, Ph.D.
Southern Illinois University, Carbondale

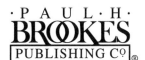

·P A U L·H·
BROOKES
PUBLISHING CO®

Baltimore • London • Sydney

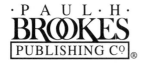

Paul H. Brookes Publishing Co., Inc.
Post Office Box 10624
Baltimore, Maryland 21285-0624
USA

www.brookespublishing.com

Typeset by BLPS Content Connections, Chilton, Wisconsin.
Manufactured in the United States of America by
Sheridan Books, Inc., Chelsea, Michigan.

The publisher and the authors have made every effort to ensure that all of the information and instructions given in this book are accurate and safe, but they cannot accept liability for any resulting injury, damage, or loss to either person or property, whether direct or consequential and however it occurs. Medical advice should only be provided under the direction of a qualified health care professional.

The vignettes presented in this book are composite accounts that do not represent the lives or experiences of specific individuals, and no implications should be inferred. In all instances, names and identifying details have been changed to protect confidentiality.

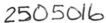

Library of Congress Cataloging-in-Publication Data

Feeding challenges in young children : strategies and specialized intervention for success / written by Deborah A. Bruns and Stacy D. Thompson.
   p.   cm.
Includes bibliographical references and index.
   ISBN-13: 978-1-59857-121-9 (paper w/cd in back)
   ISBN-10: 1-59857-121-4 (paper w/cd in back)
   1. Children—Nutrition.   2. Diet therapy for children.   3. Children—Nutrition—Psychological aspects.
I. Bruns, Deborah A. (Deborah Andrea)   II. Thompson, Stacy D.

RJ206.F416 2012

618.92—dc23   2012004344

British Library Cataloguing in Publication data are available from the British Library.

2016   2015   2014   2013   2012

10   9   8   7   6   5   4   3   2   1

Contents

I   Foundations

II   Feeding Process

III   Strategies and Specialized Interventions

Contents of the Accompanying CD-ROM

Appendix E

Breastfeeding

Developing Feeding Plans

Enteral Feeding

Feeding Strategies and Specialized Interventions

Feeding Team Requirements

Mealtime Considerations

Meeting Sensory Needs

Positioning Strategies and Equipment

Specialized Bottles, Utensils, Bowls, Plates, and Cups

Swallowing Disorders

About the Authors
End User License Agreement

About the Authors

Deborah A. Bruns, Ph.D., is Associate Professor in the Department of Educational Psychology and Special Education at Southern Illinois University in Carbondale, specializing in early intervention. She serves on the editorial boards of the *Journal of Early Intervention, Early Childhood Research & Practice, Neonatal Network,* and *Young Exceptional Children*. Dr. Bruns is active at the state and national levels in the Division for Early Childhood. She is also a member of the National Association for the Education of Young Children. Dr. Bruns' research interests include play-based assessment as a teaching tool, examining feeding development of young children with and without disabilities, and parent-professional relationships in early intervention. She is also Principal Investigator of the Tracking Rare Incidence Syndromes project, which raises awareness of outcomes for children with genetic conditions such as trisomy 18 (Edward syndrome) and trisomy 13 (Patau syndrome).

Stacy D. Thompson, Ph.D., is Associate Professor in the Department of Curriculum and Instruction at Southern Illinois University in Carbondale, specializing in child development. Dr. Thompson is a member of the Society for Research on Child Development, the Division for Early Childhood, and the National Council on Family Relations. She served as vice president and president for the Oklahoma Family Resource Coalition. Dr. Thompson's research interests include feeding and interventions for families and caregivers, risk-taking behaviors in adolescence, fathers of infants born to adolescent mothers, and quality care for young children.

Foreword

The degree to which babies and young children are developing physically, emotionally, and cognitively depends, to a large extent, on their nutritional intake and eating habits. As a young mother of an infant daughter with gastroesphogeal reflux, I watched with great concern as her weight slipped from the 50th percentile to the 20th percentile in a matter of months. We were living far from extended family at the time and whenever I mentioned my concern during phone calls to my mother, she assured me that "babies just spit up a lot." The nurse at the doctor's office said the same thing. My mother's opinion of the problem changed when she came for a visit and watched my daughter vomit after breastfeeding! We scheduled a visit to the doctor and what followed were uncomfortable tests and anxiety for all. Thankfully, the issue resolved itself by the time she was about 8 months old and she's now a mother of a toddler with a nut allergy. We are all learning about the lifestyle changes which we need to make to make sure my granddaughter never has another anaphylactic reaction like the one she had when she ate a little bit of peanut butter off of a spoon. (Luckily, she never had any problems with reflux!)

I share this story to reinforce the authors' assertion of the importance of feeding and nutrition, not only to a child's health and development, but to the healthy functioning of families as well. My husband and I became very tense whenever she was nursing, certain that she was going to vomit up everything she had consumed. She was irritable and cranky because she was not getting enough to eat. Bruns and Thompson emphasize the degree to which nutritional intake and healthy eating habits affects overall family functioning—I could not agree more! Not only did her medical problem cause insufficient weight gain, it caused stress for all us which influenced our abilities to provide the supportive, loving environment that she needed.

Of course, my story is trivial compared to the struggles that many families face when their children have feeding difficulties. This is evident in the comprehensive treatment of this issue by Bruns and Thompson. The table of contents reflects a book that will serve as an important reference for all who work with young children, for those whose development is typical, and for infants and children with special needs. This book provides important theoretical information, as well as practical strategies, that parents, teachers, and therapists can use to support children's healthy eating.

I would suspect that in a very short time, this book will be on the bookshelf of many childcare providers and early childhood teachers who provide meals and snacks to young children in their care. Not only does it provide important information about supporting effective eating habits for young children, it also provides critical resources about how professionals can work together to support successful feeding and mealtimes. It will be on my bookshelf and will be an important resource as I work with preservice early intervention (EI) specialists and early childhood special education (ECSE) teachers who will one day work with young children who have disabilities and possible feeding issues. I am certain that it will also be an important resource for parents of young children, both typically developing and those who have special needs. In short, this is an important book for the field.

In addition to the comprehensive scope of the book, it is organized in a way to make sure that the information is accessible and useable by a wide variety of audiences. Vignettes, personal experiences, and examples provide context for readers and enable them to engage in meaningful discussion and dialogue about the topics reflected in the table of contents. It was not until I was asked to write this foreword and review the table of contents and accompanying text, that I became aware of the need for this book. However, once I became familiar with the scope and goals of the text, I quickly became aware of just how needed this book is to the field and what a helpful resource it will provide anyone who works with or on behalf of young children and their families. In addition to the comprehensive text, the appendixes provide a range of very useful and practical resources including developmental milestones, feeding protocols, data sheets, and specialized materials and objects.

In sum, Bruns and Thompson provide a great service to the early childhood community through the publication of this book. At a time when information abounds from a variety of sources, this book will provide a solid reference of evidence-based practices that help adults support young children's optimal feeding development.

Laurie A. Dinnebeil, Ph.D.
Author, A Guide to Itinerant Early Childhood Special Education Services

Foreword

Feeding children is one of the most important things a parent or provider does multiple times a day. On the surface it looks like a simple task. An infant cries, a parent feeds the child; the child stops crying, repeat. However, any parent or caregiver will tell you it is not that easy. The feeding and care of young children is not always trouble free because children have different demands as they grow and develop, parents have different styles in feeding their children, and challenges can present themselves when a child has special needs or a parent has limited experience caring for young children. Bruns and Thompson tackle all of these thorny issues in this important volume.

Bruns and Thompson set the stage by recognizing that feeding is a developmental process between the child and provider. Sometimes the provider is a parent, sometimes the provider is a child care worker, and sometimes the provider may be a grandparent or sibling. Food is at the center of many social interactions. For young children, the back and forth exchange during early feeding helps to cement close relationships crucial for social development. As children are able to take part in family mealtimes they engage in routines that provide predictability and order to their daily lives, learn rules of social interaction, and begin to communicate as part of the larger group. These interactions then lay the foundation for regulating health and well-being later in childhood.

Bruns and Thompson point out important variations in feeding practices and mealtime routines. Cultural heritage certainly plays a role. Traditional dishes are passed down from one generation to the next, providing a sense of continuity to countries of origin as well as to relatives who came before us. There are also variations by parenting experience. The ways in which an adolescent mom may approach feeding her young infant may be very different than an experienced mother of three.

Why is this important? We know that good nutrition is important for children's physical health and brain development. We are also beginning to appreciate that how children are fed in the early years may have important consequences for their social and emotional development in later childhood and adolescence. While the obesity epidemic has raised awareness of poor nutritional habits, we are also aware that poor feeding practices and lack of regular family mealtimes places children at risk for poor school performance, mental health problems, and other physical health problems.

Bruns and Thompson have provided an easy-to-read and accessible guide for parents and practitioners. The activity-based interventions recognize that real families need real solutions. This volume opens opportunities where food and family can be connected in positive ways to promote resiliency during challenging times. Kudos are extended to Bruns and Thompson who offer a full course sampling of the complexities of feeding children and positive ways to approach one of the most important activities of the day.

Barbara H. Fiese, Ph.D.
Author, Family Routines and Rituals

Preface

"Why can't he keep his formula down?"

"He needs to eat more vegetables and fruit. All he wants is bread and cheese."

"He eats bananas, strawberries, and peaches at home, but he won't eat them at
child care or when we're out."

"She has low tone in her mouth and can't move her tongue very well. It's difficult
to feed her, no matter what I try. I tried a new cup and that was a disaster."

"I can't keep her attention long enough for her to finish a meal."

"I thought he would drink from a cup by now but he'll have nothing to do with it."

"Why does he only eat jelly sandwiches and gag on everything else?"

"I've worked with her to search for food using a spoon but she only wants to use
her hands to find food on her plate."

These comments are examples of feeding-related concerns heard from parents,
caregivers, early childhood practitioners, and professionals working with young
children. They also reflect some experiences the authors have had with young children they have worked with, as well as their own sons and daughters. Feeding is
a critical part of a young child's development. Learning to self-feed, for example,
offers opportunities for the acquisition and use of new fine-motor and cognitive
skills (e.g., eye-hand coordination and sequencing, respectively). In addition, feeding times offer social interaction between the infant and toddler's parent or other
caregivers, which include childcare providers and classroom teachers.

The context of feeding development should be examined within theoretical
models to better understand contextual factors influencing oral intake, parent–child
feeding interactions, and behavior issues related to feeding or during feedings. For
example, the family systems theory describes families as "interactive, interdependent, and reactive" (Seligman & Darling, 2007, p. 17) with each subsystem within
a family being influenced by and influencing other subsystems (Turnbull, Erwin,
Turnbull, Soodak, & Shogren, 2010). Sometimes a young child's feeding difficulties
affect all family members. For example, a 3-year-old with autism refuses all fruits,
vegetables, and meats. His limited diet directly affects his parents as they argue over
how to address his selectivity. His limited diet also affects his older brother who
dislikes mealtimes because of the stressful atmosphere.

A young child's nutritional intake is closely tied to his or her development
and growth, which further highlights the need to closely examine typical feeding development and be aware of the "red flags" or warning signs of feeding

problems, such as extended mealtimes, texture avoidance, and food sensitivities. Knowledge of feeding difficulties for infants, toddlers, and preschoolers with and without developmental delays or disabilities can positively influence the selection of appropriate strategies and specialized interventions to address them.

It is surprising that this critical area of development receives scant attention in the child development (CD), early childhood education (ECE), and early intervention/ early childhood special education (EI/ECSE) literature. The information that is available either emphasizes broad applications, examination of general problems, or very specialized interventions. Other disciplines address feeding (e.g., speech-language pathology [SLP], occupational therapy [OT], nutrition), but much of the available literature is limited with regard to modifying day-to-day feeding experiences or providing practical information from a developmental perspective.

Parents, caregivers, early childhood practitioners, and professionals from related disciplines seek strategies to effectively work with infants, toddlers, and preschoolers in a range of settings and at varying points in feeding development. There is also a need to address a range of feeding difficulties including oral-motor problems, cleft palate, and sensory-based issues (e.g., Arvedson, 2008; Bruns & Thompson, 2010). This book offers guidance and practical strategies and interventions to address these areas within the context of evidence-based practice. Buysse and Wesley (2006) stated that evidence-based practice "represents a process by which parents and professionals can make practical decisions that are tailored to the needs and priorities of individual children, families, and programs" (p. 6) and "viewed as a process that integrates empirical evidence, experience, and values to inform decisions about policies, services, supports, or instructions for young children and their families and the personnel who serve them" (p. 36). The authors emphasized how evidence-based practice can be utilized by early childhood professionals to address a range of applied situations.

Goal and Scope

This book offers readers a comprehensive examination of 1) feeding development milestones for children from birth to age 5, theoretical frameworks, models of feeding interactions, and cultural considerations; 2) detailed information about the feeding process (assessment, planning, and progress monitoring); 3) general strategies, special groups, and interventions including young children with anatomical anomalies (e.g., cleft palate), as well as those needing tube feedings and specialized feeding techniques; and 4) recommendations and conclusions. In addition, there are vignettes, personal experiences, examples, and resources for supplemental information ("Food for Thought," "Table Talk," and "Feeding Nuggets"). These materials are included to encourage discussion as well as to add a "real-life" perspective to chapter content. Appendixes are included with a variety of applied materials to draw on by preservice students and professionals in disciplines including CD, EC and EI/ECSE, SLP, and OT. These materials are intended for individuals who work with both typically developing infants and toddlers, and young children with developmental delays or diagnosed disabilities. They are also intended for other audiences including teachers, those working in child care centers, and home-based child care providers.

Uses

This book is first and foremost a teaching and professional development tool intended for a broad audience encompassing preservice and inservice professionals in CD, EC, EI/ECSE, and related disciplines. Feeding is typically not a focus in coursework or workshops, yet practitioners and professionals are routinely involved in planning and providing snacks and mealtimes to young children. Parents and caregivers also may have questions or concerns about feeding that are not addressed because feeding is typically not a large instructional focus or area of remediation in early childhood programs. The theoretical and developmental frameworks are not the focus of instruction in preparation programs or professional development opportunities.

It becomes necessary to be knowledgeable about the breadth and depth of available feeding-related adaptations, general strategies, and specialized interventions. Program and agency administrators also will find the information helpful for daily programming as well as staff development and training activities. Parents, family members, and caregivers can gain knowledge and strategies to better meet the feeding needs of young children in their care. The applications described in this book provide a range of techniques and methods that can be implemented with young children with feeding difficulties. The strategies also provide a range of factors affecting feeding development, such as sensory processing and parent–child interaction. Finally, empirically proven interventions are necessary to inform practice (Buysse & Wesley, 2006).

Additionally, this book is intended for professionals in related disciplines who are part of young children's feeding teams, including SLPs, OTs, physical therapists, dietitians, social workers, and neonatal and pediatric nurses. As previously mentioned, the responsibilities of these individuals may not focus exclusively on oral intake, but feeding difficulties or concerns are often among the areas requiring their services.

It is anticipated that feeding team members will share information in this book with families and caregivers. We feel that the scope of information necessary for practitioners to effectively address feeding development and difficulties is sizable. Therefore, it becomes critical to have a reliable and complete resource. The book is meant to accomplish this purpose.

We invite you to sample specific chapters or all of the materials to increase your understanding and to find practical strategies and specialized interventions in this critical developmental area.

Acknowledgments

We would like to acknowledge all of the individuals who gave their time in a variety of ways to help us prepare this book. Our passion for this book is due to all of the children and families that we worked with when we did not have a resource like this. We wanted to provide information to help, families, caregivers, early childhood practitioners, and professionals who address feeding issues on a daily basis.

We had a wonderful team of students who worked with us over 2 years—affectionately called "The Feeding Team." For helping us locate literature, going to classrooms to take photos, finding chapter resources, and sharing their experiences, we thank Jessica Clayton, Kelly Bault, Evelyn Barrientos-Perkins, Julia Irwin, Jessica Sanchez, and Katlin Chumbley. We also thank all of the students who submitted their feeding experiences to us in our respective courses.

There are several teachers and child care professionals to whom we would like to express our gratitude for their input and for allowing us entrance into their classrooms to observe mealtimes. Robyn Rogers is an early childhood special education teacher like no other. She has worked with so many children with feeding challenges and found strategies and materials to address each unique one. Thank you for sharing your expertise and homemade adaptations. Melanie Hamilton showed us several novel approaches to encourage feeding in young children with autism. Nicole Zavala welcomed us into her child care classroom and encouraged parents to share their feeding stories. Special thanks for Lori Van Horn and the staff, children, and parents of Southern Illinois University's Child Development Laboratories. We enjoyed spending time with the children in all of these settings as they helped us make progress with this book.

There are also many parents to thank who shared their children with us in their homes and who shared their feeding stories. We especially want to express our thanks to Laura Bishop, Jacki Ruebke, Morgan Chitiyo, and their children. Special thanks are also extended to parents from the Tracking Rare Incidence Syndromes project for sharing their children's unique feeding experiences, especially Carolyn Cockburn, Marie Donaldson, Kelly Freeze, Penny Victor, and Jude Wolpert. We also want to thank our own children for a limitless array of anecdotal feeding stories and for reminding us of our own childhood feeding experiences.

We are grateful for input from experts who provided feedback on early versions of chapters including Maureen Flanagan, Valerie Boyer, and Gail Durkota. We are also indebted to authors—notably William Crist and Anne Napier-Phillips, Winnie Dunn, Corinna Jacobi and colleagues, Colleen Lukens, Thomas Linscheid, and Sheena Reilly and colleagues. They shared their assessment instruments with us through personal contact and published materials, and collectively, they broadened our understanding of the interrelated areas of feeding development, assessment, and intervention.

Last, and definitely not least, we are indebted to the wonderful individuals we've worked with at Brookes Publishing. Johanna Cantler believed in us and the importance of this book from the very beginning. She was always available by e-mail, cell phone, and for the occasional dinner when schedules allowed. Julie Chavez helped us get started and worked to keep us on track. The marketing and production teams have also worked with us to develop our vision for our book.

To my husband, Bill, for supporting me throughout this process, and to my children, Marlie and Will, for supplying inspiration in so many ways. Finally, I dedicate this book to the children I worked with when I was in the classroom; they taught me the importance of feeding as a means to facilitate development.

Debbie

I am grateful to my family, Steve, Gabriel, Karalyn, and Shayla, for their enduring support, patience and creative motivation and to my parents for their suggestions, feedback, and guidance. This book is dedicated to them and to all the professionals, parents, and children who asked challenging questions about feeding.

Stacy

Foundations

INTRODUCTION

"The implicit (and sometimes explicit) ethnocentrism that underlies much of the pediatric, nutritional, and psychological literature on infant feeding results in findings that apply only to middle-class Anglo-Americans and yet are written as though they refer to 'human development' or 'human behavior.'"

(Dettwyler & Fishman, 1992, p. 172)

Section I discusses the foundations related to feeding development, aspects of feeding risk, and the corresponding strategies and specialized interventions that address feeding difficulties.

Chapter 1 discusses feeding milestones. It describes the progression in feeding development, including breastfeeding and bottle feeding, the introduction of solid foods, and the development of healthy eating habits. In addition, "red flags" related to feeding development are discussed in order to convey the depth and breadth of possible feeding difficulties.

Chapter 2 introduces a number of theoretical frameworks, including attachment, family systems, social cognitive, and bioecological theories to better elucidate the direct and indirect impact of relationships on feeding development.

Chapter 3 focuses on feeding interactions. The chapter examines feeding opportunities between young children and their parents, family members, and caregivers in a variety of child care settings.

Chapter 4 delves into many aspects of diversity that influence feeding. It includes a cross-cultural overview of choices that parents make for children during the first year and a description of each culture's mealtimes. The chapter also discusses at risk groups, such as families in poverty and parents with limited knowledge of feeding development (e.g., adolescent parents). Several of the chapters in this section include "Feeding Nuggets" which offer a listing of resources such as topic-specific books and web sites.

1

Feeding Development

What You'll Learn in This Chapter

This chapter provides

- An overview of feeding milestones for typically developing children
- An overview of the progression of feeding development and related research
- Red flags that may indicate feeding problems

■ ■ ■ FOOD FOR THOUGHT ■ ■ ■

"We had a hard time feeding our newborn, Mallory. We struggled to find a formula that would settle in her tummy. We tried Similac, and she became constipated. Soy milk never filled her. When she reached 2 months, the doctor said to try some cereal. I mixed it very thin but fed it to her using a spoon. This helped her get full and not have stomach issues."

Kathy, Parent

"My 2-month-old daughter eats about every 4 hours. Around the time she usually eats, she becomes fussy. I mixed her water and formula. I sat on the couch with her in my arms. I gave her the bottle. She ate 2 ounces while I sang 'You Are My Sunshine.' After she finished the 2 ounces, I sat her on my chest and lightly patted her back. She let out a quiet burp. Then I began feeding her again. After 1 ounce, she fell asleep."

Lisa, Parent

The previous examples are snapshots of typical feeding development; this chapter's focus. The chapter describes typical feeding milestones, as well as other developmental milestones that happen in synchrony with feeding milestones. The feeding development of young children is a complex process, and a full understanding of this process must include an awareness of both physiological development and cultural issues, which often underlie the development of food preferences. As more is learned about various influences on young childrens' eating and feeding, better strategies can be developed to help solve feeding issues and to encourage acceptance of a variety of foods and textures (Mennella, Nickbus, Jagolino, & Yourshaw, 2008).

TYPICAL FEEDING DEVELOPMENT

The feeding development of most young children progresses in the same sequence, beginning with an all-liquid diet and progressing to a diet that includes both liquids and solids. The transition to solids includes acceptance of semisolid foods (such as infant cereals mixed with formula, breast milk, or water), then chewy foods, and finally (when children have the ability to bite, chew, and swallow) crunchy foods. Toddlers demonstrate food preferences at approximately 18 months, with some children accepting only limited foods for several months to a year (Chatoor & Macaoay, 2008). By age 2, most typically developing children have eating abilities similar to those of adults, although some foods continue to pose a choking hazard and others (such as nuts and honey) present allergic reactions and health issues. Handouts listing typical feeding milestones for infants and toddlers are available in Appendix 1.

Feeding Milestones

Each infant proceeds through a predictable and invariable progression of feeding milestones (see Table 1.1). Most parents receive information from their pediatricians concerning when to start solids and how to introduce new foods, but parents rarely receive information regarding the way that certain foods or aspects (such as textures) may affect the infant's feeding abilities. Educating parents about feeding milestones and issues that might arise improves feeding interactions with their infants.

Suckling   From birth to about 4 months of age, infants have strong oral reflexes for suckling and swallowing, and they should be solely breastfed and/ or bottle-fed. Because gravity helps to move liquids down to the stomach, infants should be held at about a 45-degree angle during feeding (Marrs, 2004–2011).

Sucking   At about 4 months to 6 months of age, infants begin sucking; they are no longer only suckling. The action involved in drinking from a bottle or breast-feeding is becoming less automatic and more voluntary, and a cup may be introduced at about 6 months of age. Many infants also are introduced to soft solid foods, such as cereals and puréed fruits and vegetables. When first introduced, these foods are usually very runny, and the child will mostly be drinking the food as opposed to chewing it.

Table 1.1. Key feeding milestones

Feeding skill	Typical age of onset	Behavioral indicators
Accepts fluids (breast or bottle)	Birth	Coordinates the suck–swallow–breathe reflex
Begins solids	4–6 months	Mouths objects Uses tongue to move foods to back of mouth Pats bottle cleans spoon and swallows pureed foods
Self-feeding from bottle	6 months	Holds bottle independently
Demonstrates some independence in self-feeding	1–2 years	Scoops and brings spoon to mouth with little spillage Brings food to mouth with spillage Holds cup by handle(s) and brings to mouth
Chews foods	16–18 months	Bites down on solids, closes lips, and chews Moves food in mouth to assist with chewing
Demonstrates food preferences	18 months–2 years	Predisposition to being selective or fearful of new foods
Distinguishes between edible and nonedible items	18 months–2 years	Puts food into mouth Does not attempt to ingest nonedible items
Eats wide range of solid foods	2–3 years	Bites, chews, and swallows Accepts textured foods
Feeds self with little spillage	3–4 years	Independent feeding

To prevent choking, infants must reach specific milestones before they are offered solid foods. Infants are developmentally ready for solids when they can hold up their head and neck, can sit upright with support, and appear to be interested in foods that others are eating. Once they reach these milestones, infants can manage thicker purées, such as banana and avocado. Forestell and Mennella (2008) found that infants are more likely to accept new foods if they are introduced slowly, with a new food being offered every 8 or 9 days instead of every 4 or 5 days. Caregivers should pay attention to both the texture and the thickness of new foods. Some infants may reject a particular food because they are sensitive to textures or thicknesses rather than because they dislike the taste of the food.

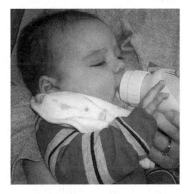

1.1 Infant sucking

Munching   Between 6 and 9 months of age, infants begin to open their mouths in anticipation of the spoon entering. They use small, rhythmic, up-and-down movements of the jaw and side-to-side movement of tongue to move food back to the molars and then to the front of the mouth. Infants at this stage can use their upper lip to clean food off the spoon, and they can manage dissolvable soft foods like graham crackers and Cheerios, as well as ground or lumpy solids such as stewed

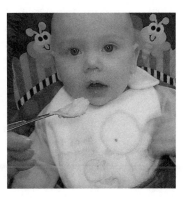

1.2 Infant opening mouth in anticipation

vegetables. At about 9 months of age, infants can drink from a straw. Also around 9 months, finger foods can be offered, giving the child practice handling food. Young children enjoy foods that dissolve in their mouths, and they take pleasure in foods, that they can squeeze between their fingers or onto another surface, such as peas (Morris & Klein, 2000).

Biting Between the ages of 9 and 12 months, an infant accepts mashed or chopped table foods with noticeable lumps. This presents a sensory change as foods change from smooth to lumpy. Although breastfeeding or bottle feeding may continue in the morning and/or at bedtime, infants begin to take most of their liquids from a cup during the day. At this age, an infant's tongue may protrude under the cup in order to add stability, and infants are likely to grab at the spoon when they are being fed. They can pick up items with a pincer grasp, so small bits of finger food, such as soft meat, pasta, cereal, and well-cooked vegetables, are an appealing addition to mealtimes. At 12 months, most infants have a controlled, sustained bite and are able to bite through cookies—hard or soft, depending on the presence of teeth.

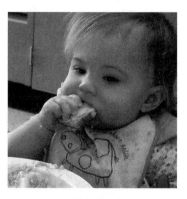

1.3 Biting bread

Chewing From about 13–15 months of age, children develop more control over their lips and tongue. The jaw is capable of grinding movement, and the rotary/diagonal movement of the tongue assists in breaking up and grinding meats. Toddlers will playfully bite on the spoon and may begin to bite on cups while drinking. They have improved their biting skills and are better able to use a controlled bite. Most infants at this age prefer to drink from a straw or regular cup instead of a bottle. At 16–18 months, toddlers can be given foods that require more chewing, such as meats and many vegetables. By 18 months, most toddlers can chew with their lips closed, keeping food from falling out of their mouths. Even when their lips are open while eating and drinking, they should not lose a significant amount of food or liquid. At 19–24 months, the toddler is getting better at drinking from a cup with little to no spillage and is less likely to bite the cup.

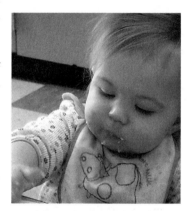

1.4 Chewing with closed mouth

Adult Feeding Pattern By the age of 2 years, children have learned all the skills they need to manage every type of food. However, they continue to fine-tune these skills over the

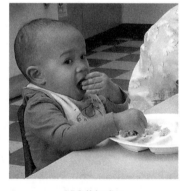

1.5 Self-feeding

next few years. A 2 year old is very busy, always moving and playing. Therefore, it is very important that caregivers realize that foods can be a choking hazard and take appropriate precautions. Foods given to a toddler should be smaller than the child's windpipe, and foods that pose a choking hazard—such as grapes and hot dogs—should be cut into small pieces to avoid danger. Having children sit down to eat also decreases the danger of choking.

As they move past these developmental milestones, toddlers become able to safely eat a wide range of foods to meet their nutritional needs, eventually learning to use utensils and feed themselves. These are skills they will further refine with practice and developmental maturity.

Oral-Motor Development

In order to further understand typical feeding development, it helps to understand the process of oral-motor development. The term *oral-motor development* refers to the child's abilities to maneuver his or her tongue and mouth. Table 1.2 shows levels of oral development (as indicated by tongue movements), along with the feeding techniques and appropriate foods for each stage.

All infants need sensory experiences to develop properly. If an infant is not given foods that meet his or her oral-motor developmental needs, he or she may chew on a parent's fingers or seek foods with more texture. For example, a child who has been given pieces of meat of various sizes may choose larger pieces, seemingly seeking more oral stimulation. Ramming, Kyger, and Thompson (2005) discuss the importance of meeting a child's oral-motor needs to prevent biting. This view challenges the widely accepted idea that aggression motivates biting. Anecdotal evidence demonstrates that children bite less if their oral-motor needs are met with foods that provide stimulating oral experiences. For example, if children eat bacon for breakfast rather than oatmeal, or if they have fruit chews available to munch on, they may bite less than they would otherwise.

THE PROGRESSION OF FEEDING

One of the first decisions that new parents make is whether to breastfeed or bottle feed their infant. Although this seems, on the surface, to be a simple choice, either option brings with it a number of issues. The following sections review the research related to various feeding decisions that parents make.

Breastfeeding

During the first few months of life, breast milk is a complete infant food, meeting all of the infant's nutritional needs. Breastfeeding also has an impact on later

Table 1.2. Oral-motor development, feeding techniques, and types of foods

Oral-motor tongue movements	Feeding method	Types of foods
Anterior and posterior	Nipple	Liquid: breast milk, formula, juice, and water
Up and down	Spoon	Puréed: oatmeal, and mashed foods with some lumps
Side to side	Finger foods	Soft: cooked vegetables, breads, and cheese
Diagonal	Self-feeding	Hard: raw vegetables, toast, and bagels
		Chewy: dried fruits and vegetables, meat

food preferences (Birch & Dietz, 2008) and can influence a child's growth and metabolism. Most health authorities, including the American Academy of Pediatrics, recommend breastfeeding until the child reaches 1 year of age, with exclusive breastfeeding (no solids) from birth to 6 months of age (American Academy of Pediatrics, 2005; Gartner et al., 2005).

A mother's decision to breastfeed is based on factors such as knowledge about breastfeeding, family history (whether family members breastfed), partner support (Shaker et al., 2004), and whether pain is involved (Wambach & Koehn, 2004). Of new mothers, 75% initiate breastfeeding (Centers for Disease Control, 2010). The number of mothers who exclusively breastfeed until starting solids and who continue to breastfeed following the introduction of solids is increasing. However, rates of breastfeeding among low-income mothers and minorities is below the national average (see Table 1.3 for breastfeeding rates by race/ethnicity, age, and education).

Healthy People 2010 set goals for breastfeeding as 75% at birth, 50% at 6 months, and 25% at 1 year. The National Immunization Survey (2005) found 73% of children were breastfed at some point, 39% were breastfed at 6 months, and 20% were breastfed at 1 year (http://www.cdc.gov/breastfeeding/data/NIS_data/data_2005.htm).

Women are more likely to breastfeed if they are older, affluent, educated, and health conscious. They are also more likely to breastfeed if they have positive attitudes toward breastfeeding and knowledge about the health and nutritional benefits of breast milk (Shaker et al., 2004). Women are less likely to breastfeed if they are younger (under 25 years of age), less affluent, less educated, employed full time outside of the home, African American, and unmarried (Grummer-Strawn & Shealy, 2009; Merewood et al., 2007).

Benefits of Breastfeeding   The benefits of breastfeeding are numerous and wide-ranging. These benefits are well-documented and continuously researched as part of the National Immunization Survey (2004–2008) as well as other studies. Benefits of breastfeeding for the infant include a decreased incidence and/or severity of a wide range of infectious diseases (Heinig, 2001; Howie, Forsyth, Ogston, Clark, & Florey, 1990). See Table 1.4 for a more specific listing of health benefits related to breastfeeding.

Breastfeeding has also been linked to better developmental outcomes. Specifically, studies have suggested that breastfed infants have improved attachment and cognitive development outcomes (Anderson, Johnstone, & Remley, 1999; Britton, Britton, & Gronwaldt, 2006; Kramer et al., 2008). Smith and Ellwood (2011) examined some of the mechanisms related to breastfeeding that might enhance attachment and cognitive development in infants. They noted that breastfeeding mothers spent substantially more time in "emotional" caring for their infants compared with mothers who chose to bottle feed.

According to Labbok (2001), and others as indicated in this section, there are several short and long-term benefits for mothers who breastfeed:

- Decreased postpartum bleeding and more rapid shrinking of the uterus to pre-pregnancy size (Chua, Arulkumaran, Lim, Selamat, & Ratnam, 1994)

- An earlier return to pre-pregnancy weight (Dewey, Heinig, & Nommsen, 1993)

- Decreased blood loss during menstruation and increased space between children due to lactational amenorrhea (Kennedy, Labbok, & Van Look, 1996)

Table 1.3. Breast-feeding rates by race/ethnicity, age, and education

Race/ethnicity	Ever Breastfed (%)	Breastfeeding at 6 months (%)	Breastfeeding at 12 months (%)
American Indian/Alaska Native	73.8	42.4	20.7
Asian/Pacific Islander	83.0	56.4	32.8
Hispanic/Latino	80.6	46.0	24.7
African American/Non-Hispanic Black	58.1	27.5	12.5
White/Non-Hispanic	76.2	44.7	23.3
Age by race/ethnicity			
Under 20 years			
Non-Hispanic White			40.0
Non-Hispanic Black			30.0
Mexican American			66.0
20–29 years			
Non-Hispanic White			65.0
Non-Hispanic Black			44.0
Mexican American			75.0
30 years or older			
Non-Hispanic White			77.0
Non-Hispanic Black			56.0
Mexican American			76.0
Education			
Not a high school graduate	67.0	37.0	21.9
High school graduate	66.1	31.4	15.1
Some college	76.5	41.0	20.5
College graduate	88.3	59.9	31.1

Adapted from "Racial and Ethnic Differences in Breastfeeding Initiation and Duration, by State," by the Centers for Disease Control. *National Immunization Survey Morbidity and Mortality Weekly Report (MMWR).* © 2010 by the Centers for Disease Control.

- A decreased risk of breast cancer (Collaborative Group on Hormonal Factors in Breast Cancer, 2002; Jernstrom et al., 2004; Lee, Kim, Kim, Song, & Yoon, 2003)
- A decreased risk of ovarian cancer (Rosenblatt & Thomas, 1993)
- More convenience and less expense

Other breastfeeding benefits are not as well known. Mothers who breastfeed expose their infants to flavors that prime them to more willingly accept new foods as toddlers and young children (Forestell & Mennella, 2008). Children fed formula are not exposed to these varied flavor experiences (Birch & Dietz, 2008). Breastfeeding provides a "flavor bridge" to promote the acceptance of solid foods later on. Mennella and Beauchamp (1991) found that infants whose mothers took a garlic or vanilla supplement fed significantly longer than those whose mothers did not take the supplement. Very early on, infants are aware of the flavors transmitted in breast milk, and they are reminded again of these flavors when they begin eating solids. These positive effects can be seen at 7 years of age, when children who were breastfed were less likely to be as picky in their eating habits as those who were fed formula (Addessi, Galloway, Visalberghi, & Birch, 2005). Furthermore, compared with bottle feeding, breastfeeding may provide a modest protective effect in later growth patterns for obesity (Dewey, 2008; Dietz, 2001), especially for children who are breastfed for at least 7 months (Gillman, Rifas-Shiman, Camargo et al., 2001).

Table 1.4. Benefits of breastfeeding

Benefits to mother and/or infant	Studies
Decrease in respiratory infections	Bachrach, Schwarz, and Bachrach (2003); Ip, Chun, Raman et al. (2007); Lopez-Alarcon, Villalpando, and Fajardo (1997)
Decrease in ear infections	Rovers, de Kok, and Schilder (2006)
Reduction of infant mortality rates by 21%	Chen and Rogan (2004)
Decreased rates of sudden infant death syndrome	Ford, Taylor, Mitchell, et al. (1993); Horne, Parslow, Ferens, Watts, and Adamson (2004); McVea, Turner, and Peppler (2000); Mitchell, Taylor, Ford, et al. (1992); Mosko, Richard, and McKenna (1997)
Reduced incidence of Type I and Type 2 diabetes	Perez-Bravo, Carrasco, Guitierrez-Lopez, Martinez, Lopez, and de los Rios (1996); Pettit, Forman, Hanson, Knowler, and Bennett (1997)
Reduced incidence of cancer	Bener, Denic, and Galadari (2001); Davis (1998); Smulevich, Solionova, and Belyahova (1999)
Reduced incidence of obesity	Arenz, Ruckerl, Koletzko, and Von Kries (2004); Armstrong and Reilly (2002); Dewey, Heinig, Nommsen, Peerson, and Lonnerdal (1993); Gummer-Strawn and Mei (2004); Stettler, Zemel, Kumanyika, and Stallings (2002)
Reduced incidence of asthma	Chulada, Arbes, Dunson, and Zeldin (2003); Gdalevich, Mimouni, and Mimouni (2001); Greer, Sicherer, Burks, and The Committee on Nutrition and Section on Allergy and Immunology (2008); Oddy, Holt Sly, et al. (1993); Oddy, Peat, and de Klerk (2002)
Pain relief for the infant	Carbajal, Veerapen, Couderc, Jugie, and Ville (2003); Gray, Miller, Phillip and Blass (2002)

Regardless of the many benefits, most women do not breastfeed as long as health experts recommend. As stated previously, about 73% of new mothers initiate breastfeeding, but only 39% still breastfeed at 6 months. According to Li, Fein, Chen, and Grummer-Strawn (2008), the number one reason mothers discontinue breastfeeding is that they do not think they are producing enough milk to satisfy their infants. Other reasons cited are related to lactation functioning or to the infant's choosing to wean.

There are very few contraindications to breastfeeding, but these do exist. The American Academy of Pediatrics (1998) recommends that a mother not breastfeed if she has HIV, or other infectious diseases, that could be transferred to the infant through her milk. Other reasons a mother should not breastfeed include active tuberculosis, herpes simplex lesions on the breast, and drug abuse (Berlin, Paul, & Vesell, 2009; Buhimschi & Weiner, 2009).

Promoting Breastfeeding To determine what can be done to increase breastfeeding rates, researchers have studied women who initiate breastfeeding and are successful. According to Backstrom, Wahn, and Ekstrom (2010), getting help in the hospital was an important factor in mothers' breastfeeding initiative and success. However, it is not just any help that predicts successful breastfeeding. Mothers want to feel respected, not manipulated. Mothers may express annoyance at nurses who touch the mother's breast, inserting it into the infant's mouth instead of teaching the mother how to breastfeed (Weimers, Svensson, Dumas, Naver, & Wahlberg, 2006). This touch is often unexpected and unpleasant, especially for adolescent mothers and those who are self-conscious. Good support by health care professionals is based on the individual needs of mothers. Specifically, mothers often feel it is important to be able to express their feelings to health care professionals in order to get appropriate support for breastfeeding (Backstrom et al., 2010). Family support, including support from the mother's partner, is another predictor of longer-term breastfeeding (Anderson, Nicklaus, Spence, & Kavanagh, 2009; Mahoney & James, 2000; Shaker et al., 2004). Having relatives who breastfed their children also predicts breastfeeding success and longevity (Corbett, 2000; Mahoney & James, 2000). These predictors are especially strong for adolescent and low-income mothers.

The Baby-Friendly Hospital Initiative (babyfriendlyusa.org) is a global program that encourages and recognizes hospitals and birthing centers that offer an optimal level of infant feeding. The purpose of the initiative is to provide mothers with the information and skills they need in order to help successfully continue to breastfeed or to formula-feed their infants in the most appropriate ways. These hospitals are sponsored by the World Health Organization (WHO) and the United Nations Children's Fund (UNICEF). The overall goal is to help support mothers to their fullest capability and to protect infants and young children from infectious diseases and malnutrition. In order for mothers to reach these goals, the WHO and UNICEF suggest that mothers initiate breastfeeding within the infant's first hour of life; breastfeed exclusively without offering other food or drink; breastfeed on demand; and avoid bottles and pacifiers. Baby-Friendly Hospitals can be found around the world. In fact, according to Baby-Friendly USA, more than 19,000 international maternity facilities have received the Baby-Friendly Award.

Breastfeeding Routines   Mothers who choose to breastfeed should feed on demand (when the infant is hungry). Usually infants who are fed on demand will eat about every 2 to 3 hours; mothers should not let more than 4 hours pass between feedings during the day, especially during the first few months. Breastfed infants play an active role in determining the frequency of feedings and the volume of milk consumed at each feeding.

Pacifiers and Breastfeeding   Infants are born with reflexes that help with survival, and one of the strongest such reflexes is sucking. Infants begin sucking in utero as early as 12 weeks gestation (de Vries, Visser, & Prechtl, 1982). Once infants are born, they continue to seek comfort through nonnutritive sucking. Brazelton (1956) noted that most infants engage in significant amounts of sucking behavior that is unrelated to feeding; they suck on their fingers, fists, and pacifiers. The debate in many newborn nurseries is whether an infant given a pacifier will experience nipple confusion and stop breastfeeding. O'Connor, Tanabe, Siadaty, and Hauck (2011) found no support for the idea that pacifier use affects breastfeeding. However, further research is needed in the area. Some parents report that when they offer a pacifier, their infants will not breastfeed; others offer pacifiers between feedings with no negative effects on breastfeeding. This is a personal decision. However, regardless of whether an infant takes a pacifier, breastfeeding infants should feed every 2 to 3 hours. Caregivers should be sure they do not offer a pacifier when an infant should be feeding.

Expression of Milk   Most breastfeeding mothers (85%) express milk, usually so someone else can feed their infant, but sometimes in order to have excess milk available or to relieve engorgement (Labiner-Wolfe, Fein, Shealy, & Wang,

2008). Pumping (expressing) milk can be helpful, especially when the infant will be in someone else's care. Pumping both breasts at the same time helps mothers express more milk and helps to maintain available milk volume for the infant.

Breastfeeding Multiples   The choice to breastfeed multiples (e.g., twins, triplets, quads) provides the opportunity for mothers to bond with each infant, but it can also be stressful for the mother. Many expectant mothers of multiples decide to breastfeed, but express concerns about time, commitment, and whether they will have an adequate milk supply (Sollid, Evans, McClowry, & Garrett, 1989). Most literature on breastfeeding focuses on mothers with only one infant; because of this limited knowledge base, professionals may struggle to support breastfeeding of multiples.

Mothers who breastfeed multiples must decide when to feed each child. With twins, mothers have the option of feeding their infants simultaneously or individually (Sollid et al., 1989). When feeding infants individually, the mother can choose to feed each infant on demand, or to feed one infant on demand and the other infant immediately afterward (Flidel-Rimon & Shinwell, 2002). Some mothers of triplets breastfeed two infants at each feeding, while bottle feeding the third infant, then they rotate for the next feeding. This ensures each infant gets breast milk at every other feeding.

Twin type, monozygotic or dizygotic, may also contribute a challenge in feeding. Mothers from a La Leche League in Cincinnati reported surprise that their monozygotic (or identical) multiples often had closely synchronized biological clocks, waking within minutes of each other for feeding (Gromada & Spangler, 1998). In contrast, mothers of dizygotic (or fraternal) multiples reported concerns "about their multiples' different styles of breastfeeding, including length of feeding and time between feedings" (Gromada & Spangler, 1998, p. 445).

Mothers of multiples have several issues to consider before deciding whether and how to breastfeed. First, the physical condition of the mother and the infants must be assessed. For the mother, the status of her recovery, her level of energy, her breastfeeding experience and preparation, her openness to new ideas, and her support system are considered. When choosing individual or simultaneous feeding, the infants' gestational age, individual weights, sucking ability, medical condition, and individual temperaments should be considered (Sollid et al., 1989). When one infant cannot nurse due to ongoing hospitalization, the mother should continue to prepare to breastfeed the hospitalized infant in addition to the infant (or infants) she has at home. If she has twins, she can nurse the healthier infant on one breast and pump the other breast, alternating sides at each feeding. Or she can breastfeed the infant (or infants) at home on both sides and follow the nursing session with pumping. Either of these choices will ensure the most abundant milk supply for the infants when the other infant begins to breastfeed.

Once both infants are breastfeeding, mothers decide whether or not to feed each infant on the same breast at every feeding. When an infant is fed on the same breast for each feeding, he regulates the amount of milk he needs (Sollid et al., 1989). However, alternating breasts provides some benefits. It ensures more milk production because the more vigorous infant increases the milk supply on both breasts. Alternating breasts also provides equal visual stimulation for the infants and allows healing time for sore nipples. Sometimes infants develop a preference for one breast and may resist being moved to the other breast (Sollid et al., 1989).

In order to be successful in simultaneous breastfeeding of multiples, a mother will need advice on positioning. Convenience and comfort are the deciding factors, but mothers should be made aware of the variety of positions available. There are five positions that can be used to facilitate simultaneous feeding of multiples, and each has advantages and disadvantages. The positions include the football hold, the cradle and football, the parallel hold, the crisscross hold, and the V position. "No one position will work for all mothers, nor will each mother use the same position each time" (Sollid et al., 1989, p. 51).

In order to promote optimum health of mother and infants, the mother must take proper care of herself by eating high-quality foods and drinking plenty of fluids. Many mothers of multiples have a greater appetite and thirst when producing milk for two or more infants. Drinking water and eating a snack during each breastfeeding session may help mothers meet their nutritional needs. In order to minimize fatigue in the mother, a husband, partner, or other family member can support the mother by helping with household chores and by providing the mother with rest time when the infants are at ease or napping. If other people are coming in to help care for the infants, a record of infant feeding (time and amount), sleeping, and diaper changes can be very useful (Sollid et al., 1989). Such a record helps to ease the transition between caregivers.

Breastfeeding an Adopted Child   Mothers who adopt, or who do not give birth to their infants, still have the opportunity to breastfeed through induced lactation. According to the Newman-Goldfarb Protocol, 31% of mothers were able to produce all of their infant's milk needs without supplementation (Goldfarb, 2011). In order to prepare for breastfeeding, mothers need to begin pumping before the infant is born. This allows the breasts to begin producing milk and helps to establish a good supply of milk for the infant. Once the infant comes home, he or she should be put to the breast to stimulate a better supply. Pediatricians caution that if a mother is adopting and plans to breastfeed her infant through induced lactation, she should seek professional support (American Academy of Pediatrics, 2005).

Bottle feeding

Literature related to bottle feeding is less abundant. Reasons parents give for choosing bottle feeding (with formula as opposed to breast milk) often include maternal discomfort with breastfeeding, fathers' desire to be actively involved in feeding their infants, and parental concern that infants do not get enough milk through breastfeeding. Bottle feeding presents unique issues—first and foremost, the need to choose the right formula.

Types of Formulas   Formula is an artificial milk substitute for human milk. Types of formula include dairy–based (cow's milk), soy–based, hydrolyzed whey–based, casein hydrolysate–based (elemental), and amino acid–based formulas. Most formulas come in ready-to-feed packaging, which can simply be topped with a nipple or poured into a bottle, and in liquid or powder concentrates, which need to be diluted with water.

Dairy–Based Formulas   Dairy-based (cow's milk) formula is most common and has a caloric density of 20 kcal per ounce, with most infants consuming about 32 ounces per day. The most widely used name brands of cow's-milk formulas are Similac and Enfamil.

Soy-Based Formulas   Soy formula provides less calcium and phosphorus than other formulas. It provides adequate nutrition for preterm infants (Committee on Nutrition, 2000) but has been responsible for hypophosphatemia (low levels of phosphate in the body) in full-term infants.

Whey-Based Formulas   Hydrolyzed whey–based formula contains whey fraction, which is cow's milk protein that is broken down by enzyme hydrolysis so it is easier to digest and less likely to cause allergic reactions. Casein hydrolysate formulas, such as Nutramigen, Pregestimil, and Alimentum, for example, are based on a hypoallergenic protein source made up of amino acids and small peptides. This type of formula is usually recommended for infants who have had damage to their gastrointestinal tracts. Damaged gastrointestinal tracts are permeable to foreign proteins, predisposing many infants to allergic reactions. Although this type of formula may improve digestion and help with a progressive change to typical formulas, it tends to be very expensive compared with typical formulas.

Amino Acid-Based Formulas   Amino acid–based formulas, such as Neocate, are often recommended for infants who have difficulties with other formulas or who have multiple food protein intolerances.

Choosing a Formula   Sometimes a particular formula is recommended to parents; at other times, parents simply choose one formula to try. If parents think their infant is fussy, they often switch to another formula. However, most physicians recommend not changing formula because doing so can lead to gastric upset. A few studies have been conducted on the parent–child relationship in relation to changes in the infant's formula (Forsyth & Canny, 1991; Polack, Khan, & Maisels, 1999). However, very little is known about this dynamic.

Issues Related to Bottle Feeding   Parents who choose to bottle feed their infants have a number of considerations not faced by breastfeeding mothers. First, they need to choose the formula itself. They must also make sure that they properly prepare the formula. If formula is diluted too much, the infant runs the risk of being malnourished. If the formula is not diluted enough, the infant runs the risk of becoming dehydrated. Also, the water with which formula is diluted must be safe for infant consumption.

Parents must also decide whether to warm their infant's formula. Many parents do so, but it has been suggested that infants are fine with formula at room temperature (France, 2007; Kidshealth, 2009). If parents choose to warm their infant's formula, they must be very careful. Warming formula in a microwave can cause uneven heating and hot spots that may burn the infant.

Formulas have different flavors. The different formulas contain different taste compounds that influence later food preferences (Mennella, Forestell, Morgan, & Beauchamp, 2009). Milk–based formula is generally considered more palatable than hydrolysate formula, which can taste bitter. Formula-fed infants have exposure to one constant flavor unless parents change formulas (Nevo, Rubin, Tamir,

Levine, & Shaoul, 2007). This is in contrast with breastfed infants who are exposed to a variety of flavors depending upon what their mothers eat.

Parents who choose bottle feeding may persuade their infants into taking more than the infants would naturally choose to take. Caregivers may see a little formula left in the bottle and, not wanting to waste it, may encourage the infant to empty the bottle, by jiggling it, thinking, "It is just a little more."

Starting Solids/Weaning

Parents do not always know the developmental importance of delaying the introduction of solids. As mentioned previously, infants need to achieve certain developmental milestones before they are ready to begin eating solids. First, they should have control of their head and neck and the ability to sit with support in a highchair or infant seat. Also, they need to have stopped thrusting with their tongue so they do not spit out the food, but rather move it to the back of their mouths to be swallowed. Infants do not usually reach these milestones until they are 4 to 6 months old, and solids should not be introduced prior to this time.

Even with these recommendations and concerns, some parents, especially African American adolescent parents, start feeding solids earlier. In one study, adolescent mothers were educated about the importance of delaying solid foods, but their mothers (the infants' grandmothers) started feeding the infants solids before 4 months of age despite the mother's objections (Bentley, Gavin, Black, & Teti, 1999). These issues are discussed in more detail in Chapter 4.

Olson, Iwanski, Horodynski, and Brophy (2010) asked mothers why they introduced cereal early. Some of the reasons cited were: 1) acid reflux; 2) getting infants to sleep through the night; 3) coping with feeding infants formula (mothers appeared to have misunderstandings about their infants' cues about being hungry or full when on formula, and therefore, might introduce solids earlier than needed); 4) belief that the child has an allergy or intolerance to formulas or breast milk (this allergy causes infants to spit up); and 5) parents, especially fathers, feel "proud" when infants begin eating solids and are therefore eager to introduce solids.

Many parents receive information at their infant's birth or well-baby visits concerning when to start solids and the types of solids to introduce first. However, they may not receive sufficient education about the importance of waiting until the infant is 4 to 6 months old to start solids, how to feed the first foods, the appropriate consistency of first foods, or issues to look for in order to make sure the infant is handling the changes. Parents should also receive the information that early food choices are important and have long-lasting consequences. Early food preferences are linked to later food preferences (Skinner, Carruth, Bounds, & Ziegler, 2002).

Newborn infants can discriminate between sweet, bitter, and sour flavors, and by 4 months of age, they demonstrate a taste for salty flavors (Birch & Fisher, 1996; Cowart, 1981). In addition, infants appear to prefer stronger flavors. Cowart and Beauchamp (1986) found that infants showed a preference for sweeter flavors over less sweet flavors and a preference for saltier flavors over less salty flavors. Infants are able to distinguish among foods that are very different from each other, such as a fruit and a vegetable or a vegetable and meat, but they are not always able to distinguish between two foods that are more similar, such as two vegetables or two fruits (Mennella & Forestell, 2007).

Developing Healthy Eating Habits

There are several ways to foster healthy eating habits in young children, and an understanding of typical feeding development and common issues can help parents and caregivers do so. The following section provides information related to these issues.

Neophobia   Between 18 months to 2 years of age, many children develop neophobia, literally "fear of the new." In other words, they "do not readily accept new foods, with the notable exception of foods high in sugar, which they automatically like" (Birch & Fisher, 1996, p. 131). Children prefer sweet and reject sour and bitter foods (Cowart, 1981).

A child's hesitance to try new foods during this developmental stage has been reported as a common occurrence and may be a protective factor passed down in our evolutionary history and common among omnivores (Rozin, 1977). Because omnivores must discover new foods including those that could be poisonous, neophobia may be an adaptive response, preventing exploring toddlers from eating items that could be dangerous. Young children are eating a diet of foods that are entirely new to them, so neophobic responses may be common as they select foods. One way to encourage children to try new foods is to offer them in social settings; children are more willing to try new foods when in the company of others (Skinner et al., 2002).

Another way to encourage children to try new foods is to offer a variety of choices. One very early study (Davis, 1939) examined food choices in newly weaned infants who were offered a variety of foods. The foods provided were healthy, having been prepared without added sugar and salt. The infants tasted several of the foods. Davis found that infants showed a preference for some foods and avoided others. She concluded that when caregivers provide a selection of healthy foods and let children choose, children are likely to find a healthy choice they enjoy.

Fruit and Vegetable Intake   Less than half of all American children meet daily recommendations for fruit and vegetable intake (Guentherer, Dodd, Reedy, & Krebs-Smith, 2006). Furthermore, about one third of children under 2 years of age consume no vegetables or fruit on a given day (Fox, Pac, Devaney, & Jankowski, 2004). In fact, most Americans eat far less than recommended amounts of fruits and vegetables (Guentherer et al., 2006). Because children are very young when they form food preferences (between 2–3 years of age), getting them to accept vegetables and fruits early forecasts better eating habits and better health as they grow and age. Several studies have focused on different ways to increase the likelihood of vegetable intake (Epstein et al., 2001; Spill, Birch, Roz, & Rolls, 2010).

Several studies by Mennella and colleagues have found links between breast-fed and formula-fed infants and their preferences for particular vegetables. One study found that infants fed hydrolysate formula, which is bitter, consumed significantly more broccoli and cauliflower than infants fed a cow's milk–based formula (Mennella, Kennedy, & Beauchamp, 2006). There was no difference between the amounts of carrots consumed by the two groups. The authors hypothesized that, over time, the infants will have a preference for broccoli, cauliflower, and similar foods because the context of bitter flavor in their milk will transfer to other settings, like solids (Mennella, Jagnow, & Beauchamp, 2001).

Another study found that infants may experience "sensory-specific satiety" (Mennella & Beauchamp, 1997). After breastfeeding mothers consumed a carrot-rich diet, their infants had lower acceptance of carrots when offered in a flavored cereal. The authors hypothesized that the infants were less receptive to the carrot flavor because they already had exposure to it through their mothers' milk (Mennella & Beauchamp, 1997). However, later on the children showed a preference for carrot flavored foods.

Although more research is needed when it comes to how infants develop food preferences, one research-based recommendation is to feed infants a particular food (or similar foods, such as broccoli and cauliflower) for 8 or 9 consecutive days so that they get the same flavor over different feedings (Mennella et al., 2006). In a later study, infants had increased acceptance of fruits and vegetables when these foods were offered for 8 consecutive days (Mennella et al., 2008). When infants were fed a variety of vegetables, including green beans, carrots, and spinach, for 8 consecutive days, they had greater acceptance of foods with the repeated exposure.

Another way to increase children's vegetable consumption may be to offer larger portions. Spill, Birch, Roz, and Rolls (2010) found that preschoolers ate 47% more carrots when the portion size was doubled. (It is interesting to note that when the portion size was tripled, there was no further increase in consumption.) Spill et al., (2010) recommended serving the large portions of vegetables as a first course (without other foods) to promote vegetable consumption.

Self-Regulation of Food Intake   Even as early as 8 weeks of age, children are able to self-regulate the amount of intake. Wright, Fawcett, and Crow (1980) found that breastfed infants had their largest meal in the morning after fasting all night. By the age of 6 months, infants showed self-regulation similar to that observed in adults, letting the size of one meal predict the interval before the next meal.

In the 1920s and 1930s, parents were told to schedule their infant's feedings, usually feeding every 4 hours. Currently, the prevailing advice is to feed infants on demand, letting them decide when and how much to eat (Satter, 1990). Fomon (1993) stated that it is important to allow infants to determine when and how much to eat in order establish "habits of eating in moderation" (p. 114). He found that 6 week old infants consumed different amounts of formula depending on whether they were given an energy-dilute or an energy-dense formula.

Le Magen (1985) found that when a child eats a great amount of food at one time, that child waits longer before eating again than when the child eats a small amount of food. Several researchers have found that after eating meals high in fat, young children choose lower-fat foods at the next meal (Birch & Deysher, 1985; Birch, McPhee, & Sullivan, 1989). In addition, Johnson, McPhee, and Birch (1991) found that children who were offered pudding or yogurt with different caloric densities adjusted the amount consumed at the next meal. Children who consumed a higher caloric-density food ate less at the next meal than children who had eaten the lower caloric-density food.

Encouraging Healthy Eating   Children over the age of 3, generally speaking, are more susceptible to environmental influences on their eating and more likely to ignore internal signals from their bodies (Birch & Deysher, 1986; Birch & Fisher, 1995; Fisher & Birch, 1995). Social cues (e.g., seeing food, anticipation of a meal) and environment begin to play a role in when a child wants to eat.

Parents can help their children make healthy food choices, and the more parents learn about this important role, the better they can promote healthy eating habits in their children. Skinner, Carruth, Bounds, and Ziegler (2002) suggest that parents should model appropriate food choices; for example, if a mother wants her child to drink milk, she should also drink milk. Another suggestion is to provide a variety of healthy foods for the child to choose from. Make sure that the child has the opportunity to try many different fruits, even if he or she has shown a preference for bananas. If a child does not eat a particular food, parents should keep offering it because children often need repeat exposure to a new food before they will accept it.

On the other hand, parents should not offer rewards or threaten punishment in an effort to encourage healthy eating. In fact, rewarding children for eating a food decreases their desire for that food (Birch, Birch, Marlin, & Kramer, 1982; Birch & Fisher, 1996; Birch, Marlin, & Rotter, 1984). Therefore, most experts suggest providing healthy choices for meals and snacks, without encouraging, threatening, bribing, or coercing children to eat.

The best advice for parents was provided by Davis in 1939 (over 70 years ago), and it still holds true today. Parents should influence their children's eating only through the foods offered. In other words, parents should offer a variety of healthy food options, without coercion regarding the specific foods children choose or the amounts they ingest. This approach will foster the child's acceptance and ingestion of healthy foods in the appropriate amounts and create a nutritionally sound diet leading to a consistently good growth trajectory.

WHAT IS A FEEDING DISORDER?

Now that typical feeding and factors that influence typical feeding have been covered, the following section discusses feeding problems among young children and red flags that indicate the need for further investigation. A feeding disorder is diagnosed when a child does not eat enough for proper nutrition, calories, or hydration. Because eating is a central part of our lives, when eating problems exist, they are central to our lives as well. The term feeding disorder is defined as "behavior of those who have difficulty consuming adequate nutrition by mouth (impaired feeding), those who eat too much (hyperphagia), and those who eat the wrong thing (pica)" (Manikam & Perman, 2000, p. 34). Rogers observed the following:

> There is increasing recognition of the range and significance of feeding disorders in childhood. In spite of this, there is a paucity of information concerning the development of feeding efficiency and the prevalence of feeding impairments in the general population. (2004, p. S28)

The reason for this discussion of red flags is to support appropriate decisions when concerns arise regarding a child's feeding and to address "waiting and watching" versus referral to a professional for assessment. It is important to note "the process of feeding is a complex, interconnected, and flowing event. No feeding problem is due to a single factor" (Morris & Klein, 2000, p. 354).

Prevalence of Feeding Problems

The prevalence of feeding issues varies across different groups. Between 30% and 80% of children with developmental disabilities have a feeding issue (Ahearn,

2001), and between 10% and 40% of children without developmental disabilities have a feeding disorder (Manikam & Perman, 2000; Mayes & Volkmar, 1993). Only 3%–10% of children experience severe feeding problems that require hospitalization (Kerwin, 1999); these situations usually involve failure to thrive, in which there is significant growth faltering and the child is not keeping up with growth trends for age and gender.

Not all problems are severe enough to warrant professional intervention. Some children eat all kinds of food, but eat a limited variety of vegetables; other children may consume only three foods that all have the same color and texture. Between 25% and 40% of toddlers and early school-age children have "common" feeding problems like food selectivity, dawdling, and issues with the texture of the foods they eat (Mayes & Volkmar, 1993). These are not long-term concerns and often disappear on their own, although some caregivers may seek information or professional help to address these issues.

Red Flags

Each child, and his or her eating issues, must be considered individually because the range of issues is broad. One child may have one feeding issue, and another child may have several. In addition, the cause of most feeding disorders is almost impossible to determine. For these reasons, treatment varies and must be developed for each individual child. Feeding issues that should be investigated include the following:

- Difficulty latching on to the breast or bottle (could be due to lack of muscle tone)
- Difficulty coordinating the suck–swallow reflex for breast or bottle
- Difficulty with breast milk and/or formula, including gagging, coughing, vomiting, and/or swallowing problems (dysphagia; see Chapter 11)
- Excessive gagging, coughing, retching, or vomiting that interferes with eating
- Lack of "mouthing" behavior (i.e., exploration with the mouth) when developmentally appropriate
- Weight loss or lack of weight gain for 2–3 months
- Severely restricted variety of foods and/or liquids
- Inability or difficulty progressing to solid foods and textures
- Regular refusal of food
- Unwillingness to drink water
- Feeding periods that last longer than 30 minutes
- Holding and/or storing food in cheeks or under tongue instead of swallowing
- Holding liquids in the mouth instead of swallowing
- Challenging behaviors and power struggles at mealtimes (e.g., throwing food, spitting, self-induced vomiting; refusing to sit in a highchair; see Chapter 10)
- Eating nonfood items (a condition known as pica; see Chapter 11)
- Crying during mealtimes
- Eating or drinking only from a bottle beyond 2 years of age

SUMMARY

Each child has unique eating patterns and behaviors. If a child has a feeding disorder, parents, caregivers, and early childhood professionals must work together to build on the child's strengths and meet the child's unique feeding needs (Johnson, Handen, Mayer-Costa, & Sacco, 2008). The best approach is for parents to educate themselves and seek professional help if needed. If the child has several feeding issues, a feeding team may be helpful (see Chapter 5). The experience of a professional is imperative in helping a child with a feeding problem, and it is important that if parents are concerned, those concerns be addressed—not dismissed with, "He'll grow out of it."

■ ■ ■ TABLE TALK ■ ■ ■

When Janie first started eating solids, she tried everything. In fact, she would eat foods that kids usually reject, like spinach, broccoli, and avocado. But Janie is 2 years old now, and things have changed. Janie's mom, Samantha, is concerned because Janie no longer eats a wide variety of foods. Samantha has tried everything, including begging, bribing, and trying to put different foods in Janie's mouth or on her lips. Janie will not eat casseroles at all and rarely eats meat. Samantha has tried to hide the foods that Janie will not eat inside other foods that she will eat. Samantha also makes Janie stay at the table to finish her food and entices her by offering dessert if Janie finishes her food.

Discussion Questions

■   Is Janie's behavior evidence of a feeding disorder?

■   Do you think Samantha should continue to use the tactics described?

■   What suggestions do you have for Samantha to get Janie to eat?

FEEDING NUGGETS

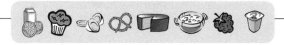

Books

Baby Bites by Bridget Swinny (2007)

Child of Mine: Feeding with Love and Good Sense by Ellyn Satter (2000)

The Family Nutrition Book: Everything You Need to Know about Feeding Your Children– From Birth through Adolescence by William Sears (1999)

The Nursing Mother's Companion, 6th Edition: 25th Anniversary Edition by Kathleen Huggins (2010)

Books for Children

How Do Dinosaurs Eat Their Food? by Jane Yolen and Mark Teague (2005)

Web Sites

"Develop Healthy Eating Habits"
United States Department of Agriculture, Feb. 2011
http://www.mypyramid.gov/preschoolers/healthyhabits/index.html

"Introducing Solid Foods"
Reviewed by the BabyCenter Medical Advisory Board, April 2011
http://www.babycenter.com/0_introducing-solid-food_113.bc

"Healthy Eating Habits Start Young"
By Cheryl Tallman and Joan Ahlers
http://www.parenthood.com/article-topics/healthy_eating_habits_start_young.html

2

Feeding in Context

■ ■ ■ FOOD FOR THOUGHT ■ ■ ■

"Ryan enrolled in our early childhood program as a 3-year-old with developmental and speech-language delays. The first issue was getting Ryan to come to the table during snack time. This took months. We eventually were able to get him to the table, but he would not push his chair up to the table. He sat a bit back, which was fine as a first step. We tried to get him to respond verbally with yes or no when asked whether he would like a snack. Once he accomplished this task, we worked on getting him to try to eat what we were offering for snack. He might say yes and then still not eat. We had multiple conversations with his parents about his food preferences, and they never indicated that he had a strong like or dislike for any particular type of food. He seemed to like crackers and animal cookies that he could pick up with his fingers. We tried both peer and adult modeling of appropriate table behavior. We demonstrated licking the food to see if we

liked the taste and would maybe want more. We demonstrated wetting our finger and then rubbing on the food (like with an apple) and then licking our finger to get the taste."
Ashley, Teacher

If a parent, child care provider, teacher, or other professional asked an early childhood professional what to do about Ryan (in the previous scenario), he or she might first consider what typical development looks like, but he or she might also consider the situation from a particular theoretical perspective. This book draws on developmental theoretical perspectives to examine feeding issues—to understand the process of feeding, to explore why we have certain associations with food, and to discuss how to approach eating issues in young children. This chapter examines several theoretical frameworks and how each can be used to better understand the dynamics of feeding and feeding issues in young children.

BEHAVIORISM

The central premise of behaviorism is that the environment is central to development. Behaviorists believe that children come into the world as blank slates and that children's interactions in the environment guide their development. Two views within behaviorism are classical conditioning by Pavlov and Watson (1927), and operant conditioning by Skinner (1938).

Classical Conditioning

Pavlov (1927) was the first to demonstrate a pattern of responses to the environment that became known as classical conditioning. He sprinkled meat powder (the unconditioned stimulus) on a dog's tongue and the dog automatically salivated (the unconditioned response). Then he paired the meat powder with the ringing of a bell. After several trials that paired the bell with the meat powder, Pavlov found that the dog salivated with the ringing of the bell only. The bell's ringing (the conditioned stimulus) elicited salivating (the conditioned response).

Classical conditioning can help parents and practitioners understand feeding issues because children develop associations between stimulus and response. For example, an aversive smell (e.g., a candle) that a child associates with food presentation may be related to a child's refusal to eat certain foods. A child who has vomited after eating a certain food may develop an aversion to that food—even if the vomiting was caused by stomach flu.

Positive associations also develop, sometimes making people want certain foods in particular situations. For example, people often associate pumpkin pie with Thanksgiving, cake with a birthday party, a hot bowl of chili with cold weather, and so forth. Sometimes when a child will not eat a certain food or will not eat in a certain place, the cause may be a negative association.

Operant Conditioning

In Skinner's theory of operant conditioning (1938), the consequences of a behavior either increase or decrease the chance of that behavior being repeated. Types of consequences include reinforcers and punishment. Reinforcement increases the likelihood that a behavior will occur again, while punishment decreases the likelihood that a behavior will occur again. Food is often used as positive reinforcement for desired behaviors. For example, a popular method of potty-training is to give a toddler candy after he or she uses the potty.

A negative reinforcer increases the likelihood that a behavior will be repeated. For example, if a child leaves the table because he becomes nauseous from the smell of a particular food, the nausea is likely to disappear. The behavior of leaving the table is reinforced by the lack of nausea (the negative reinforcer). The child's behavior alleviates something that is negative to him.

Punishment decreases the tendency of a behavior to occur. On the other hand, punishment can involve either an unpleasant experience, such as a spanking, or the end of a pleasant experience, such as when a toy or dessert is taken from the child or denied. A child being made to stay at the table until he finishes his food is punishment. It decreases the behavior (e.g., eating a disliked food) rather than increasing it.

Behaviorism techniques are commonly used by caregivers to increase desired behaviors, but these techniques do not always have the intended effect. For example, as discussed in Chapter 1, studies have shown that rewarding children for eating a food decreases their desire to eat that food (Birch, Birch, Marlin, & Kramer, 1982; Birch & Fisher, 1996; Birch, Marlin, & Rotter, 1984).

The principles of operant conditioning (reward and punishment) clearly demonstrate that children respond to rewards. Often, children are offered a reward (e.g., dessert, a preferred activity) for eating a food they would rather not eat. Inadvertently, children also may be rewarded for undesirable behaviors. For example, negative behaviors during snacks and meals can be linked to rewards parents do not realize they are providing. Parents may cajole, nag, and threaten a child who refuses to eat, and while these parental behaviors may seem negative, they are still a form of attention. As such, they may reinforce the behavior of not eating. Throwing food may also be indirectly rewarding for the child because the caregiver's reactions cause excitement and stimulation for the child. It is important to pay close attention to the child's environment and watch for unintended reinforcement of undesireable behavior.

SOCIAL COGNITIVE THEORY

Bandura's social cognitive theory (1965) departs from the thinking of the behaviorists, positing that children learn through observation, imitation, and modeling. In other words, children can learn by observing other people's behavior and the outcomes of that behavior (Ormond, 1999). A child will repeat actions, words, and behaviors that he or she has observed and is even more likely to imitate the behavior if the model's behavior is reinforced. An individual's behavior is based on interactions within his or her environment. However, Bandura believed that cognition plays a role in learning. He stated that children think about what action they should take rather than, as behaviorists believe, simply react to their environment. This is triadic reciprocal determinism wherein three key factors—behavior, environment, and cognition—interact.

Triadic reciprocal determinism exemplifies Bandura's social cognitive theory (2001; Figure 2.1). Again, behavior, internal events (such as cognition, biology/genetics), and the external environment interact; furthermore, these interactions are bidirectional. What a person thinks, believes, or feels directly affects how he or she behaves. For example, when a person likes a food, she eats it. When a person is in a new place and offered a new food, her thoughts about foods (accepting or not) determine how willing she is to try something new.

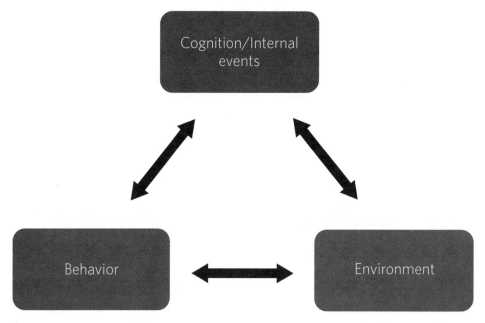

Figure 2.1. Bandura's triadic reciprocal determinism, the factors that influence a child's behavior and how those factors are interrelated.

The environment represents another important factor in Bandura's model. Each child evokes different responses from the environment, depending on age, race, sex, attractiveness, actions, and so forth. A talkative child may evoke more interactions than a quiet child of the same age. A child who is a picky eater may invite more attention during meals than a child who is not. The bidirectional influences between the behavior and environment shown in Bandura's model represent how behavior changes the environment and vice versa. Children change their environments, and they are products of their environments. A parent provides a variety of foods for the child, but the child selects the foods that are more delectable to her. The child's interactions with her parents are affected by how the parent interacts with the child.

Bandura's most famous experiment was the "Bobo doll" experiment (Bandura, 1965). In this experiment, children observed a model interacting aggressively with a Bobo doll with three different outcomes. The first group of children observed the model being rewarded with a sweet drink and a treat. The second group of children observed that the model's aggressive behavior was ignored. The third group of children observed the model receiving a spanking. The children were then placed alone in a room with a Bobo doll and observed to see if they imitated the physical aggression. The children who saw the model rewarded or ignored (the first two groups) were most likely to imitate the model's aggressive behaviors; the children who saw the model being spanked after the aggressive behaviors (the third group) still imitated the model, but the number of imitated behaviors was lower. The study helped to predict situations in which children were more likely to imitate a model.

Social cognitive theory stresses the importance of modeling the behaviors that you want a child to imitate. Support for this can be seen in a study where children were found to be more likely to eat fruits and vegetables if they observed their mother eating them (Horodynski, Stommel, Brophy-Herb, Yan Xie, & Weatherspoon, 2010).

According to this theoretical view, a child makes decisions about his or her behaviors and cognitively represents the behaviors observed. Children model parents' behaviors, including those that happen during mealtimes. Therefore, a parent who wants a child to eat certain foods, such as peas, should eat them too. According to social cognitive theory, this increases the likelihood of the child eating the food as well. This theory also supports the importance of modeling appropriate manners and mealtime routines.

ATTACHMENT THEORY

The term *attachment* is defined as an emotional bond with another person that endures over space and time (Bowlby, 1969). John Bowlby, an attachment theorist, stated that attachment is a "lasting psychological connectedness between human beings" (Bowlby, 1969, p. 194). Attachment theory evolved out of ethology, the study of animal behavior. Ethology stresses that animal behavior (including human behavior) is influenced by biology, tied to evolution, and characterized by sensitive periods in which certain developmental tasks need to be accomplished. Ethologists assert that specific behaviors emerge during a critical period. Before being applied to attachment, this theory rarely had been applied to human development. Bowlby (1969, 1989) applied ethological theory to human development and stated that attachment between an infant and a caregiver develops during the infant's first year and that the quality of that attachment has long-term consequences for the rest of the child's life.

Attachment has a profound impact on development during the first year and over the life course. For securely attached infants, feeding is a positive experience. When they are hungry, they are fed, and their mothers or fathers look into their eyes with affection during feedings. A secure infant has a caregiver who is sensitive (can read infant cues), consistent (responds in the same manner) warm (shows affection), and responds promptly.

On the other hand, insecurely attached infants are less likely to have positive feeding experiences. Their caregivers are likely to be inconsistent, unresponsive, and/or lacking in warm interactions. These caregivers are less likely to respond promptly to their children's needs, often delaying feeding until the infant is past the point of hunger. When they do respond, there is little interaction or positive affect between caregiver and child (Murray, Fiori-Cowley, Hooper, & Cooper, 1996). These interactions inform the child's feeding later on, creating a negative feeding relationship, possibly leading to feeding disorders. The formation of attachments and how their quality affects feeding will be discussed in the following section.

The Internal Working Model

Bowlby (1973) believed infants develop an internal working model (IWM) built on interactions with their caregivers through the cycle of attachment to protect them from external threats or danger, promoting security (see Figure 2.2). An IWM is developed during the first year of an infant's life and represents the child's view of the world based on interactions with caregivers and the environment. The child views current interactions or relationships based on his or her past. Therefore, a child develops a positive IWM if his or her caregivers are sensitive, warm, and consistent (Figure 2.2). The positive IWM is wired into the child's brain as a result of the interactions and the feelings that arise from them. This positive IWM guides the child in present and future interactions.

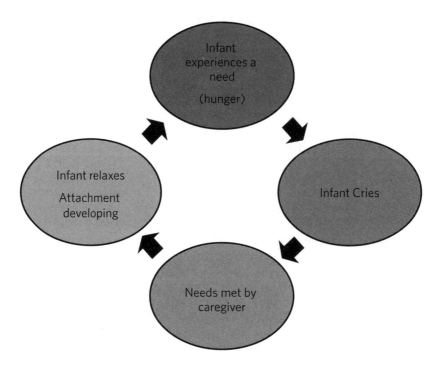

Figure 2.2.   This cycle represents the development of a secure attachment through an infant's interaction with caregivers which is integrated into the internal working model. Positive interactions between a child and caregiver translate into a secure attachment and positive associations with feedings..

Compared with children of warm, consistent, and responsive parents, children whose caregivers are insensitive, inconsistent, and/or unresponsive and children who have suffered the loss of a caregiver or experienced abuse and/or neglect are more likely to develop a disturbed IWM (See Figure 2.3). The responses of these parents may be inconsistent or delayed because the parents are unable to read the infant's cues or unable to meet their child's needs. This may be due to immaturity, lack of support, poor parenting models, or a mental disorder. For example, depressed parents are less likely to respond promptly, responsively, and consistently. These poor interactions inform the IWM which provides the child with a premise that shapes his expectations of interactions. In this case, the IWM is disturbed; the child has a negative cognitive model of how others are likely to behave in interactions with him. If negative experiences happen again and again over the course of the infant's first year, infants in these situations may develop an insecure attachment or an attachment disorder. (For more information on insecure attachment, see Hughes, 2006, Cassidy & Shaver, 2008.)

Attachment theory may seem like it has more to do with relationships than with feeding. However, feeding is critical to relationships because feeding meets the infant's needs and helps the infant to feel contented. Infants whose hunger is not consistently satisfied or whose meals are not enjoyable (because they are not held and talked to or because they do not have a nutritious meal served in a clean and safe environment) are more likely to have feeding difficulties, compared with infants who have positive relationships and positive mealtime experiences. Children with a disturbed attachment cycle may develop failure to thrive, rumination, swallowing problems, or other feeding issues (Sacrato, Pellicciari, & Franzoni, 2010).

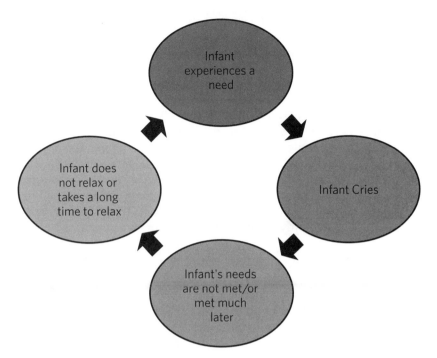

Figure 2.3. A representation of how a disturbed attachment cycle is developed during the child's interactions and integrated into his or her internal working model.

It should be noted that children who have eating difficulties—even if they are not at the low end of their growth trajectory and do not require medical attention—could still be having feeding issues tied to their relationships with caregivers. According to attachment theory, the relationship between parent and/or caregiver and child is critical to later outcomes and provides a framework within which professionals and caregivers can address the child's feeding issues. The next section discusses the different characteristics of attachment and how they affect parent and child.

Attachment Classifications

Children demonstrate two types of attachment: secure attachment and insecure attachment. Children with each type of attachment are likely to have parents that exhibit specific behaviors.

Ainsworth (1979) developed an assessment of attachment called "the strange situation." In the strange situation, an infant is observed during a series of introductions, separations, and reunions with the primary caregiver and a stranger. The process occurs in a specified order, and the infant's behaviors upon separation and reunion provides information about the infant's attachment to the caregiver. Based on the infant's behavior during the strange situation, infants can be described as either secure (65%) or insecure (35%).

Secure Attachment Secure base, maintaining proximity, and separation distress are characteristics of healthy attachment. A secure base is displayed when the caregiver provides a safe place from which the child can explore the environment. Maintaining proximity is when the child stays near the caregiver, which provides safety for the child and protects him from harm. A child shows separation distress when she becomes upset during separation from the caregiver.

Securely attached children—due to interactions during their first year—feel safe and protected and are able to depend on their adult caregivers to meet their needs. When entering the strange situation, secure infants viewed the caregiver as a "secure base" from which to explore the setting, and the infants sought physical proximity with the caregiver. When the caregivers left the room, the securely attached infants were distressed; when the caregivers returned, the infants were happy to see them and settled down relatively quickly. The infants sought out the caregiver, relaxing when held, actually sinking into the caregiver's arms. When the caregiver left, the securely attached children might have been upset, but they also felt assured that the parent or caregiver would return. When frightened, securely attached children sought comfort from their caregivers. These children know their parents or caregivers will provide comfort and reassurance.

Insecure Attachment   Insecure attachment is broken down into several classifications, however only two will be discussed for the purpose of this section. They are: ambivalent/resistant attachment and avoidant attachment. Infants who fit into either classification have parents or caregivers who are not meeting their needs consistently, warmly, and/or sensitively.

Ambivalent/Resistant Attachment   Infants who exhibit ambivalent attachment have parents who respond to their needs inconsistently (often because of a lack of knowledge, a lack of maturity, or issues related to their own upbringing) or parents who are emotionally or psychologically unable/unavailable to meet the infant's needs. Only about 7%–15% of children fall in this classification (Cassidy, J. & Berlin, L.J., 1994). In the strange situation, these children usually became very distressed when parents or caregivers left the room. However, when caregivers returned, the ambivalently attached children did not relax and accept comfort from their caregiver; instead, they fluctuated between clinging and pulling away, "often crying excessively." These children could not depend on their caregivers to be available when they need them.

Avoidant Attachment   Children who are classified as avoidant tend to avoid parents and caregivers and generally show no preference between caregivers and complete strangers. Research has suggested that this behavior could be in response to a caregiver who has been abusive or neglectful (Prior & Glaser, 2006). During the strange situation, avoidant children appeared as if they were unconcerned when caregivers left; they did not seem to notice. However, physiologically, these children experience signs of stress such as an increased heart rate and/or blood pressure, but they have learned not to show their stress because they will not get the support and sensitivity they need and may suffer negative consequences if they show a need for being nurtured. These children have learned *not* to depend on their caregivers; they have been punished for relying on a caregiver, so they *avoid* relying on them in the future.

Caregivers whose children exhibit insecure attachment often had an insecure attachment with their own caregivers: The cycle repeats itself because people usually parent in the same way they were parented. Furthermore, failure to form a secure attachment as a young child can lead to negative outcomes in later childhood and adulthood. Research suggests that the attachments created early in life impact later relationships and other areas of development (Crockenberg & Leerkes, 2005).

Some researchers have studied a link between nonorganic failure to thrive (in which infants do not gain weight as appropriate for their age and sex) and the attachment relationship between the infant and caregivers (Brinich, Drotar, & Brinich, 1989; Chatoor, Ganiban, Colin, Plummer, & Harmon, 1998; Ward, Kessler, & Altman, 1993). Early studies in the attachment field focused on the lack of weight gain (and sometimes death) of infants in orphanages who had appropriate amounts of milk but did not gain weight (Oates, 1984). Those who dealt with underweight infants assumed that growth faltering was caused by maternal deprivation, neglect, or physical abuse (Call, 1984; Kotelchuck, 1980). Working with parents to help them become more sensitive to the infant's cues and needs may lead to the weight gain and more appropriate growth trajectories.

Feeding and Attachment Theory   Attachment theory demonstrates the importance of caregiver–infant interactions and how the foundation of this relationship leads to a cognitive representation of attachment. This cognitive representation influences later interactions and predicts behavioral outcomes in several areas. Depending on the research that is consulted, attachment is understood to be indirectly and/or directly linked to feeding. This chapter has explored how a typically developing child's relationship with a caregiver can be linked to feeding issues. In children with disabilities, some studies have shown that maternal sensitivity and maternal representations of relationships may impact the care of the infant with special needs (Sayre, Planta, Marvin, & Saft, 2001). Disabilities themselves sometimes interfere with attachment. In other cases, issues with the caregiver's feelings toward the child could interfere with feeding; attributes of children with disabilities may overwhelm the parent's representation of the attachment with the young child and change behavior or care of the child.

FAMILY SYSTEMS THEORY

The family is a complex unit, involving interactions that influence all family members. In other words, one family member's behavior affects all the others in the family. This fact can be especially evident during mealtimes. "Families are viewed as interactive, interdependent, and reactive," and the "emotional functioning of every family member plays a part in occurrence of medical, psychiatric, or social illness in one family member" (Seligman & Darling, 2007, p. 17). It stands to reason, then, that a child's feeding difficulties affect the rest of the family and that in order to understand what is happening with one member, it is important to study the family as a whole. Furthermore, treatment must be focused on the family system, not on a single individual. To exemplify family systems theory and each of its related tenets, the following paragraphs explore a family that includes a child with a disability that leads to disordered feeding. Each family is unique and culture often plays a role in each family system.

According to family systems theory, a child with a feeding difficulty is not operating in isolation; she exists in the context of the family. A family is comprised of three central subsystems: 1) the spousal subsystem (the two parents), 2) the parental subsystem (each parent along with each child, and 3) the sibling subsystem (among siblings).

Among subsystems, there are boundaries that are permeable or impermeable. Most nuclear and extended families have boundaries that are permeable. However, this is not always the case, and even established boundaries can change. For example, a child's feeding issue may seem to invite extended family members to give advice; if the parents resent that input, an impermeable boundary may be created, with the parents refusing to take advice from the extended family.

There are also boundaries between the family and those outside of the family, such as the physicians and early intervention team members with whom the family works to address a child's feeding issues. In this sense, family systems can be open or closed. Open systems accept information from the outside and also provide information to the outside. Closed systems have impermeable or rigid boundaries that are not easily crossed. There are disadvantages with both open and closed systems. An open system can get too much help and become overwhelmed. A closed family may feel that they can solve their child's feeding difficulty without help; such a family then may become isolated from community supports and from other families. Families that fare the best maintain a balance between being open and being closed.

A child with no feeding issues, for example, may be in a family with a balance between permeable boundaries (open) and impermeable boundaries (closed). On the other hand, a child with feeding issues may live in a family that is on either end of the continuum. Lack of balance with regard to permeable versus impermeable boundaries may be linked to the cause of the feeding issues (e.g., too much advice and care from too many people or not enough advice and not enough support-seeking) or the lack of balance may be linked to the outcome (e.g., the child may have more difficulties with feeding because the family needs more help but is not seeking it or the family gets too much help and does not know what to do with the information). Inappropriate boundaries can hinder a family's development.

Cohesion

Cohesion is another aspect of systems theory. This term refers to the level of emotional closeness or independence within a family. Family members often struggle to learn how to be close within a family yet separate individuals. A typical two-year-old is striving for a sense of individuality when he begins independent feeding. Some families have weak boundaries within the family, resulting in members who are enmeshed, such as when a parent is overprotective of a child. For example, the parent may not allow anyone else to feed the child.

On the other end of the spectrum are families whose members are disengaged from one another; these families have rigid boundaries and are not involved with one another. An example of disengagement causing feeding issues is the child whose parent is overly involved with work and not spending enough time with the children, especially the child with a feeding issue. In this situation, the other parent may be overly involved with the infant, and the parents may not be engaged with each other to solve their children's issues. One parent may be involved in the parental subsystem, but not in the spousal system. Families that are functioning well have achieved a balance between enmeshment and disengagement. Cohesion can also be seen when a family does not let anyone from the outside, like a grandparent or child care provider, into the family system. As you can see, it is difficult to determine whether the overly cohesive or under-cohesive family leads to more problems with feeding or whether feeding issues lead to disturbances in these families.

To demonstrate cohesion, let us examine one family that has a child with a feeding issue compared to another family that does not. The family with the feeding issue may have a mother and young child who are enmeshed, having become so close to one another that they will not allow other family members to become involved. The enmeshed parent feeds the baby every time, not allowing the other parent any feeding opportunities. The child might also resist the other parent's attempts to offer food by throwing a tantrum. Other children in the family are also left out of the enmeshed parental subsystem. The family without the feeding issues is more balanced. This family is likely to have parental subsystems that are not preferred over the spousal subsystem. Both parents feed the child and make feeding decisions. Also, the parents are likely to be appropriately engaged with their children, but not enmeshed.

Adaptability

Adaptability is the family's ability to change in response to a stressor (Olson, Russell, & Sprenkle, 1980). When considering adaptability, families exist on a continuum that stretches from rigid to chaotic. Rigid families have a lot of rules that make it difficult to adapt to stress. Chaotic families have few rules and members are not dependable, making adaptation difficult. The best case is to be in the middle of the continuum. This position creates families with shared leadership, role sharing, democratic discipline, and the ability to adapt as necessary. These families are loyal and strike an even balance between dependence and independence.

Let us put this into the context of feeding. A child who has a feeding issue may come from a family that is chaotic. Chaotic families lack leadership; there is no member who provides direction. There also may be shifts in roles that add to the child's developmental issues, feeding in particular. The parents may provide little guidance about what the child should eat and when, instead letting the child decide to set his own limits. Parents may punish the child for playing with his food at one meal and laugh at the behavior the next time. Chaotic families cause a great deal of confusion for the child and contribute to disordered eating. A chaotic family might move from enmeshment to disengagement and back again.

A rigid family is on the opposite end of the continuum with a clear and constant leader, strict discipline, and too little change. This type of family would be unlikely to work with the needs of the child, instead expecting the child to adjust to the demands and rules of the family. Neither the chaotic nor the rigid family is likely to adapt well to stressors. Consider the following child and how she might fit into each family type.

> Willa, who is 7 months old, was born addicted to methamphetamine. Her development has been delayed 4 to 5 months. It is hard feeding her because she doesn't like most table food. She eats mashed potatoes, soft bread, and puréed fruits and vegetables. She lives with two parents and has two older siblings, who are 5 years and 4 years of age. (Sharon, undergraduate in early childhood)

If Willa is in a rigid family, the father might be the person in charge who dictates how Willa will be fed, who will feed her, and when she will be fed. In a rigid family, Willa would be fed in the same manner at each meal because rigid families do not like change. In this system, if Willa will not adapt and eat more solid foods, then she will not eat.

If Willa were part of a chaotic family, she would not experience consistency, and she would not be able to develop expectations for how she will be fed. For example, one day her mother might feed her using a technique that the speech-language pathologist suggested; the next day someone else may feed Willa without knowledge of the new technique introduced. In the chaotic family, there is no consistency from meal to meal and no consistent timing of meals.

If Willa were in a flexible family, there would be more consistency, but also flexibility to make changes in a logical, thought-out manner as needed. The structured family also exhibits consistency and more flexibility than rigid families. Flexible and structured families—with their consistency, adaptability, and good communication, are beneficial for children in general, and they are especially helpful for those with feeding issues.

BIOECOLOGICAL FRAMEWORK

Bronfenbrenner's bioecological framework (1993) provides another model for understanding children's development in the context of the system within which they develop (See Figure 2.4). The individual's development and his or her biological characteristics are central to development within his or her ecological context. According to this theory, all social systems are reciprocal, and there is diversity in the contexts in which children live.

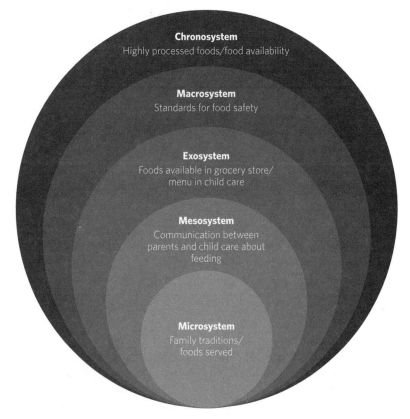

Chronosystem
Highly processed foods/food availability

Macrosystem
Standards for food safety

Exosystem
Foods available in grocery store/
menu in child care

Mesosystem
Communication between
parents and child care about
feeding

Microsystem
Family traditions/
foods served

Figure 2.4.   Bronfenner's bioecologic framework, which includes several subsystems: the microsystem, the mesosystem, the exosystem, the macrosystem, and the chronosystem.

Bioecological Subsystems

The ecological system includes several subsystems: the microsystem, mesosystem, exosystem, macrosystem, and chronosystem. Each of these will be discussed with examples of how each relates to feeding young children.

The Microsystem   The bioecological system most immediate to the child is the microsystem:

> a pattern of activities, roles, and interpersonal relations experienced by the developing person in a given face-to-face setting with particular physical, social, and symbolic features that invite, permit, or inhibit, engagement in sustained, progressively more complex interaction with, and activity in, the immediate environment. (Bronfenbrenner, 1993, p. 15)

In the microsystem, there are "two kinds of processes that promote development: 1) interactions with people, and 2) activities in which children engage" (Thomas, 1996, p. 385). The microsystem encompasses, but is not limited to interactions at home, at school, in the neighborhood, and within the peer group. With regard to feeding, for example, a child may eat different foods in the home, at school, and with peers. In addition, the extended family may provide different foods, such as when a child's grandmother provides more candy and less emphasis on healthy eating compared with the child's parents.

The Mesosystem   The next subsystem of the bioecological framework is the mesosystem. The mesosystem includes interactions among the microsystems as explained above. A mesosystem comprises the linkages and processes taking place between two or more settings containing the developing person (Bronfenbrenner, 1993, p. 22). When it comes to feeding, for example, the grandmother and the parent may be in conflict. The parent might express disapproval at what the child is eating at grandma's house. Or a child may be excited to eat something at home that they tried at a friend's home. Both of these examples involve the mesosystem.

The Exosystem   According to Bronfenbrenner, the third subsystem of the bioecological framework is the exosystem, which

> comprises the linkages and processes taking place between two or more settings, at least one of which does not contain the developing person, but in which events occur that indirectly influence processes within the immediate setting in which the developing person lives. (Bronfenbrenner, 1993, p. 22)

The exosystem impacts the child, but the child has no impact on the exosystem. Food-related examples of exosystems include the menu at the child's school, or child care and television programming that provides images of foods that are low in nutritional value. The child cannot change the menus outside the home or what is seen on television. However, these food-related experiences do affect the child. For example, when the child goes grocery shopping with a parent, the child might ask for the cookies shown in a television advertisement.

The Macrosystem   The subsystem of the bioecological framework that is most removed from the child is the macrosystem, which includes the expectations held by society, such as laws and customs. American society has food on almost every corner, and people eat all times of the day in public spaces. These customs are part of the macrosystem. In contrast, many other societies have more structured ways of eating, including precise mealtimes and rituals. The French have several courses for dinner and longer mealtimes than Americans. Other aspects of the United States' food-related macrosystem are programs that assist people without resources to obtain foods for their families, like Temporary Aid for Needy Families (TANF) and similar programs.

The Chronosystem   The final subsystem of Bronfenbrenner's bioecological framework is the chronosystem, which includes the sociohistorical conditions and events that occur over the course of a lifetime. Societal change—such as the production of food moving from personal (e.g., a garden) to removed (e.g., buying foods in a grocery store)—is a chronosystem change. The fact that most foods are produced and processed by industries and that they are likely to be low in nutritional value compared with foods in the past, is another example of a chronosystem change.

Feeding and Bioecological Theory

Feeding takes place in a context that is unique for every child. The bioecological framework helps us understand each child and his or her behavior within the context of each system. Consider Willa (from the previous section):

- Willa's family is her microsystem.
- Willa is in child care, and her mother speaks with the caregiver about her feeding issues. This communication helps to ensure that there is consistency across settings: Willa's mesosystem.
- The director of the child care is held to standards set by the United States Department of Agriculture (USDA) regarding the foods served by the child care, affecting the foods offered to Willa. (Willa does not have an effect on the USDA or the child care menu.) These are aspects of the exosystem.
- The USDA's food program is part of the larger society's goal to have nutritional standards for children in child care; this goal is part of the macrosystem.
- Willa is part of a society whose attitudes toward feeding difficulties have changed over time. These changing attitudes are part of the chronosystem.

SUMMARY

Each of the theories reviewed in this chapter provides a unique way to view a child's feeding development and provides a range of perspectives through which to examine a feeding issue. Every individual has perspectives that have been guided by interactions with others and by families of origin. To better understand and assist children and parents in improving a child's eating and feeding behaviors, practitioners should understand the dynamic process of interactions in light of various theoretical frameworks. Each theory provides a perspective to better understand children and the environments that affect their development in general and that affect their feeding in particular.

▦ ▦ ▦ TABLE TALK ▦ ▦ ▦

Aidan, who is 8 months old, lives with his mother, father, and twin sister, Emily. Aidan eats at the same time as his twin sister, which appears to be increasing the likelihood that he is becoming an aggressive eater. In fact, Aidan often grunts to express hunger and impatience. Aidan has always wanted to be fed first, and he will start yelling if he is not. He gets the first spoonful of food, but as soon as it is gone, he gets very upset. It seems as though he wants his caregiver's undivided attention. Emily is more relaxed and patient at mealtime, perhaps because Aidan is so dominant.

When Aidan gets angry because too much time elapses between bites, he occupies himself with another activity. If he is barefoot, he chews on his feet. He will cross his legs until they get stuck and he cannot get them down. He bothers Emily if she is close by.

Aidan is also a very picky eater. If he does not want a particular food, his parents have a difficult time finding an alternative that is acceptable to him. He is loud and energetic and wants all of the family's attention. When he is done eating, he seems to feel that Emily should be done as well. Every time the twins eat, Aidan controls who gets fed first as well as when mealtime is over.

Discussion Questions

▪ How would Aidan's feeding behaviors be addressed by each of the theories?

▪ What theory do you think works best for solving the issue?

FEEDING NUGGETS

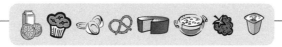

Books

Building the Bonds of Attachment: Awakening Love in Deeply Troubled Children by Daniel A. Hughes (2006)

Handbook of Attachment, Second Edition: Theory, Research, and Clinical Applications by Jude Cassidy and Phillip R. Shaver (2010)

I Love You Rituals by Becky A. Bailey (2000).

Understanding Families: Approaches to Diversity, Disability, and Risk by Marci J. Hanson and Eleanor W. Lynch (2003)

Web Sites

Attachment Theory
http://www.essex.ac.uk/armedcon/unit/
projects/wwbc_guide/wwbc.chapter.1.english.pdf

Attachment Theory
http://dhs.georgia.gov/DHR-DFCS/DHR-DFCS_
CommonFiles/Module%209%20Attachment%20Handouts.pdf

Family Systems Theory
http://www.genopro.com/genogram/family-systems-theory/

Bioecological Theory
http://www.psy.cmu.edu/~siegler/35bronfebrenner94.pdf

3

Feeding Interactions

■ ■ ■ FOOD FOR THOUGHT ■ ■ ■

"While visiting with a friend, I observed her 13-month-old son Ben during lunch. His mother put him on a mat on the floor because he refused to sit in a highchair and was not stable enough to sit at the family table, which had a bench for seating instead of chairs. The table was also too high for Ben to reach if seated on the bench. His mother put his food in front of him, and Ben fed himself, refusing any attempts at assistance. He was very content, ate a variety of food, including macaroni and cheese, sliced fruit, and graham crackers. Ben predominantly used his hands but made several attempts to keep food on his spoon. He did not show concern over the mess or stickiness until he was done. Then he allowed his mom to assist him with a wipe."

Melissa, pre-K Teacher

"At 4 years of age, Noah loved going to McDonald's. He loved their hamburgers so much that he started refusing to eat hamburgers I cooked at home. We finally had to stop letting him eat at McDonald's until he started eating what I cooked at home. One evening, I cooked a nutritious meal, and he refused to eat. He cried to go to McDonald's. I would not give in to him, so he got on the phone and called his grandma (my mother) and told her I wouldn't feed him. We had a good laugh over this, but he still didn't get McDonald's that night."

Cheryl, Parent

"When my daughter, Adrianna, was 8-months-old, it was difficult to feed her. She wouldn't eat table food, so I was still feeding her baby food. I didn't know that I was supposed to feed her table food at that age. The child care facility said she wouldn't eat lunch. They were trying to feed her table food. I decided to take a 4-day weekend and get her used to table food. I would put the food in her mouth, and many times she spit it out. No matter how small the pieces were, she would not eat. Every time she spit the food out, I would put it back in her mouth. The 4 days didn't work with her. I explained to the child care what I was doing so that she could eat at school as well. It took a few weeks before she ate table food. She is almost 9 years old now and she still smashes some food before eating it."

Sherre, Parent

"When my godson Ryan was born, his mother was a new, inexperienced mother. She wanted to breastfeed but was not sure how. The day after he was born his mother was in the hospital trying to breastfeed him. She could not get him to latch on, so I attempted to help. Neither of us knew what to do, so we called the nurse. After the nurse showed her what to do, she had it. After about a week at home, Ryan would no longer take her milk, so she went to a bottle, which he took with no problem."

Jamaya, Godmother

As the previous scenarios illustrate, there are many types of mealtime interactions and many different expectations and ways of handling mealtimes with young children. Family mealtimes can be a great way to share family unity and discussion. For some families, dinner is the only time they have to reflect on and share their thoughts about the day, but other families' schedules may not allow them to enjoy even one daily mealtime. This chapter covers the changes in society that have affected families and mealtimes, a discussion of the developmentally appropriate feeding expectations at different ages, child care providers' roles in feeding young children and working with families, and a discussion of the feeding needs of young children who have a disability.

As our society changes, so does the family mealtime experience, which has evolved dramatically over the last century (See Table 3.1). In the 1950s, for example, a family meal would often take a fair amount of time to prepare. Generally, meal preparation was the woman's responsibility, and she was expected to have the evening meal ready for the man when he returned home from work. The family meal

Table 3.1.   Comparison of mealtime in 1950 verus today

1950s	2010
Whole and fresh foods	Large quantities of processed foods
Not rushed	On the run
Sit together and each member has his or her own place to sit	Technology is usually around at dinner (TV, cell phones, computers, etc.)
Proper table manners	Dinner time is irregular (never a set schedule)
Dinner was served at the same time every day	Majority of dinners are a variety of take out

was structured and routine, often with assigned seating for family members and enforcement of proper manners.

With increased employment rates for women, increased involvement in extracurricular activities for children, and longer work hours and commutes for both parents, today's family mealtime experience is far different from that of the 1950s. According to Larson, Branscomb, and Wiley (2006), mothers continue to shoulder most of the responsibility for mealtimes; however, instead of cooking they often resort to fast food or eating out. Also, the television is on more than ever during dinner time; in a survey of children ages 8–18 years, 63% revealed that television is "usually" on during their meals (Larson, Branscomb, & Wiley, 2006). The nutritional value of meals has also changed. Meals in the 1950s were usually home-cooked, wholesome, and eaten at home, but modern families often eat relatively unhealthy take-out food in front of the television or in restaurants. Research suggests that families with a positive mealtime atmosphere—in which shared meals are a priority and include rules and structure—have adolescents who are less likely to get involved with unhealthy dieting and disordered eating habits (Larson et al., 2006). These dramatic changes in family meals have affected families and their young children in subtle but very important ways.

MEALTIME AND ITS EFFECTS ON EARLY CHILDHOOD DEVELOPMENT

Eating is a social activity. Celebrations and social gatherings often include specific foods as part of the tradition. Family mealtimes are embedded in a social, cultural, and economic context that is associated with a variety of indicators of children's health and well-being (Fiese & Schwartz, 2008). There are slight variations in regularity and frequency of reported mealtimes across income and ethnic groups. These variations are due primarily to lower reported numbers of family mealtimes in poor families, associated in part with the added strain of juggling shift jobs and longer commutes (Fiese & Schwartz, 2008).

Mealtimes last an average of 20 minutes and are loaded with expectations, rituals, and interactions that are associated with positive or unfavorable child developmental outcomes (Fiese & Schwartz, 2008). Mealtimes provide nutritional sustenance, but they also establish and reinforce expectations for acceptable behavior at the table, a process that begins when children are very young. Although family mealtimes don't last long, they are nevertheless very important for children's development, and the importance of mealtime interactions should not be underestimated. Assuming positive mealtime interactions, the benefits of a family mealtime include:

- Enhancing children's language development and literacy skills (Snow & Beals, 2006)

- Socializing children into the family culture (Ochs & Shohet, 2006)
- Teaching children manners (Fiese, Foley, & Spagnola, 2006)
- Indirectly enhancing children's emotional development (Fiese et al., 2006)
- Lowering the incidence of risky behaviors and emotional problems among adolescents (National Center on Addiction and Substance Abuse, 2010; Eisenberg, Olson, Neumark-Sztainer, Story, & Bearinger, 2004)
- Providing children with a feeling of belonging (Fiese et al., 2006)
- Increasing the likelihood that meals are nutritious

As mentioned previously, these benefits are likely to be gained during positive mealtime interactions. In fact, the family climate during mealtimes can either support or derail positive child and adolescent health and well-being. Considering that infants and toddlers spend about 11.5 hours per week eating in their homes, pleasant and predictable mealtimes are important (Fiese & Schwartz, 2008). Fiese et al. (2006) described the social and interactive components of mealtimes in order to demonstrate the dynamic process that takes place in those crucial 20 minutes. Their findings are described in the following section.

First, families differ in the amount of structure in their mealtimes, ranging from highly structured to *laissez-faire*. Highly structured mealtimes have distinct features: They occur at a designated time, each family member has clearly defined roles, all members understand that there are appropriate (and inappropriate) mealtime conversation topics, and all family members know the rules for being excused from the table (Fiese et al., 2006). In comparison, a *laissez-faire* mealtime may seem chaotic; few requirements are made of members in terms of attendance and roles.

Family mealtimes are extremely important because mealtime social interactions teach children a number of different skills (Fiese et al., 2006). These interactions help foster a sense of group identity, help children develop beliefs about relationships, and promote or hinder the emotional well-being of children. Fiese et al. (2006) studied communication between family members, how tasks are carried out, and the continuity between meals that help to explain the significance of a meal. They found that mealtimes vary across families with regard to three important factors: communication, commitment, and continuity. Each of these factors is incorporated into mealtimes through routines and rituals.

Communication

During mealtimes, families communicate about a variety of topics, including what happened during the day, future plans, manners, and feelings about other family members. There are two main types of communication: routine communication and ritual communication.

Routine Communication   Routine communication is something that children and other family members can expect at each meal. Direct and indirect communication are the two types of routine communication.

Direct Communication   When families engage in direct communication, information is clearly stated. There is no confusion among members about the routines surrounding the meal. For example, a parent might explicitly state an expectation for children to sit during the meal or to use utensils instead of their hands to pick up food. In families that use direct communication, roles are clearly defined and expectations are clearly understood (Fiese et al., 2006).

Indirect Communication   On the opposite end of the spectrum is indirect communication. Indirect communication does not make expectations clearly known, and members are often confused about their roles. Because of this ambiguous interaction, indirect communication may have a negative impact on a child's mental health (Fiese et al., 2006). Children may be more distressed in situations involving indirect communication; however, the impact is not clear. Other variables may contribute both to indirect communication and to the child's mental health and well-being.

Ritual Communication   In contrast with routine communication, ritual communication is the focus of family conversation during mealtimes. According to Fiese et al. (2006), "Mealtimes are opportunities for members of the family to work together to solve problems of a sensitive nature, building on personal knowledge of past experiences" (p. 78). Ritual communication is also observed in insider information, information that only members of the group will know. For example, a family might discuss what happened at a parent's workplace, a child's routine during his day at child care, or an issue that a family member is having. It is conversation that the members expect, a ritual.

Commitment

Commitment refers to the behaviors or tasks surrounding a meal that accomplish the goals of a meal.

Routine Commitment   Commitment is demonstrated in the ways tasks are accomplished, and it can be either rigid or chaotic. With rigid commitment, the mealtime becomes overly focused on accomplishing a task, such as having a child eat a certain amount of food or eat a particular kind of food. This rigidity can have a negative effect on the social interactions that would otherwise occur during mealtime. No flexibility leaves no choices, and choices are important to young children. Also, rigidity can make meals uncomfortable if expectations are not developmentally appropriate. On the other hand, meals that have little routine commitment can become unruly. Children may get up from the table many times, and they may not have a clear understanding of when the meal begins and ends (Fiese et al., 2006).

Ritual Commitment   Ritual commitment is demonstrated through family members' responses to problems that are expressed by other family members; when these responses are positive, family cohesion is demonstrated. For example, during a meal, parents can give children encouragement and validation for positive behaviors, and family members can demonstrate concern for each other (Fiese et al., 2006).

Continuity

Continuity is seen in the frequency of meals and in consistency across meals. Like communication and commitment, continuity can be routine or ritual.

Routine Continuity   Routine continuity is demonstrated through meal-time roles played by each family member. Dinner conversations in Western culture usually include children's activities that occurred during the day, children's peers, plans for the next day, and plans for the future, such as an upcoming family celebration. These conversation topics result in members' taking on roles such as child care attendee, parent, chauffer, and party planner. The repetition of these roles results in a positive influence on behaviors outside of the home, peer relationships, and planning for future events (Fiese et al., 2006).

Ritual Continuity   Ritual continuity is demonstrated through the planning and passing of rituals from one generation to the next. Planning for future events validates to the group that it will endure over time. For example, when planning a party, parents discuss what is needed. Once the children understand the different parts of the ritual, they can start helping to plan their own parties by suggesting a particular kind of birthday cake, various party activities, and a location for the event. Ritual continuity reinforces the value of individuals within the group and the value of the group as a whole. Ritual continuity is also displayed when meals are held at specific times, when traditional recipes are used, and when dishes from a parent's childhood are served and passed from one generation to the next (Fiese et al., 2006).

A family's mealtime rituals and routines can affect a child's well-being positively or negatively. Although some mealtime factors (e.g., indirect communication; Fiese et al., 2006) may negatively influence a child's well-being, shared family mealtimes are overwhelmingly associated with positive outcomes, such as academic achievement, language development, physical health, and reduced risk for substance abuse (Fiese & Schwartz, 2008).

DEVELOPMENTAL FEEDING NEEDS OF YOUNG CHILDREN

The feeding relationship begins very early—even before birth. Mothers make food choices that reinforce family preferences and that introduce her fetus to her culture. Additionally, a healthy diet during pregnancy is more likely to lead to a healthy infant. "The child's natural feeding environment can provide critical information in understanding the parents' priorities, available resources, and the settings that affect the child's feeding behaviors" (Manikam & Perman, 2000, p. 37). Ellen Satter (1986) wrote about the "feeding relationship" and the "complex interactions" that are inherent within that relationship. According to Satter, one of the most important factors in a positive feeding environment is trust; infants and toddlers should have an intimately positive and enduring connection with their caregivers for a good feeding environment. For example, when infants are hungry, they want to be fed until they are satiated. If the caregiver misreads the infant's signals and tries to play with the infant instead of providing food, the infant's immediate needs are not met, which may affect the establishment of trust between the infant and caregiver. After all, the infant is learning about the environment and what to expect; when the infant's needs are not met or when they are met inconsistently, this provides information that the environment cannot be trusted. Positive responses are consistent, warm, and sensitive. In addition, the caregiver's appropriate and timely response to the infant's needs helps the infant learn regulation. A parent soothes an infant who is upset and excites an infant who wants to play. This regulation is important in helping the infant to regulate behavior; it is also important in the relationship the infant forms with the parent. All of these positive interactions enhance the feeding relationship.

Feeding Infants

Infants are totally dependent on their caregivers, especially for feeding. Feeding includes more than just food choices, it also includes the feeding environment. In general, infants should be fed promptly when they are hungry and before they begin to cry. Infants should be held during feedings; bottles should not be propped because the interaction during feeding is as important as the nourishment the infant receives. Infants should be in charge of when they eat and how much they eat; in other words, they should be in control of their eating pattern. From the very beginning, infants let caregivers know when they are hungry and full. It is important for professionals and parents to be aware of these cues and to respond accordingly. An infant may root around and fuss to show that he or she wants to be fed and may move away from a nipple, spit it out, or shut his or her mouth tightly to demonstrate satiety. Because the infant is in charge of the feedings, the caregiver must be attentive to the infant's cues, while at the same time recognizing that there will be variation in how much food infants take across feedings because infants self-regulate the amount of they consume.

Synchrony makes a feeding interaction more positive. When the child and the parent are "in sync," they engage in an intimate dance in which each partner anticipates the other's next motion. A parent who anticipates when an infant needs to eat, feeds the infant, burps the infant, and rocks and soothes the infant in concert with his expressed needs demonstrates synchrony with the infant. "Feeding is a concrete demonstration to the child of parental attitudes and expectations" (Satter, 1986, p. 352). An infant smiles, and Mom or Dad smiles back. The infant opens his or her mouth for food and very shortly receives food. Synchrony sometimes takes practice; it shows the intimate relationship between the infant and all caregivers, not just parents. A caregiver who robotically shovels food into a child's mouth is providing the infant with a significantly different experience than the caregiver who patiently waits for the infant to show that he or she is ready for another bite by looking toward the caregiver with an open mouth. Synchrony is a relationship built on trust and respect.

Breastfeeding   Professionals who work with parents and young children need to support mothers who breastfeed because this is a wonderfully nutritious feeding method. Mothers who are supported in the decision to breastfeed maintain it longer. Breastfeeding is a very personal choice, and many factors influence a mother's decision to breastfeed. Consider Nicole's experience breastfeeding her infant:

> I had decided that I wanted to breastfeed long before I found out I was pregnant. I had heard and read many things that indicated how important it was. I learned that it is important to have a strong commitment to breastfeeding because there will be difficult times. It is also important to have a support system, such as a spouse, partner, family, and friends. (Nicole Zavala, personal communication September 29, 2010)

In a review of qualitative studies on breastfeeding support, the authors found that mothers who breastfed felt that "good social support was essential" (McInnis

& Chambers, 2008, p. 422). Mothers with good social support appeared to have less guilt, to deal with issues regarding breastfeeding better, and to be less likely to doubt their abilities. Breastfeeding mothers need support that is informational, practical (e.g., when a friend helps with the house) and emotional (e.g., when a grandmother listens when the mother feels overwhelmed). It is interesting to note that social support usually came from grandmothers and rarely from the mother's partner in this particular study (McInnis & Chambers, 2008).

The way support is conveyed is important. When health professionals provided information, even good information, in a pressuring and judgmental manner, mothers found that the method of delivery made the information more difficult to follow. Therefore, health professionals and others should provide information in a "relaxed manner, within a trusting relationship, and individualized according to need" (McInnis & Chambers, 2008, p. 421). This was especially important when mothers were learning to breastfeed. When first putting their babies to the breast, mothers felt that instead of the health professional putting the infant on the breast themselves, they should show the mothers how to do it.

Mothers who breastfeed in public are sometimes viewed as violating public morality (Van Esterik, 2002). Requiring a breastfeeding mother to conceal her infant's feedings from others can make a mother feel uncomfortable rather than allowing her to embrace her role as a mother providing the best possible food for her infant. In the workplace, a mother may be forced to pump her breasts in a restroom, which is unsanitary and uncomfortable. Support for a mother means that there will be opportunities to feed her infant or pump without discomfort.

Practitioners who work with families must consider the roles that other members of the family have in supporting the mother's feeding practices. In the past, fathers were excluded from the birth process and the decisions involved in caring for young children (Finnbogadóttir, Crang Svalenius, & Persson, 2003). It was believed that breastfeeding was not a father's concern. Pontes, Osorio, and Alexandrino (2009) studied the role of the father in breastfeeding. Although the father's role in the family is often viewed as provider and head of the home, active participation of the father is very valuable for breastfeeding mothers and their infants. Fathers can support breastfeeding by staying close and helping whenever possible. One father described his participation in breastfeeding by saying, "I used to wake up at dawn with my wife…sat on the bed, looking at the baby being breastfed…placed the baby on my shoulder to make it burp" (Pontes et al., 2009, p. 200). By being active participants in and supporters of breastfeeding, "Fathers will be able to develop parenthood (i.e., to help their wives or companions to provide for their children's needs, in every phase of their lives)" (Pontes et al., 2009, p. 196).

Abby, the mother quoted in a previous section, stated, "Having a supportive partner/spouse was very important during those first few days" (Nicole Zavala, personal communication, September 29, 2010). Grassley and Eschiti (2007) said that "Grandmothers are important to successful breastfeeding because their knowledge, attitudes, and experiences influence their daughters' decisions to initiate and continue breastfeeding" (p. 23). Mothers who choose to breastfeed want the grandmothers to be advocates in their decisions, even if breastfeeding conflicts with the grandmothers' personal opinions. When grandmothers offer unsolicited advice, a mother interprets the advice as a criticism of her parenting efforts (Reid, Schmied, & Beale, 2010). Grassley and Eschiti (2007) studied 35 grandmothers and concluded that the grandmothers' role in encouraging breastfeeding includes being helpful, updating their knowledge, and having the desire to learn together with the mother. Grandmothers' knowledge about breastfeeding may be outdated and in conflict with current information. Practitioners can provide classes, handouts, or Internet resources that are specifically designed for grandparents (Grassley & Eschiti, 2007). Other ways in which a grandmother can be helpful is through emotional and practical support. She can provide emotional support by affirming that the mother's choice, whatever it may be, is the right one. By supporting the mother's choices, even when they differ from her own, a grandmother provides the mother with loving encouragement.

Bottle Feeding   Other mothers choose to bottle feed. They choose bottle feeding for a variety of reasons, such as working outside of the home and the fact that bottle feeding allows others to feed the infant. From interviews conducted with 200 young women, Dix (1991) found that young mothers who chose not to breastfeed did so because they saw breastfeeding as embarrassing and inconvenient. Other factors included work or school intentions, the influence of friends and family, the mother's knowledge base, and lack of support from health care professionals. Some mothers combine bottle feeding and breastfeeding; their infants are breastfed while the mothers are home, and they are bottle-fed while in another person's care.

When an infant is bottle-fed, all practitioners should be aware that the infant will take the amount of formula (or pumped breast milk) she needs and should not be encouraged to take more by jiggling the bottle. In addition, the feeding environment should not be too stimulating. Sometimes if the environment is too loud, an infant will not eat. Specific formulas are chosen by parents, their health providers, or the hospital where the infant was born. Formulas are not interchangeable, so the infant must be fed the same formula at each feeding.

Introducing Solids   Solids are typically introduced between 4–6 months of age, as discussed in Chapter 1. The developmental readiness of each child should be evaluated before solids are introduced, and professionals should work with parents to introduce solids slowly, one new food at a time. Also, professionals and parents should be aware of signs that might indicate an allergic reaction. As new foods are introduced, there must be good communication among all caregivers and professionals in order to ensure consistency between foods served at home and those served away from home. The schedule for the introduction of solids usually progresses from very thin cereals, to vegetables, fruits, and meats (see Chapter 1 for more information).

Each caregiver influences the introduction of solids, and the introduction of solids may cause in each caregiver different feelings or perceptions of meaning. In a study conducted by Anderson, Nicklas, Spence, and Kavanagh (2009), infants' fathers (or men who acted as father figures), began feeding solids earlier than medically recommended. Fathers' perceptions of infant feeding were acquired through sources such as prior experience, advice from experts, and from reading books, magazines, and online articles. Fathers were most likely to accept advice from people with experience as well as advice in written form or retrieved from the Internet. Advice received from pediatricians or others without children was not highly regarded by fathers. One reason fathers introduced solids earlier than medically recommended was to modify the infant's undesirable behaviors, such as spitting up, not sleeping through the night, and not seeming to be full after a bottle. Fathers influence the introduction of solids by being sources of information, but the ultimate decisions about feeding the infant are made by the mother (Anderson et al., 2009). Other studies have suggested that the maternal grandmother has the most influence on the mother with regard to the early introduction of solid foods (Alder et. al., 2004; Reid et al., 2010).

Feeding Toddlers

Toddlers are learning how to assert their independence and autonomy. This is a major task and may be dreaded by caregivers and parents, but it is also an opportunity for parents and caregivers to learn about the uniqueness of each child through the choices he or she makes. Autonomy is often first noted in children's food choices. Often to the dismay of their caregivers, toddlers now make decisions about what, when, and how much to eat. Within the bounds of proper, healthy nutrition, it is important to allow toddlers to make their own choices. Allowing toddlers to make food choices from a group of healthy possibilities sets the stage for good eating habits. Positive guidance shows toddlers that they are valued, encourages cooperation, and helps toddlers learn problem-solving skills. Adults who set appropriate limits, provide a pleasant eating environment, and offer choices while supporting children's behaviors are creating a safe and positive environment for development.

Toddlers are picky eaters, and food neophobia (i.e., fear of the new) is common among 2-year-olds. Because breastfed children experience a variety of flavors through breast milk, they may not be as neophobic in their food choices as formula-fed children (Addessi, Galloway, Visalberghi, & Birch, 2005). In this way, breastfeeding continues to have a positive influence on children's eating behaviors. To help a child who is experiencing food neophobia, caregivers should continue to offer foods that were previously rejected; children often try a new food several times before accepting it (Savage, Fisher, & Birch, 2007). Providing a social setting in which a child can observe others eating a new food will also help the child accept it (Addessi, Galloway, Visalberghi, & Birch, 2005).

Toddlers may also go on a food jag in which they request and eat only one food, such as macaroni and cheese, peanut butter and jelly sandwiches, or chicken nuggets. Food jags may be related to the neophobia or just familiar flavors that comfort the young child. Sometimes children are sensitive to specific flavors in foods and reject those with phenylthiocarbamid, which is a chemical that can cause a bitter flavor experience. It is found in foods such as strawberries, green beans, broccoli, and apples (Gamble, 2004). The eating behaviors described here are typical, so it is important to be patient with children when they exhibit these behaviors.

A toddler's appetite may be sporadic. For example, one day a toddler may consume a large amount of food, including extra servings at meals. The next day, the same toddler might just nibble. It is best to consider a toddler's diet over the course of a week rather than day by day; this provides a better picture of the general nutritional content of the child's diet. Like infants, toddlers should be allowed to self-regulate their eating to meet their nutritional and caloric needs. However, around the age of 3 years, children's eating is influenced by parental and environmental cues rather than physiological cues of hunger and satiety (Klesges, Stein, Eck, Isbell, & Klesges, 1991; Koivisto, Fellenius, & Sjoden, 1994).

Because adults feel responsible for a child's eating behavior and nutrition, they may try to control the toddler's eating habits. However, this creates an unnecessary power struggle. Toddlers seek independence and are perfectly able to regulate their own food intake. In addition, eating struggles may promote negative feeding behaviors and support behaviors that are counter to the parent's actual preferences.

Professionals receive little training on how to handle feeding issues in young children and how independence may affect feeding. Only 42% of teachers working with young children are trained on how to feed young children (Sigman-Grant et al., 2008). Children must be allowed to have some control, but caregivers should provide clear consistent limits. Adults can ensure that the child is provided meals, that the foods offered are healthy, and that the child is provided with good modeling and consistent expectations regarding mealtime manners. Children need to be left as the decision makers for how much they eat and whether they eat at all.

Toddlers love to do things for themselves, and they learn how to do things by actually performing the action. Allowing children to feed themselves may lead to a mess, but the child's process of learning to eat independently is much more important than avoiding a mess. For example, a toddler might create a huge mess by independently eating spaghetti and pudding, but the skills learned outweigh the mess. As gross motor skills improve, children will move food from plates to their mouths more smoothly. Improved fine motor skills will allow them to use a spoon, getting most of the food in their mouths. It is important for caregivers to be flexible, allowing children to make mistakes, such as taking too much for a serving and dropping foods off of their spoons. Toddlers learn a great deal from these experiences.

Toddlers are developing their own likes and dislikes, often influenced by family, caregivers, and their social environment. Mealtimes are significant because of the feeding skills and the social skills they allow children to develop. Adults should engage in mealtime conversations with children about what they have done prior to the meal or events at home. These conversations help children realize that they are important, and they enhance enjoyment of meals. Serving meals "family style" (allowing children to select what and how much to eat) is a developmentally appropriate practice for toddlers and young children. Sigman-Grant et al. (2008) reported that less than half of child care centers studied engage in family-style meal service. Benefits of family-style meals include the opportunity for children to self-regulate their food intake, the presence of adults acting as role models, the opportunity for children to learn social skills like sharing and taking turns, and the opportunity for adults to teach nutrition and prevent accidents such as choking (Sigman-Grant et al., 2008).

Toddlers are a unique group. They are learning so much at such a fast pace that working with them can be thrilling. Flexibility and consistency on the part of caregivers allow toddlers to thrive developmentally in their feeding environments.

Feeding Preschoolers

Preschoolers are learning the skills and customs that surround meals and snacks. Developmentally, preschoolers are recognizing that they are separate individuals who can make their own choices. They understand the difference between acceptable and unacceptable mealtime behavior. Preschoolers have the ability to be patient and pay attention to processes. For example, preschoolers can learn to sit still while a meal is being served, they can make decisions about what foods to take, and they can recognize the importance of using utensils (instead of fingers) for feeding.

Preschoolers are influenced by their environment. Teachers, friends, parents, and television all influence the foods preschoolers will eat. Most children feel comfortable eating familiar foods, but some will try new foods if encouraged. Wardle, Herrera, Cooke, and Gibson (2003) found that children were more likely to try a new food when it was offered without the enticement of a reward. Children are more likely to try new foods without coercion and without a lot of attention being paid to their reactions. The introduction of a new food can also be a learning experience for preschool-age children. Children can learn about the food, including where it comes from and how it is prepared.

Parenting Styles and Children's Eating Behavior

Parents are a big influence on children, and their style of parenting has an impact on children's eating behavior. Hughes, Power, Fisher, Mueller, and Nicklas (2005) studied African American and Hispanic families involved in the Head Start program and found that parenting style influenced feeding. Two dimensions of parenting were studied: demandingness (parental expectations) and responsiveness (parental sensitivity to children's feeling, thoughts, and beliefs). These are comparable to the parenting styles described by Baumrind (1971), and Maccoby and Martin (1983). The Hughes et al. (2005) study revealed ways in which each parenting style affected eating behavior.

Authoritarian Parenting   Approximately one third of the African American and Hispanic parents in the sample were "authoritarian," including high levels of restrictive feeding and pressure to eat (Hughes et al., 2005). Authoritarian parents are very demanding and have high expectations; furthermore, compared with other parents, authoritarian parents are not as responsive or sensitive to children's needs and wants. Previous studies have shown that an authoritarian style is related to problems with self-regulation of energy intake and reduced responsiveness to energy density of foods (Birch, McPhee, Shoba, Pirok, & Steinberg, 1987; Johnson & Birch, 1994).

Authoritative Parenting   Compared with parents who have an authoritarian feeding style, parents with an authoritative feeding style showed more support and involvement but still exerted appropriate levels of control related to the children's consumption of healthy foods. Authoritative parents have expectations for their children and are responsive to their children's needs. If parents and other caregivers maintain appropriate control (such as that exhibited by authoritative parents), children will develop self-regulation of food intake and a healthier body mass index. Authoritative parents have good parental control in that they balance demands and expectations with sensitivity and responsiveness.

Permissive-Indulgent Parenting   Two permissive styles of feeding were identified, and ethnic differences can be observed between the two. Permissive–indulgent parents are high in responsiveness, but low in demandingness.

Permissive–Uninvolved Parenting   Permissive–uninvolved parents are low in both demandingness and responsiveness; they are viewed as neglectful. Hispanics are more likely to be permissive–indulgent, and African American parents are more likely to be permissive–uninvolved (Hughes et al., 2005).

CAREGIVERS AND FEEDING DECISIONS

Leaving a child in the care of trusted caregivers may be difficult, but it is necessary for most families in today's society because most parents work. In 2010, nationwide statistics indicated that 35% of infants and toddlers needed child care and 30% of preschool-age children needed child care (National Association of Child Care Resource and Referral Agencies, 2010). Of these children, 80% were enrolled in child care full time and 20% were enrolled part time.

Parents must develop good relationships with their child's caregiver in order for the child to get the best possible care, and constant communication is the key to forming a trusting relationship. Regular communication is necessary in order for the parents to inform the caregiver about matters that concern the child. By opening this line of communication, the caregiver and parent will become a team caring for the child.

Feeding Infants in Child Care Settings

When a child is enrolled in child care as an infant, many decisions must be made. One of the most challenging decisions for parents is whether to feed the child breast milk or formula at the child care. As described previously, breast milk provides many benefits to infants. However, many challenges arise when mothers try to juggle breastfeeding with a return to work. Fein, Bidisha, and Roe (2008) studied a subsample of mothers who were concurrently working and breastfeeding. They found that the four most common ways in which the mothers continued to provide breast milk after returning to work were as follows:

1) directly breastfeeding the infant,

2) pumping milk for later consumption,

3) using a mixed strategy of pumping and feeding directly, and

4) not providing breast milk during the workday (either discarding pumped breast milk or not pumping).

Ways in which direct breastfeeding was supported by the workplace included allowing the mother to keep the infant at work with her, providing on-site or near-site child care and breastfeeding breaks, allowing mothers to telecommute, and allowing the infant to be brought into the workplace for feeding (Fein et al., 2008). In order for mothers to pump at work, the employer must allow them to take breaks when they feel it is necessary to pump. For a mother to both breastfeed and pump, she needs an opportunity to take breaks and a flexible schedule in order to leave the workplace to feed her infant according to the infant's schedule. These accommodations demonstrate manageable strategies to support breastfeeding mothers in the workplace; however, "most employers do not have formal breastfeeding support programs" (Fein et al., 2008). In order to compensate for the lack of breastfeeding support in the workplace, some mothers have used an alternative approach: delaying a return to work until the infant is older and taking some solids.

Breastfeeding mothers who have jobs that are not flexible have a different kind of challenge. To have an infant fed solely on breast milk while attending child care puts a high demand on the mother to provide enough milk to last throughout the day. Some women produce an abundance of milk, while others produce less. To support mothers who choose to feed their infants only breast milk after returning to work, child care centers are required by the Department of Child and Family Services (DCFS) to have a refrigerator that is accessible to infant classrooms (Department of Child and Family Services, 2010). This allows parents to bring in a full day's supply of breast milk. In addition to the classroom refrigerator, some child care centers have a freezer where breast milk can be stored for up to 12 months. The milk stored in the freezer gives parents a sense of security because they know their infant has a good supply of milk.

An additional difficulty with breastfeeding and having an infant in child care is the concern over whether the child will accept the bottle. Based on the experiences of an infant child care provider, there is a particular challenge in feeding infants who received only breast milk prior to enrolling in child care (Nicole Zavala, personal communication, September 29, 2010). For example, one infant had been solely breastfed before starting child care. When she was offered the bottle at child care, she cried and refused to latch on to the nipple, turning her head away from the bottle. The caregiver tried every type of bottle and every type of nipple, but the infant refused to take her mother's milk from a bottle. Infants in this situation must wait for their mothers to feed them, causing stress for the infants, the caregivers, and the mothers. Consider the experiences of Carrie, an early childhood student:

> Anna is 3 months old. She has been breastfed since she was born, and she continues to get breast milk. Her mom has recently gone back to work, and she is now fed a 5-ounce bottle of breast milk about every 3–4 hours while her mother is at work. The breast milk is frozen in bags and needs to be thawed before feedings. Anna gets very impatient if she is hungry and the milk does not thaw fast enough. She usually cries and starts sucking on her fist when she is hungry. She takes about 30 minutes to finish her bottle. When she is eating, her eyes close as if she is really relaxed. Sometimes she falls asleep, and when I move the bottle from her mouth she continues sucking. If you pull the bottle out too soon, she begins to cry. She knows when her bottle is done, and she doesn't cry if you pull the bottle out when it is empty. I sit her up after feeding and usually get about 2–3 good burps from her.

In a child care setting, breastfed infants pose a challenge. Formula-fed infants typically have an eating schedule and eat approximately the same amount at each feeding. In contrast, infants who are fed breast milk may become hungry sooner than the schedule suggested by parents. An infant on breast milk may also vary in the amount he or she consumes from one feeding to the next. To provide a formula-fed infant with a bottle is simple in comparison: The caregiver measures the appropriate amount of water and adds the appropriate amount of formula. Providing an infant with a bottle of breast milk may take more time. The caregiver must first warm the cold or frozen milk, so there may be waiting period for an infant who was not scheduled to eat but wanted to eat. During this time the infant may get upset and require soothing before feeding, thereby creating even more wait time.

When a mother decides to give her infant formula instead of breast milk during the child's day in child care, the parents incur an expense. A young infant typically eats 4 ounces every 2–4 hours, and the amount of milk given at each feeding increases steadily as the infant gets older. A can of formula for an infant who attends child care full time typically lasts one week. Formula can get very expensive, especially if the infant needs a special type of formula due to gastrointestinal complications such as acid reflux.

Caregivers are able to nurture a sense of emotional well-being in infants. When a caregiver perceives an infant's cries to mean that he or she is hungry, the caregiver is initiating responsive feeding. Responsive feeding is the perception, interpretation, and appropriate response to an infant's hunger or fullness cues (Branscomb & Goble, 2008). Caregivers' responses to these hunger cues (rather than a schedule) have a lasting effect on the child. Infants who are fed when they are hungry and stop feeding when they are full are less likely to overeat later in life; as a result, they are less at risk for obesity (Branscomb & Goble, 2008). A caregiver who cradles and/or sings to an infant while the infant eats is helping to promote the emotional well-being of the infant and helping to strengthen the bond between the caregiver and the infant.

Feeding Toddlers in Child Care Settings

Mealtimes are often more difficult with toddlers. Typical eating behaviors of toddlers include decreased appetite, picky eating, and food refusal (Branscomb & Goble, 2008). It is important for caregivers to help toddlers develop their independence by providing a variety of healthy foods and allowing toddlers to choose what they eat. Allowing toddlers to make such choices supports the development of lifelong healthy eating habits (Parlakian & Lerner, 2007). Caregivers can further assist toddlers with mealtimes by engaging in conversation with the toddlers, being flexible, being attentive to signs that the child is done eating, and having toddlers eat at the same time so that they can see other children eating food they may be hesitant to try (Parlakian & Lerner, 2007). Communication between parents and caregivers is very important in helping to develop mealtime practices that are similar at home and at child care (Branscomb & Goble, 2008).

Feeding difficulties can cause concern in families; however, most of these issues are temporary in typically developing children. Concerns about children's eating usually are related to one of the following areas: self-restricting food intake, selectivity about which types of food are acceptable, undesirable behaviors during meals, and taking too long to eat a meal (Sisson & Van Hasselt, 1989). These disruptions in feeding can be linked to several causes, such as the child's temperament, incompetent parenting, disruptions in the child's environment (e.g., divorce, loss of parental employment), and sensory processing issues. For example, when toddlers are picky (e.g., about which foods they eat, about the feeding environment) and caregivers do not make adjustments, more feeding issues can arise. Professionals who work with parents who are experiencing these issues need to be aware that picky eating is typical for infants and toddlers. To help young children overcome picky eating, caregivers should consistently offer a variety of foods, not just those the child prefers. In fact, caregivers should repeatedly offer foods that children have rejected before. The repetition helps with familiarity, and as the child becomes more familiar with the food, he or she may eat it. Often a food must be offered over a dozen times before a child will accept it. Children benefit from an environment in which their caregivers are patient and accepting.

FEEDING CHILDREN WITH SPECIAL NEEDS

Children with disabilities are a unique population whose needs are so individualized that professionals have to be especially careful not to make assumptions
about what their care entails. This may be especially important when it comes to
feeding. The Americans with Disabilities Act (ADA; 1990) requires that certain
provisions be made in early childhood environments to accommodate children
with special needs. A plan must be in place, and that plan must include expectations related to the child's developmental needs. Feeding should be included in
these plans because it plays a central role in a child's development and health. For
each child, there are several areas that should be addressed as caregivers and other
professionals consider the child's feeding needs.

Physical difficulties are a primary concern because if a child does not have
the skills to feed him- or herself, special accommodations need to be made. Some
children may need special chairs to help them maintain the posture needed for
eating. Often young children need a chair that is similar to a highchair but at a
lower level so the child can interact with peers. Some types of furniture help the
child to control bodily movements by holding down feet or arms and preventing
movement that may interfere with feeding. (Chapter 8 covers more specifics about
the selection of equipment for children with special needs.) Utensils often need
modifications, sometimes as simple as bending the handle, to assist children in
getting foods to their mouths as independently as possible. It is important to make
sure that children with special needs develop and maintain their independence as
much as possible.

Some children with special needs have metabolic disorders or allergies requiring changes in and attention to feeding practices. These children are likely to
have special dietary limitations that may not fit nutritional guidelines. Children
with metabolic disorders include those with cystic fibrosis, diabetes, and Phenyl-
ketonuria (PKU) as well as many other disabilities. Children with PKU are not able
to metabolize the amino acid phenylalanine. A diet including this amino acid can
cause intellectual disability, but when a child's diet is free of phenylalanine, intel-
ligence is in the typical range.

Children who have food allergies also need special attention. Allergic reactions may result in hives, digestive problems, or swollen airways that can result in
death. Food allergies are "an abnormal response to food that is triggered by a specific reaction in the immune system and expressed by certain, often characteristic,
symptoms" (MedicineNet, 2011). Common foods that children may be allergic to
are eggs, milk, peanuts, and fruits, particularly tomatoes and strawberries. Some
children outgrow allergies. Staff education and clear communication practices are
imperative in child care centers attended by children with allergies.

Children with disabilities may require more time to eat than typically developing peers. Eating for these individuals might also be messier than it is for same-age,
typically developing peers. It is not surprising that many people who care for children with special needs do not have training on how to feed each child according
to specific requirements. Many caregivers get on-the-job training (after all, the child
has to be fed), or they may be educated by the parents or another caregiver. Caregivers need intervention and outside help to be able to provide the best feeding
situation for young children.

SUMMARY

All children, including those with special needs, should be respected for their abilities, nutritional needs, and food preferences. Although feeding young children appears to be a simple and straight-forward task, it has huge implications with regard to relationships across caregivers. It is important to recognize and support these important relationships because they provide the foundation for a child's later feeding behaviors. A child should receive care that demonstrates respect and that allows the child freedom to make feeding decisions within developmentally appropriate boundaries.

■ ■ ■ TABLE TALK ■ ■ ■

Katye and Jack have a 6-month-old son, Sam, who has been breastfed since he was born. They also have a 5-year-old son, Stefan. Jack feels as if it is time to start Sam on solid foods. When the family sits down for a meal, Katye feeds Sam only cereal, but she is starting to add baby food fruits and vegetables. Sam tends to pay attention to the solid food that his family is eating. He reaches for his parent's plates from his highchair. Jack attempts to give Sam bits of food that are easy for Sam to eat. Katye gets upset and states that Sam is still too young. When she is asked when they should introduce solid foods, she dismisses the question. Katye works late 2 days a week and on those days at dinner, Jack feeds Sam solid foods along with his baby food. It is not mentioned to Katye, but Sam eats everything that is given to him.

Discussion Questions

- ■ Should Sam be eating table foods?
- ■ What would you tell Katye and Jack about starting Sam on solid foods?
- ■ What additional suggestions do you have for improving Sam's eating habits?

FEEDING NUGGETS

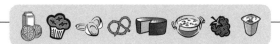

Books

Family Mealtime as a Context of Development and Socialization Edited by Reed W. Larson, Angela R. Wiley, and Kathryn R. Branscomb (2006)

Secrets of Feeding a Healthy Family: Orchestrating and Enjoying the Family Meal by Ellyn Satter (2008)

Websites

Family Day: A Day to Eat Dinner with Your Children"
The National Center on Addiction and Substance Abuse at Columbia University (CASA)
www.casafamilyday.org

"Make Mealtime Family Time" by David Lynn (2007)
www.makemealtimefamilytime.com

"Family Meals: More Than Just Eating at Home" by Dairy Council of California (2011)
http://www.mealsmatter.org/Articles-And-Resources/Healthy-Living-Articles/
Family-Meals.aspx

$$\boxed{4}$$

Diversity
and Feeding

What You'll Learn in This Chapter

This chapter provides

- An overview of several cultures with a description of mealtimes and cultural expectations for feeding young children
- A discussion about populations whose children may be at higher risk of feeding issues
- Strategies and specialized interventions to address the issues faced by high-risk groups

■ ■ ■ **FOOD FOR THOUGHT** ■ ■ ■

"When Maci was 4 years old, we went to a Passover Seder at the temple. When the matzo ball soup was served, she looked at me and said, 'Is everyone here sick?' This story is one of my absolute favorites!"

Starla, Parent

"The feeding experience I observed was with a child that came from a family where English was not their first language. While Chuck sat for snack, he was unable to convey what he wanted. The only word he got out was 'juu' for juice. He would repeat it over and over and over and get louder and louder until you gave him juice. Then you would have to hold the cup or he would tip it too high and spill it on himself. After he was finished with his two glasses of juice (the maximum allowed), he was given water and became upset. He did not eat at this sitting."

Maria, Child Care Worker

"Manuel is my baby brother. He was born in the Dominican Republic in 1988, when I was almost 14 years old. As the older sister, I was many times responsible for caring for him, and that included feeding him. In the Dominican Republic, we tend to start babies on solids early, at about 3 months of age. We feed them our staple foods of rice and beans mashed up, and we force feed them sometimes. I remember when I would feed him, I was told by his mom to make sure he ate his food, so I would make him cry in order to get him to open his mouth and I could insert the food in his mouth. Today I know that doing this is very inappropriate and not healthy for the baby. But back then, I was just following tradition and doing what I was told to do."

Ava, Early Childhood Student

Many parents base their feeding practices on experience, family history, socioeconomic circumstances, and cultural beliefs. Fiese and Schwartz (2008) pointed out, "Family mealtimes are embedded in a social, cultural, and economic context that are associated with a variety of indicators of children's health and wellbeing" (p. 1). This chapter focuses on mealtime experiences across cultures; it discusses foods, flavors, methods of food preparation, and mealtime expectations for young children. Other topics covered are at risk families, including low-income and adolescent parents, and the affects of at risk status on young children and their feeding.

CULTURAL CONSIDERATIONS

A great many of our beliefs come from our relationships with family and friends. Feeding practices, in particular, are influenced by culture, ethnic, and racial origins (Birch & Fisher, 1995). "Food habits are the most enduring aspect of a culture" (Birch & Dietz, 2008, p. X). Every culture includes different foods, usually those that are available in the group's original geographic region. Also, each culture also has specific ideas about feeding young children, including whether infants should be breast-fed or bottle-fed, when infants should transition to solids, when children should be weaned, and which solid foods should be introduced first. In fact, our earliest flavor influences occur while still in utero, where we get our first taste of the culture we will be born into through the amniotic fluid (Mennella, 2008; Mennella, Jagnow, & Beauchamp, 2001). What a mother eats during pregnancy and while breastfeeding passes on her culture's food choices to her infant. Once the infant begins to eat solids and table foods, these early influences are reinforced.

Food choice is the result of a complicated set of factors that can be categorized in different ways. In 1956, Yudkin argued that "food choice was influenced by physical factors (e.g., geography, season, economics and food technology), social factors (e.g., religion, class, education, and advertising), and psychological factors (e.g., hereditary, allergy, and nutritional needs)" (as cited in Ogden, 2010, p. 32).

Food choices can also be categorized as internal or external to the individual (Shepherd, 1989). Internal food choices include those motivated by factors such as personality, sensory needs, and genetics. External food choices are governed by the individual's cultural context, social environment, or available foods.

Steptoe, Pollard, and Wardle (1995) studied why people make various food choices. The top reasons were health, sensory appeal, cost, and convenience. Each person makes different foods choices taking these factors into account either consciously (e.g., reading labels) or unconsciously (e.g., buying the foods that have always been in their home).

Mealtime Expectations

Each family has a unique constellation and unique constraints that contribute to the selection of foods that are consumed and preferred. Meals shared at celebrations include specific foods, flavors, preparation methods, and behavior expectations. For example, celebratory foods eaten at the New Year vary from culture to culture. In Greece, New Year celebrations include a pastry with a coin baked inside. In Japan, foods are prepared a week before the holiday and represent a wish for the New Year; for example, seaweed represents a wish for happiness. For each culture, different foods and preparations are made for weddings, funerals, holidays, and other life events, demonstrating the uniqueness of each culture's beliefs and each culture's rich history. Rituals are passed down through generations and have cultural ties to the past. Often as a younger member is helping with celebration preparations, he or she will ask, "Why are we doing this?" and get the response, "Because this is the way my grandmother did it."

As Denham (2003) pointed out, "Family dietary rituals and routines vary based upon things such as family type, children's ages, cultural practices, social resources, and other factors" (p. 319). Single parents have different constraints compared with parents who have partners; single parents generally have less time to prepare meals and less money to purchase food, resulting in diets that contain more processed foods and fewer fresh fruits and vegetables. Additionally, families with infants have different expectations for mealtime behaviors and manners compared with families with school-age children.

Often, the foods we eat are determined by what is available in a particular region. In the past, food availability varied regionally in the United States. For example, in the South, citrus fruits such as oranges and lemons, along with vegetables such as peppers, broccoli, green onions, and sweet corn, were widely available. In the North, diets relied more heavily upon grains, such as barley and buckwheat, and on root vegetables, such as sugar beets and potatoes (Economic Research Service, 2002). Today, however, reliable systems exist to safely move foods from one area of the country to another, which means more choices and some changes in our preferences. Rozin (1982) asserted that information about a person's culture or ethnic group is the best predictor of food preferences, feelings about foods, and routine eating practices (as cited in Ogden, 2010, p. 32). Because of the incredible amount of diversity in food preferences, the choices we make about foods are part of a complex process; they are not merely a preference we are born with.

The main point of reference for feeding milestones is the impact of parenting behaviors on the eating habits of young children (Birch et al., 2001; Wardle, Sanderson, Gutherie, Rapoport, & Plomin, 2002). Information on "feeding norms" is stated as a developmental norm, but has an ethnocentric bias because "norms" are generally based on one ethnicity, usually the middle-class (Dettwyler & Fishman,

1992). For example, in the United States, parents encourage children to finish the food they are eating and may use a reward, such as a dessert, a toy, or a television show as an incentive. They may also employ guilt. A parent may say to the child, "There are children starving in Africa!" or "Your mother spent a lot of time and energy preparing the food!" Americans are also are more likely to use highchairs or booster seats with straps to restrain a child. Thus, parents have control over when the child leaves the meal (Dettwyler, 1989).

Because culture plays an intricate and dynamic role in our food choices, this chapter discusses several different cultures. Rozin (1982, as cited in Rozin, 1996) stated there are "three indirect influences on the foods we eat: 1) basic ingredients (e.g., rice, potatoes, fish), 2) characteristic flavors employed (flavor principles; e.g., a combination of chili pepper with either tomato or lime for Mexico), and 3) particular modes of food preparation (e.g., stir frying in China)" (p. 236). In addition, there are different expectations for mealtime behavior.

For each of these influences, the following cultures will be discussed: African, Asian, European, and American Indian/Alaskan Native. It should be noted that there are gaps in our knowledge about certain cultures. Therefore, information is not available regarding each of the influences for every one of the cultures discussed. Also, we must be careful not to make broad generalizations about the information and remember that what is true for a larger culture is not necessarily true for an individual member of that culture. Table 4.1 summarizes each type of information, as available, for each culture.

African Foods and Mealtime Expectations

Typical foods in the African American diet are located in Table 4.1. (Poe, 1999). *Soul food*, a term that arose in the 1960s, refers to foods commonly found in the African American diet (Opie, 2008). Beef, pork, rabbit, and seafood are typical meats used in soul food, which can include gumbo, e'toufee, and Cajun cuisine. Other foods that are typically included in soul food are vegetables, okra, black-eyed peas, tomatoes, peaches, broccoli, watermelon, eggplant, sesame seed, sorghum, collard greens, and sweet potatoes. Children are expected to eat plenty of food because it gives them strength and health. Mealtimes are important, and foods are often "left on the stove" for family members to eat at their convenience (Lynch & Hanson, 2004, p. 162).

Asian Foods and Mealtime Expectations

The foods eaten by Asians are driven by the concept of yin and yang, a belief system that seeks balance in all things. Foods in the Asian diet can be found in Table 4.1. (Gordon, Kang, Cho, & Sucher, 2000). Asians believe that an improper diet leads to imbalance. Each food has a hot or cold property that turns into air after being eaten (Lynch & Hanson, 2004). Cold foods consist of fruits and vegetables such as cabbage, melon, and seaweed. Juice and water are also served cold. Hot foods consist of meats, fried foods, cereals, nuts, and beans; coffee and alcohol are served as hot beverages (Lynch & Hanson, 2004). Foods vary according to the region; wide cultural variation across Asian regions leads to variations in foods served. In Asian cultures, the foods are relatively low in calories and cooked for a time to achieve a flavor and consistency that is appealing to the senses. In most Asian cultures, ingredients are cut into smaller pieces to reduce cooking times because of limited fuel resources.

Table 4.1. Preferred foods, characteristic flavors, and preparation methods by culture

	African American[a]	Asian	Asian Indian	French	Italian	Irish	Swedish	Hispanic[l]	Native American
Preferred foods	Greens Yellow vegetables Legumes Beans Rice Meat stew Soul food[b]	Rice[c] Vegetables[c] Fruits[c] Little meat[c]	Vegetables Chicken Fish Fruit	Fruits Vegetables Meats Fungus	Antipasti Soup/sauces Breads Pasta Rice Fish Meat dishes/cured meats	Irish stew Boxty[f] Coddle[g] Colcannon[h] Fresh vegetables[i] Seafoods[i] Handmade cheeses[i] Soda bread[j]	Breads Pastries Dary products Potatoes Fruit soups Game	Rice Beans Non-meat foods of vegetable origin (dried beans, whole grains) Tortillas	The Three Sisters[k] Frybread Cornbread Turkey Fish Cranberry/blueberry Hominy Mush Nuts
Characteristic flavors	Salt Peanut butter (e.g. for flavoring greens) Tomatoes Onion Curry	Ginger[d] Black pepper[d] Soy sauce[d] Rice-wine vinegar[d] Sesame oil[d]	Stocks[e] Ginger[e] Cumin[e] Celery[e] Onion[e] Garlic[e] Chutney[e]	tarragon rosemary thyme fennel sage marjoram herbs de Provence	Garlic Bay leaves Basil Onion Fennel Mint Oregano Chili pepper Parsley Rosemary Sage Thyme	Leeks/onions Salt/pepper Caraway seeds Nutmeg/mace Butter Bacon fat	Simple seasonings Butter	Garlic Oregano Chili (mild or hot)	Ramps Wild ginger Juniper Salt Sugar
Preparation methods	Frying Boiling (slow cooking) Sautéing	Stir fry Deep fry Steaming Stewing Roasting Paper-wrapped frying	Breading Frying	No specific methods	No specific methods	No specific methods	No specific methods	No specific methods	Roasting Baking

[a]Poe, 1999. [b]See text for more details regarding soul food. [c]Gordon, Kang, Cho, & Sucher, 2000. [d]Kittler & Sucher, 2008 [e]Misra, 2009. [f]Boxty is a potato pancake. [g]Coddle is a dish made with boiled pork sausage. [h]Colcannon is a potato dish made with kale or cabbage. New additions to the Irish diet. [l]Hispanic preferred foods and characteristic flavors vary by region. [k]The Three Sisters are corn, beans, and squash.

In some Asian cultures, foods provide more than just sustenance. For example, the Chinese do not eat just to alleviate hunger; rather, foods are "for health promotion, treating diseases and, most importantly, building relationships among people and enhancing family values" (Li-Jian-rong, 2004, p. 147). Gender and age often play a role in Asian cultures in who gets to eat and when people eat. In North Vietnam, boys are able to select their own food, but girls may be scolded for being greedy, for using chopsticks incorrectly, and for failing to show respect (Ochs & Shohet, 2006; Rydstrom, 2003). However, women are the primary persons in charge of meals (Pan, Dixon, Himburg, & Huffman, 1999, p. 56).

For the Chinese, older family members eat before the younger ones, and children may not eat with others during formal occasions. "During more intimate family mealtimes, adults and children may eat at the same time" (Ochs & Shohet, 2006, p. 38). Children are to eat everything, including every grain of rice and, to demonstrate respect, refrain from taking more food than others take. Yen (1955) and her brothers were "cautioned to eat all of our rice lest we marry pockmarked persons" (p. 11–12). The Japanese have a less structured mealtime with less conflict than Anglo Americans (Martini, 1996).

Asian Indian Foods and Mealtime Expectations

Asian Indians believe that food can be hot (garmi) or cold (sardi). Garmi food (e.g., dates and grapes) "thickens the blood and speeds the metabolism," whereas sardi food (e.g., plums and oranges) "dilutes the blood and slows the metabolism" (Lynch & Hanson, 2004, p. 393). Garmi and sardi foods should be eaten in balance for good health. Foods in Asian Indian culture are usually high in fat (Misra, Khyrana, Isharwal, & Bhardwaj, 2009). Typically, vegetables, fish, and chicken are spiced with ginger, cumin, chopped onion, and garlic. These ingredients are then blended with flour, shaped into small patties, and deep fried. According to Misra et al. (2009) common Asian Indian foods include the following (see also Table 4.1):

- Parantha, a flat bread from India
- Bhatura, a deep-fried, leavened bread often eaten with a chickpea curry
- Pulao, also called pilaf, which is rice cooked in aromatic spices or stock
- Pakora, small, deep-fried snacks with chick-pea flour as an ingredient in the mixture
- Dosa, a thin South Indian pancake made from fermented lentils and rice blended with water, that is typically served with chutney or sambar, a Southeast Asian deer

Many Asian Indians eat with their hands, using a flatbread to pick up foods, and meals are eaten with the right hand, never the left hand. (Hand washing before and after meals is expected.) Asian Indians discourage too much talking or loud speaking during meals. Parents do not impose discipline on children when eating. A common practice in India is to walk infants during meals to distract them when they stop eating, in the hopes that they can be persuaded to take more food.

> Parents like to make the baby sit and feed but after a certain stage the baby refuses to sit in one place like a gentleman. The mother's intention is somehow to stuff into him whatever portion of food she has taken for him, so she walks around to distract his attention (Raphael & Davis, 1985, as cited in Dettwyler, 1989, p. 60)

Anglo European Foods and Mealtime Expectations

Europe is the epitome of diversity. Each of the many countries in Europe has unique foods and eating traditions. This section provides a brief glimpse into European mealtime customs, but cannot capture all of Europe's foods or food-related rituals.

The French eat a variety of foods (see Table 4.1). Dinner is usually a three-course meal. The first course is the hors d'oeuvre (or introductory course), the main course is a *plat principal,* and the final course is a dessert or cheese. Mineral water, wine, and bread are served with the meal.

In Italy, lunch is the main meal, while dinner is usually lighter. The meal begins with antipasti, which consists of cold meats and ham, small sandwiches, and sauces. The first course consists of pasta, spaghetti, soup, or crepes. The second course is meat or fish, followed by dessert and fruit. Italian children usually eat mid-afternoon snacks, consisting of various foods, ranging from raisins to biscuits to yogurt. After a light dinner, Italian families usually do not have dessert. Also, parents do not expect their children to finish meals. Instead, parents expect children to develop their own tastes and preferences. Both adults and children show appreciation for the food and the person who prepared it (Ochs & Shohet, 2006). During meals, Italian parents share memories of meals that were particularly pleasing in their own childhoods, bringing to mind family members who are no longer alive and thus linking generations (Ochs & Shohet, 2006).

In Ireland, foods have been influenced by crops and farm animals suited to the climate. The potato has been central to Irish cuisine ever since its introduction during the second half of the 16th century.

In Sweden, breads are central to the culture and are available in many forms. Pastries are popular, especially sweet pastries. Sweden has one of the highest rates of coffee consumption in the world, and milk is a common drink for both adults and children.

The main meal of the day is consumed at noon in many parts of Europe (Kittler & Sucher, 2008). Also, independence is emphasized early, including feeding. In general, families have meals together, but cultures differ in the role of children during meals. For example, in Sweden parents, especially mothers, dominate conversations during dinners (Ochs & Shohet, 2006 p. 42). Similarly, in New England, parents dominate conversations, with children contributing only about a third (Ochs & Shohet, 2006). Italian parents show pleasure in meals and model this pleasure for their children, emphasizing food as a pleasure, not expecting or pushing their children to finish all the food on their plates. Italian parents are likely to serve children foods first.

Hispanic Foods and Mealtime Expectations

Hispanics comprise the largest minority in the United States (U.S. Bureau of the Census, 2011) and Hispanic/Latino population includes individuals from Mexico, Cuba, South or Central America, Puerto Rico, and other Spanish cultures (U.S. Bureau of the Census, 2001). The diversity represented by these countries and their feeding traditions rivals the diversity found in Europe; therefore, only a sampling will be provided (see Table 4.1).

Preferred foods eaten (noted in Table 4.1) make up about half of the Hispanic diet. Fruit, vegetables, and dairy products are not particularly common in Hispanic diets (Levy-Costa, Sichieri, dos Santos Pontes, & Augusto-Monteiro, 2005), which may be due to limited accessibility because dairy and vegetables are less available in the north and northeast Brazil while eggs are scarce in the southeast (Levy-Costa et al., 2005).

Because Hispanics hail from so many different places, their food preferences vary. For instance, the U.S. Department of Agriculture (USDA, 2002) found that Mexicans prefer corn and amaranth. Rice is common in the Caribbean and coastal areas of Latin America, and South American diets include wheat, potatoes, and quinoa. Different beans are popular in different areas. For example, red kidney beans are preferred by Cubans and Central South Americans, while Venezuelans and Southern Mexicans use black beans. One might think Hispanic foods are spicy. However, Cuban, Puerto Rican, and Dominican cultures have foods that are mild, using tomato, garlic, oregano and only mild (not hot) chilies for seasoning. The preparation of foods also varies; for example, tortillas are prepared differently in different areas.

Food is important to Hispanic culture. Foods have properties of "hot" and "cold" and must be balanced. Many people in this ethnic group do not value independence; this also relates to expectations during meals (Heise, 2002). There is leniency in children's eating in that children are not forced to eat certain foods. In fact, preschool age Latino children may be allowed to drink from a baby bottle (Lynch & Hanson, 2004). Also, negative emotions are discouraged and positive emotions are acceptable (Lynch & Hanson, 2004). In some families, only the children are to remain quiet, but in the Peruvian Amazon everyone is to remain silent during a meal (Ochs & Shohet, 2006).

American Indian/Alaska Native Foods and Mealtime Expectations

There are about 576 tribal entities recognized in the United States. Nearly half of all Native Americans have an annual household income under the poverty level, only 8% have a college degree, and few Native Americans obtain prenatal care. Each tribe has a unique history and a unique culture regarding foods and mealtime traditions. Although there is variation across tribes, some generalizations can be made (see Table 4.1.)

FEEDING YOUNG CHILDREN ACROSS CULTURES

This section examines the cultural differences in breastfeeding and bottle feeding, the age of children when each culture generally weans them and starts introducing solids, and typical first foods. Our cultural beliefs directly and indirectly influence decisions to breastfeed or bottle feed, when to wean, what foods to feed an infant, and other decisions regarding the care of young children (Pak-Gorstein, Haq, & Graham, 2009). Again, not all of this information is available for every culture that is discussed. Additionally, some variation exists within each group, so this section offers general insight into each culture's beliefs and practices.

In many countries around the world, most infants are breastfed (World Health Organization & UNICEF, 2010). In rural areas of Africa (Buskens, Jaffe, & Mkhatshwa, 2007) and Latin America (Perez-Escamilla, 2003), it is assumed that mothers will breastfeed. However, in industrialized countries, where mothers have a choice, mothers breastfeed at much lower rates. Minorities in the United States are less likely to exclusively breastfeed than if in their country of origin (Anderson, Damio, Chapman, & Perez-Escamilla, 2007). They all refer to rates at 6 months Asian and Pacific Americans have the highest breastfeeding rates at 53% at 6 months, Hispanics have the next highest rates (45%), with non-Hispanic White and non-Hispanic Blacks (27%) the lowest rates, who prefer to bottle feed (Forste, Weiss, & Lippincott, 2001).

African and African American Practices for Feeding Young Children

In most African countries, all infants are breastfed—except when the mother is suffering from diseases such as advanced AIDS, in which case breastfeeding is not advisable (Buskens et al., 2007; F. Mumba, personal communication March 4, 2011). In fact, in some rural areas of Africa, a husband can seek divorce if his wife refuses to breastfeed (F. Mumba, personal communication, March 4, 2011). By contrast, in the United States, non-Hispanic African American mothers have the lowest rate of breastfeeding compared to other minority groups.

Many African mothers feed their infants water, because for them water is life and their babies need it, and others may feed their infants herbal concoctions and enemas used for various months to clean the newborn (Buskens et al., 2007). Due to work demands, some mothers in urban areas of Africa stop breastfeeding after 6 months when they start the introduction of solids. However, most mothers continue breastfeeding well into the second year of life, even though breastfeeding is not always exclusive.

Mothers in many areas of Africa begin to feed infants porridge when they are around 2 months of age. They do so by cupping the porridge in their hand and pouring it into the child's mouth. Porridge is made from corn flour mixed with sorghum and milk or butter and sugar or salt; ingredients vary by region. Many African mothers breastfeed until the infant loses the taste for milk. The child is given thicker porridge at 6 months, sometimes with peanuts added. Many African children are fed from the hands of adults and then from their own hands as they get older. By 1 year of age, children are expected to eat by themselves and spend a great deal of time eating with peers with a mother looking on.

Many African American mothers tend to introduce solid foods earlier than recommended. Some mothers introduce porridges as early as 10 days after birth because they believe that breast milk is not enough (Bronner et al., 1999; Buskens et al., 2007). In a study of low-income African American mothers, 32% of mothers had introduced some solids by 7–10 days postpartum. By 16 weeks, 93% had introduced their infant to solid food. Most often, cereal is added to the infant's bottle, and fruits and cereal are given by spoon (Bronner et al., 1999). On the other hand, in the African countries of Nigeria and Ghana, most mothers wait to introduce solids until 7–9 months or beyond (Steve, 2006; Nti & Lartey, 2007). The most common first foods have different names in the different countries, but are cereals made from corn meal or sorghum, and porridges (Buskens et al., 2007; Nti & Lartey, 2007; Steve, 2006).

Asian Practices for Feeding Young Children

Most mothers in Asian countries breastfeed their infants, and many continue to breastfeed into the second year (Dibley, Senarath, & Agho, 2010, Sinhababu, Mukhopadhyay, Panja, & Biswas, 2010). However, in many Asian countries it is common practice for mothers to wait 24 hours after birth to put the infant to the breast and to feed their infants some other liquid like tea or water, instead of colostrum.

They believe that breast milk does not contain water (Saha et al., 2008). Asian Indians are less likely to feed the newborn the colostrum because of a general belief that it is harmful and that a prelacteal feeding is helpful to the infant (Kannan, Carruth, & Skinner, 1999). This is especially true among Asian women living in their country of origin, but somewhat common among Asian women in the United States. In rural Bangladesh, the infant is fed water, milk products, honey, mustard oil, sugar, glucose, or jaggery (an unrefined sugar made from the juice of crushed sugar cane stalks) as prelacteral feedings (Saha et al., 2008).

Breastfeeding rates are high throughout Asia, but many mothers do not exclusively breastfeed their infants. Many mothers offer water in addition to breast milk. Some mothers also tend to introduce solid foods before the recommended age of 6 months, many as early as the second month. Some Asian mothers bottle feed; usually these women live in urban areas and have sufficient means to do so (Dibley et al., 2010; Sinhababu et al., 2010). As far as the type of foods introduced to infants, every Asian country has particular foods and forms of the foods, but in general, the first foods offered to infants are some sort of rice cereal or porridge. In some countries (Japan, for example) they also start with noodles (Sakashita, Inoue, & Kamegai, 2004).

Some Asian groups believe that once the infant can walk or reaches 1 year of age, the child is capable of making his or her own choices about eating. For instance, Malay children are nursed on demand until 1 year of age, then they are expected to feed themselves, even if their health suffers (Wolff, 1965). In the Asai Valley of Papua New Guinea, children nurse on demand until about 6 months of age, but then are at a disadvantage because they are expected to get food for themselves, and usually lack the ability to do so until 18–24 months (Malcolm, 1974). Similarly, in the Phillipines, when children are about 1 year of age, they begin to eat with the rest of the family (Dettwyler, 1989).

European and European American Practices for Feeding Young Children

Of Europe's many cultures, only a few are discussed here. Giovannini et al. (2004) interviewed 2,450 Italian-speaking mothers about infant feeding throughout the first year. In Italy, infants are fed water-based fluids like sugar water in the first 48 hours after birth. Italian mothers breastfeed an average of 5 months. At that time, they begin to feed the infant formula, switching to cow's milk at 9 months (Giovannini et al., 2004). About half of the mothers interviewed stopped breastfeeding before 6 months with only about 30% exclusively breastfeeding 4 months after the child's birth. Fruit juice is introduced at around 4 months with some infants being offered fruit juice as early as 1½ months of age. At the age of 6 months, 81% of the infants whose mothers were interviewed had been given fruit juice.

Ninety-six percent of Norwegian mothers breastfeed their infants initially (Lande et al., 2003). This percentage slowly decreased to 85% at 4 months and to 80% at 6 months. However, the numbers were different for mothers who breastfed exclusively: 70% at 3 months to only 7% at 6 months.

According to Kudlova and Rames (2007), most Czech infants in Prague (98.7%) are breastfed when discharged from the hospital; about 37% are still breastfed at 12 months, 4% to 5% are still breastfed at 2 years. At 5 months, most infants in the study were introduced to solid foods and nonmilk fluids. Higher education was significantly correlated with longer duration of breastfeeding and the later introduction of solids. Single parents were more likely to breastfeed for shorter periods of time. First foods that Norwegians feed their infants are fruits and cereals. Lande et al. (2003) found that 21% of infants were introduced to solid foods before 4 months of age, with formula-fed infants being more likely to be introduced early (52%) compared to 17% of breastfed infants. Iron-fortified infant cereals are common first foods.

Hispanic and Hispanic American Practices for Feeding Young Children

About 80% of Hispanics in the United States initiate breastfeeding; 45% still breastfeed at 6 months, 24% still breastfeed at 1 year (Gonzalez-Cossio, Rivera-Dommarco, Moreno-Macias, Monterrubio, & Sepulveda, 2006). Hispanic infants are the infants most likely to be breastfed (Mennella, Kennedy, & Beauchamp, 2006). In Latin American countries, mothers with lower levels of education in rural areas are more likely to breastfeed compared with educated women who live in urban areas because the urban women are more likely to work outside of the home (Perez-Escamilla, 2003). An initiative that may be responsible for part of the increase in breastfeeding duration from the mid-1980s to the mid-1990s is the Baby Friendly Hospital Initiative (BFHI; see Chapter 1). BFHI was launched by the United Nations Health Fund (UNICEF) in the late 1980s, and the initiative may have a stronger impact in urban than in rural areas and by consequence among women with higher levels of education (Perez-Escamilla, 2003).

Hispanic infants are introduced to solids between 2 and 18 months of age. When compared to other cultures, Hispanic infants are more likely to have been fed puréed foods than other infants (Mennella et al., 2006). By 6 months, most Hispanic infants are getting infant cereals on a daily basis, even rice. Fruit and fruit juices are commonly fed to almost half of 4- to 5-month-olds, and at 6–11 months. Hispanic infants are more likely to be eating puréed vegetables compared to non-Hispanic infants. Meats, eggs, cheese, and beans are also more common in the diet after 6 months of age. Compared with other infants, Hispanic infants are more likely to be eating sweet treats, such as cookies and drinks daily at 6–11 months.

Native American/Alaska Native Practices for Feeding Young Children

There are 576 federally recognized Native American tribes in the United States, and each one has its own culture with differing beliefs, values, and practices. Therefore, it is difficult to have a cohesive picture of infant feeding practices (Rhodes, Davey, Hellerstedt, Pirie, & Daly, 2008). In general, Native American breastfeeding rates meet the goals set by Healthy People 2010 for initiation (77%), but not at 6 months (42%; National Immunization Survey, 2010; Rhodes et al., 2008).

Complex sociocultural, political, historical, and economic changes in the United States have drastically affected the infant feeding practices of Native Americans (Banks, 2003; Dodgson & Struthers, 2003). For example, family and custom are no longer as central to the birthing process as they once were. Instead, health care providers take a primary role. In addition, the diet of many Native American groups is becoming similar to the majority culture perhaps because many Native Americans are now living in urban areas (Dodgson & Struthers, 2003). These changes have had a long-term impact on breastfeeding and bottle feeding rates for American Indians. Among urban Native Americans, breastfeeding was discouraged because "it wasn't the right thing to do" while formula feeding was encouraged because it was the "best way" (Dodgson & Struthers, 2003, p. 55–56). Native American mothers are less likely to breastfeed and do so for shorter durations than White mothers (Houghton & Graybeal, 2001). Native American women are often separated from relatives who might support them in making the decision to breastfeed. The loss of this support relates to lower breastfeeding rates and the loss of a traditional practice as it relates to their culture (Houghton & Graybeal, 2001). Also, Stevens, Hanson, Prasek, and Elliot (2008) cited lower rates of breastfeeding due to high rates of smoking among Native Americans and Alaska Natives, who have some of the highest smoking rates in the United States. However, according to Stevens et al. (2008), breastfeeding is the preferred method of feeding even if the mother is smoking.

Houghton and Graybeal (2001) found that when compared to White mothers, Native American mothers were less likely to breastfeed their child, and the duration of breastfeeding was shorter than it was for non-Hispanic White mothers. Socioeconomic risk factors and several cultural changes affected the mother's choice to breastfeed. About 70% of mothers made their decisions on how to feed their infants before pregnancy or during the first half of pregnancy, and only 36% stated that their cultural heritage played a role in that decision (Houghton & Graybeal, 2001). Once the infant is born about 70% (29 out of 41) initiate breastfeeding. Support is the key to breastfeeding, but only a little over half of Native American women who initiate breastfeeding are still breastfeeding at 6 months (Houghton & Graybeal, 2001). In contrast with other groups, Native American mothers with less education and those who were single breastfed longer than those with at least a high school education and those who were married (Houghton & Graybeal, 2001).

Some researchers have noted that a sense of connection to her culture increases the chances that a woman will breastfeed (Macaulay, Hanusaik, & Beauvais, 1989). Additionally, Stevens et al. (2008) noted, "Among Navajo Indians, breastfeeding is seen as a superior method of infant feeding that helps produce well-behaved children" (p. 449). For Native American mothers who breastfed, the average length of time was 21 weeks, with work or school negatively affecting the duration of breastfeeding (Houghton & Graybeal, 2001). Native American mothers noted the following reasons for bottle feeding formula: the mother's lifestyle (including returning to work or school), convenience, ease of preparation so that others could feed the infant (Houghton & Graybeal, 2001), and because breastfeeding was too difficult and cumbersome (Dodgson & Struthers, 2003). Milk is reserved for infants in some Native American cultures because it weakens adults (Kittler & Sucher, 2008). Some of the first foods given to infants are soups; jerky is provided for teething infants (Dodgson & Struthers, 2003).

AT RISK GROUPS

This section focuses on populations in which children may be more likely to have issues related to feeding. At risk groups include those living in poverty and adolescent parents. Early childhood professionals are likely to come into contact with children from these groups and should therefore have a good understanding of the variables related to feeding issues found among these populations. Factors that affect feeding and programs that address feeding issues will be discussed.

Low-Income Families and Families Living in Poverty

About 11% of households in the United States are food insecure, which is to say that they do not know where or when their next meal may be (Nord, 2006). The amount of money a family earns has a direct relationship to food budgets. Meal-times vary in regularity and frequency across income groups. Differences among income groups could be due to shift work, juggling more than one job, and trans-portation time between home and work (Fiese & Schwartz, 2008).

Food insecurity is not the only issue faced by low-income groups in the Unit-ed States. The food that is available in low income areas is likely to be of lower quality than that found in higher-income neighborhoods. Food markets in low-in-come areas may sell foods that are less than safe because the foods are exposed to temperature fluctuations and less protected from excess handling and pests (Koro, Anandan, & Quinlan, 2010). In addition, Baker, Schootman, Barnridge, and Kelly (2006) found that fresh fruits and vegetables are not as plentiful in lower income neighborhoods, but that fast food restaurants are more available. Families living in poverty are more likely to be eating processed foods, foods high in carbohydrates and fewer fruits and vegetables (Dong & Lin, 2009). It is not surprising, then, that researchers have found that food insecurity is linked to an increased risk of obe-sity (Bronte-Tinkew, Zaslow, Capps, Horowitz, & McNamara, 2007). In addition, Gunderson, Lohman, Garasky, Stewart, and Eisenmann (2008) examined obesi-ty in young children and reported that food insecurity combined with maternal stress increases the risk of obesity.

The effect of lower income on the diet of these groups extends to other areas of their lives as well. Fiese and Schwartz (2008) cautioned that the lower quality of foods and irregular mealtimes associated with low-income families could be disrupting the opportunities to enhance language development and socialization in young children.

Very early decisions about feeding correlate with income. For example, Af-rican American women under the age of 20 who live in the southeastern part of the United States, and have a lower income, are the least likely of any group to breastfeed their infants. Mothers from a low-income background state that male support is crucial in their decision to breastfeed (Ryan, & Zhou, 2006; Schmidt & Sigman-Grant, 2000). In addition to income, education plays a role in breastfeed-ing. Compared with women who graduated high school, mothers with less than a high school education are less likely to breastfeed—unless mothers and/or part-ners support and encourage breastfeeding (Mahoney & James, 2000).

Assistance Programs   The USDA has looked at programs to lower the costs of fruits and vegetables for those in lower income brackets to increase con-sumption (Dong & Lin, 2009). They found that to provide a 10% subsidy to in-crease consumption would cost a great deal, but would not necessarily meet dietary recommendations. Farm and Food Policy Project has published recom-mendations that argue that "all Americans, regardless of income, deserve access to an affordable, healthy diet" (Dong & Lin, 2009, p. 2). Some of the recommenda-tions are to provide transportation for low-income groups so they can shop where higher-quality food is available and increasing the minimum amount of benefits from food stamps (Farm and Food Policy Project, 2007). Lower income popula-tions need better access to healthy foods, more resources to get those foods, and information about how to plan meals and prepare those foods (Farm and Food Policy Project, 2007; McDermott & Stephens, 2010). Currently, there are programs designed to provide foodstuffs for families in need. Two public programs in the United States are WIC and TANF.

Special Supplemental Nutrition Program for Women, Infants, and Children (WIC)   The U.S. government created WIC (the Special Supplemental Nutrition Program for Women, Infants, and Children) to provide low income mothers with the resources necessary to attain proper nutrition for infants. This program promotes the health and well-being of mothers and children, and it provides nutritious foods and referrals to health services. Although federal rules require the WIC program to promote breastfeeding, "breastfeeding rates among WIC participants have remained depressed" (Jiang, Foster, & Gibson-Davis, 2010, p. 264). Some claim that the reason that WIC participants are less likely to breastfeed is because the WIC program provides free formula.

WIC enrollment depends upon socioeconomic disadvantage. Participants must meet the income guidelines, a state residency requirement, and be individually determined to be at "nutritional risk" by a health professional (Food and Nutrition Service, 2011). WIC recognizes two types of "nutritional risk." One type is medically based risk, indicated by the presence of conditions such as anemia, underweight, overweight, history of pregnancy complications, or poor pregnancy outcomes. The second type is dietary risk, indicated by the presence of conditions such as failure to meet the dietary guidelines or inappropriate nutrition practices. Compared with the general population of mothers with young children, WIC mothers are younger, have less education and lower incomes, are less likely to be married, and engage in more risky health behaviors (Jiang et al., 2010, p. 265). Also compared with other mothers, mothers who participate in the WIC program are less likely to initiate breastfeeding and likely to breastfeed for a shorter period of time. WIC benefits are affected by the mother's choice of whether or not to breastfeed. Women who are not breastfeeding may only receive WIC for 6 months, while breastfeeding mothers may participate for up to 1 year. Breastfeeding mothers also receive additional benefits such as peer counseling and support, education about the benefits of breastfeeding, and access to free breast pumps and nursing supplements.

WIC is available in all 50 states, 34 Indian Tribal Organizations, American Samoa, the District of Columbia, Guam, the Commonwealth Islands of the Northern Marianas, Puerto Rico, and the Virgin Islands. According to USDA statistics, WIC served approximately 9.3 million women, infants, and children in the fiscal year 2009. The program has grown tremendously since serving 88,000 people in its first year, 1974. Children have been the largest group of WIC participants throughout the years. In the fiscal year 2008, 4.33 million were children enrolled (Food and Nutrition Service, 2011).

Temporary Assistance for Needy Families (TANF)   Begun under welfare reform legislation in 1996, the Temporary Assistance for Needy Families (TANF) program became effective on July 1, 1997 and was reauthorized in February 2006. TANF replaced the welfare programs known as Aid to Families with Dependent Children (AFDC), the Job Opportunities and Basic Skills Training program (JOBS), and the Emergency Assistance (EA) program. TANF is a block grant that provides states, territories, and tribes with federal funds. TANF is designed to help needy families become self-sufficient. It encourages work by providing care for young children, and by promoting job preparation and job-search activities. In addition, it tries to encourage the formation and maintenance of two-parent families through the prevention of out-of-wedlock pregnancies and the support of marriage.

In order for families to receive this aid from the state, they are required to participate in work-related activities. TANF suggests that recipients must work as soon as they are job-ready or no later than 2 years after accepting the assistance. The amount of work required by TANF recipients is broken down depending on marital status. For instance, a single parent must participate for an average of 30 hours per week unless they have children under 6 years old, in which case the requirement is dropped to 20 hours. Two parents must work an average of 35 hours a week unless they are receiving federal child care assistance, in which case they must work 55 hours a week. However, the state cannot penalize single parents for not meeting their work requirements if they do not find adequate child care for their children. There are a variety of work activities that the state qualifies as active participation. Those include work experience, on-the-job training, community service, education related to employment, job search and job readiness assistance, and child care services.

TANF also includes Tribal Programs. If the Native American Tribes are federally recognized, they may apply directly to Health and Human Services (HHS) to operate a TANF block grant program. Tribes have the same responsibilities as States do; they may use their TANF funding in any manner that is in keeping with the purposes of TANF. The Federal government does approve tribal plans. The work program proposed for the Tribal groups is referred to as the Native Employment Works (NEW) Program. This program provides funding to tribes and inter-tribal groups to design and administer tribal work activities, while still allowing Tribes and States to provide other TANF services (U.S. Department of Health and Human Services, 2008).

Adolescent Parents

Adolescence is a time of rapid physical, emotional, cognitive, and social development. Having a child interrupts this developmental progression, and young parents frequently are not prepared for the decisions and responsibilities that come with having an infant. Adolescents often do not have good eating habits, thus dietary choices that they make for their children may be questionable (Furstenberg & Brooks-Gunn, 1986).

Much of the available research centered on adolescents and the choices they make about feeding their infants includes samples of low-income minorities (African American and Hispanic), and focuses on breastfeeding (Hannon, Willis, Bishop-Townsend, Martinez, & Scrimshaw, 2000; Nelson, 2009; Wambach & Koehn, 2004). Young parents do not initiate breastfeeding as often; 43% of mothers under 20 years of age initiate breastfeeding compared with 75% of mothers over 30 years of age (McDowell, Wang, & Kennedy-Stephenson, 2008). Young mothers who do choose to breastfeed do not continue to breastfeed as long as older women (Dennis, 2002; American Academy of Pediatrics, 1997). One source cited about 20% fewer adolescents breastfeed (Centers for Disease Control and Prevention, 2011b). At 6 months, adolescent breastfeeding rates drop to about 18% compared to 42% of older mothers.

Several studies, most with qualitative research designs, interviewed mothers about their choices to breastfeed or bottle feed. There were many similarities across the studies for reasons why adolescents breastfeed and the barriers that prevent them from breastfeeding. Researchers have studied why adolescents are less likely to breastfeed and cited several reasons including "perceptions of the benefits and problems with breastfeeding, supportive persons to help with breastfeeding (Hannon et al., 2000), lack of information about breastfeeding, unsupportive behaviors and attitudes of maternity nurses, advice that is inconsistent, and low levels of prenatal education and encouragement (Lewinski, 1992; Patton, Beaman, Csar, & Lewinki, 1996; Sable & Patton, 1998). A couple of the benefits mentioned most in research are: health benefits for the infant, and bonding between mother and child. In most studies, adolescents believed that breastfeeding was good for the infant, stating that it was "good" or "best" for the infant. Those mothers who thought breastfeeding had more benefits than barriers were more likely to have chosen to breastfeed (Radius & Joffe, 1988). However, these beliefs did not necessarily predict that a mother would breastfeed. All of these many factors must be considered when working with adolescents because the issue is complex.

Adolescents cite more barriers than benefits to breastfeeding. Barriers to breastfeeding according to adolescents are pain, embarrassment of exposure when having to feed the infant in public, inconvenience (e.g., getting up at night, leaving the infant with others), and mechanics and physiology of breastfeeding (e.g., latching on, having enough milk, changes in the breasts; Hannon et al., 2000; Nelson, 2009; Wambach & Koehn, 2004). A common worry is that the infant will be too attached to the mother, making it difficult to continue to live the lifestyle she wants (Hannon et al., 2000). Additional reasons cited are concerns about the difficulty of weaning, such as the possibility that infants might not take a bottle (Nelson, 2009). In one study of Latina and African American mothers, researchers interviewing adolescent mothers about breastfeeding found that some mothers believed that breastfeeding would cause the bonding with her infant to be excessive so that others could not feed the infant when the mother went back to school, and misconceptions about breastfeeding, such as the possibility that foods or emotions may 'taint' their milk.

Adolescents believed that "breastfeeding is a mother's choice" (Nelson, 2009, p. 252). However, it appears that the grandmother (the adolescent mother's mother) has a very strong influence (Bentley, Gavin, Black, & Teti, 1999; Moran, Edwards, Dykes, & Downe, 2007; Nelson, 2009). This is not surprising because the grandmother has experience taking care of infants and may be someone her daughter looks up to (Bentley et al., 1999). The influence can be either positive or negative. In one study, authors interviewed an adolescent mother, and the adolescent stated that her mother did not want her to breastfeed because the grandmother did not want the inconvenience of waiting on the mother to feed the infant. Other influential people are the adolescents' partners and health care professionals. Partners' support was important in the decision to breastfeed (Radius & Joffe, 1988).

The Chicago Doula Project exemplifies the issues and complexities involved in providing breastfeeding information to young parents. The project was modeled as an extension of support beyond labor and delivery for low-income, African American mothers to provide child development information and support young mothers in their parenting role. The doulas were lay people from the community with no medical experience who provided support to young mothers. Doulas had breastfed their own children and provided the young mothers information and support in making the decision to breastfeed. The outcomes of the project demonstrated the great challenges for the promotion of sustained breastfeeding with this population (Wambach & Koehn, 2004). The adolescent mothers appreciated their doulas support and did listen to the information provided. However, it was often difficult for the doulas to navigate feeding issues between the adolescent mothers and the grandmother, the most influential family member. Similar to other studies involving this population, the majority of the grandmothers did not breastfeed and would be caring for the infant and did not want to worry about the complications and inconveniences of feeding an infant when the mother was not there.

Young parents must also decide when to begin feeding their infants solids. Several studies have shown that it is common in the African American culture to start solids early (Bentley et al., 1999; Brodwick, Barnaowski, & Rassin, 1989; Bronner et al., 1999; Pao, Himes, & Roche, 1980; Parraga, Weber, Engel, Reeb, & Lerner, 1988). In fact, low-income African American adolescents were found to be more likely than other groups to feed their infants solids within the first month after birth (Bentley et al., 1999). Bronner et al., (1999) found that within 7–10 days after birth, about one third of infants born to low-income African American adolescent mothers had been fed juice or solids. Some infants were placed on puréed foods in the first month and were eating table foods by 3 months of age (Bentley et al., 1999).

Bentley et al. (1999) performed an ethnographic study in which low-income adolescent African American mothers were interviewed four times and the grandmothers were interviewed twice. The grandmothers made most of the decisions about feeding solids, even when the adolescent mothers' protested that it was too early. For example, one grandmother put cereal in her grandson's bottle without her daughter's knowledge or consent against her wishes. As reasons for starting solids early, grandmothers stated that the infant was "greedy," cried a lot, was smaller than expected, and slept better after receiving solids (p. 1091). Reasons adolescent mothers stated for starting solids early were the grandmother's advice and the infant reaching for food. Since the adolescent mothers relied on the grandmother to provide care for the infant, the grandmothers were able to make the decision of when to begin solids.

Strategies and Specialized Interventions for Young Parents

Those who work with adolescent parents must address the issues faced by this group. To dispel misconceptions, adolescent mothers need to be provided *prenatally* with factual information about breastfeeding. It is critical that information be consistent and nonjudgmental (Bentley et al., 1998; Lavender, Thompson, Wood, 2005). Some researchers have found that adolescent mothers' perceptions of support from friends, family, and especially their partners were related to a higher intent to breastfeed (Radius & Jaffe, 1988; Lavender et al, 2005). Often mothers, especially minority mothers, are misinformed and do not seek out information about breastfeeding (Hannon et al., 2000). Additionally, friends, mothers, and other relatives often relate their own negative experiences with breastfeeding, thus biasing the young mothers against making this choice. This, combined with a lack of information from health professionals, often leads adolescent mothers, especially minority mothers, to bottle feed their infants. Results from the Chicago Doula Project reveal how important it is for professionals not only to know the information relevant to development and feeding, but also to know its importance for each family and the parent-child dyad (Korfmacher, 2008). The information from the study highlights the difficulties in overcoming some barriers to breastfeeding, including family and cultural biases.

Supporting adolescents in the decision-making process is complicated. They are at a stage in their life where they strive to make decisions for themselves. One of the best ways to help them is to provide information so they can make an informed decision with regard to breastfeeding (Wambach & Koehn, 2004). They need to feel respected. That said, there were no clear answers in one of the above-mentioned stories of how to support adolescent mothers in breastfeeding, and more research is needed in this area (Moran et al., 2007; Wambach & Koehn, 2004). One study that focused on nurses' attitudes, knowledge, and beliefs about breastfeeding mothers found that these professionals felt that adolescents should be encouraged to breastfeed. However, almost a quarter felt that breastfeeding information should not be provided in public school settings (Spear, 2004). The support of nurses and physicians increases the chances adolescents will breastfeed (Lu, Lange, Slusser, Hamilton, & Halfon, 2001; Wiemann, DuBois, & Berenson, 1998). Nurses need to understand the unique needs of adolescents in relation to breastfeeding (Nelson, 2009). For example, one of the barriers to breastfeeding is embarrassment; knowing this, nurses can be especially respectful by not touching the young mothers when teaching them to breastfeed. Also, the fears and myths that adolescent mothers have about breastfeeding need to be addressed. Adolescents, like other mothers, need supportive people including their own mothers, teachers, health professionals (especially those trained in lactation and working with adolescents), partners, and so forth (Moran et al., 2007). Finally, they want to feel respected and "cared for," so each adolescent should be treated uniquely and respectfully (Dykes, Moran, Burt, & Edwards, 2003).

In general, when a professional is working with an individual whose background differs from his or her own—in age, culture, or socioeconomic factors—it is important to do the following:

- Examine your personal attitudes and knowledge about the persons in this group
- Use culturally sensitive interview tools (e.g., by asking "Is there anything I need to know about you that will help me in better understanding your needs?")
- Demonstrate comfort with differences
- Develop communication techniques that show respect for each and every individual
- Demonstrate a willingness to relinquish control and respect individual parenting practices, integrating them into the child's care and feeding
- Demonstrate RESPECT (Adapted from Bazaldua & Sias, 2004; U.S. Department of Health and Human Services Office of Minority Health, 2001.):

  Rapport should be developed by understanding the person's point of view (AVOID ASSUMPTIONS).

  Empathy is important. Remember that parents may be seeking advice.

  Support parents by understanding their social context and involve their family. Children are not raised in isolation and we need to recognize the influence and strength of the family

  Partner with parents regarding their feeding plans and negotiate if necessary.

  Explain or teach them and verify their understanding.

  Competence of each parent's diverse background should be achieved and each parent's beliefs respected

  Trust is essential and can be achieved by demonstrating patience and taking time.

▦ ▦ ▦ FOOD FOR THOUGHT ▦ ▦ ▦

Becky was sitting in the front row at church with her husband and children, 3-year-old Anna and 1-month-old Teddy. Anna loudly asked to be nursed. The next week, Becky and the children were at a park with a play group. Anna came up to Becky wanting to nurse. Becky nursed Anna then nursed Teddy. Several other mothers in the group appeared uncomfortable.

Discussion Questions

- ▦ Is it okay for Becky to nurse two children? Why or why not?
- ▦ Should Becky have weaned her older child before the birth of Teddy?

FEEDING NUGGETS

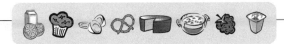

Books

Let's Eat: What Children Eat Around the World by Beatrice Hollyer (2004)

Our Babies, Ourselves: How Biology and Culture Shape the Way We Parent by Meredith Small (1999)

Infant Feeding Practices: A Cross-Cultural Perspective by Pranee Liamputtong (Ed.), (2010)

Food & Nutrition: Customs and Culture by Paul Fieldhouse (1995)

Web Sites

"Food Pyramids for different cultures"
http://www.semda.org/info/#pyramid

Cultural Diversity in Food
http://www.ca.uky.edu/HES/fcs/factshts/FN-SSB.076.pdf

http://www.007b.com/breastfeeding_public.php

Feeding Process

INTRODUCTION

"Feeding is a reciprocal process that depends on the specific abilities and character-istics of both the caregiver and the child. ...Clinicians must appreciate the sequences in normal development to be involved with assessment and management of children demonstrating disruptions that can occur in any one of those stages."

(Arvedson & Brodsky, 2002, p. 564, 567)

Section II focuses on the feeding team and the feeding process. Chapter 5 examines the key components of teaming for young children with feeding difficulties. Multi-disciplinary, interdisciplinary, and transdisciplinary team structures are described. In addition, necessary skills for team communication, collaboration, coordination, documentation, and training and professional development are provided.

Chapter 6 discusses screening and assessment methods. Descriptions, includ-ing brief summaries and examples of assessment instruments, are offered. Recom-mended key questions about a child's medical history and components of a physical examination are provided. Informal approaches such as a food diary, mealtime ob-servation, interviews, and parent report are also described. An overview of feed-ing checklists and rating scales are included, for overall feeding development and specific feeding components (e.g., parent–child interactions during mealtimes). A brief overview of functional analysis is provided. Criterion-referenced, as well as standardized, assessments with feeding-related items are examined. Commonly used describe diagnostic tests to identify conditions that interfere with oral intake are described.

Chapter 7 offers an overview of methods for including feeding needs in an in-fant or toddler's Individualized Family Support Plan (IFSP), and in a preschooler's

Individualized Education Program (IEP). An overview of instructional approaches such as activity-based intervention and environmental considerations are described. The chapter also addresses progress monitoring and methods of data collection to document feeding gains and make data-based decisions with the feeding team such as anecdotal records, food diaries, and observational recording procedures.

5

Teaming

What You'll Learn in This Chapter

This chapter provides

- A description of multidisciplinary, interdisciplinary, and transdisciplinary team structures
- Overview of key components of effective feeding teams
- An explanation of the importance of and guidance regarding ongoing training and professional development for feeding team members

■ ■ ■ FOOD FOR THOUGHT ■ ■ ■

"Emma, who has a mosaic form of trisomy 18, will eat just about anything now. Her eating problems began when we started introducing solid foods (around 10 months). She very, very slowly began to eat more solid and textured food. We had lots of help from her speech therapist and a dietician. I think she was around 24–30 months old when she ate her first bag of chips, and that was a milestone!"

Lena, Parent

"Nolan has Down syndrome. I worked with him from the time he was 43 months old until he was 79 months old. For the first 2 years, the only things he would eat were pudding, applesauce, some baby foods, and occasionally mashed potatoes. We used things like curved spoons, bowls with a lip to help with scooping, and built-up forks to encourage self-feeding skills. Once these were mastered, we moved on to drinking from a straw and an open cup. When he was able to use all of these skills across environments (home included), we moved on to solid foods. At first, we taught him simply to allow solid food near his plate. We gradually moved the food closer until the food was on his plate and he no longer pushed it away or threw it. The next step was getting him to pick up the food and play with it. Finally, when he was 5 and a half years old, he touched a solid food (carrot) to his lips for the first time."

Addie, Early Childhood Special Education Teacher

Lena and Addie describe advances in Emma's and Nolan's feeding skills. These changes were due, in large part, to collaboration among professionals. Feeding problems are multifaceted, and their treatment requires input and expertise from individuals with various backgrounds. Team structures vary. For example, Emma's mother described working with a speech therapist and a dietician, while Addie focused on her classroom team and Nolan's parents. Regardless of the configuration of the feeding team, ongoing communication and coordination of efforts is necessary to ensure optimal outcomes.

WHAT THE LITERATURE SAYS

Cooperation among parents, caregivers, and professionals is necessary in order to promote and achieve improved feeding outcomes for children. All team members must engage in meaningful activities, collaboration, and careful monitoring of progress. In order to address feeding issues, a team with varied areas of expertise and the common goal of promoting the acquisition of age-appropriate skills and enjoyment of feeding interactions is necessary. This team must include parents and caregivers as members. Rapport, McWilliam, and Smith (2004) stated that team members must

> know child functioning and intervention strategies, family and classroom functioning, and collaborative consultation skills. When professionals have this wide array of knowledge and skills, they are respected and highly valued by their colleagues from other disciplines, and they add to the outcome of effective and efficient early intervention for young children with disabilities and their families. (p. 42–43)

Along with families, a team of colleagues from various disciplines has the skills and expertise to develop a feeding plan that builds on a child's strengths, emerging skills, and unique needs. (See Chapter 7 for a full description of feeding plans.)

All efforts must be made to collaborate with a child's caregivers about all facets of feeding: adequate nutritional intake, the acceptance of textured foods, and the development self-feeding (Arvedson, 2000; Bruns & Thompson, 2010; Field, Garland, & Williams, 2003; Rudolph & Link, 2002). Accomplishment of these tasks requires that appropriate professionals are included on the child's team. For example, Manikam and Perman (2000) discussed how a feeding team should include, at a minimum, a gastroenterologist, a nutritionist, an occupational therapist (OT), and a speech-language pathologist (SLP). (See Table 5.1 for a brief description of feeding team members and their contributions.) The authors also note that in order to support coordination and consistency, strategies must address all aspects of the child's difficulties and offer training to all team members.

Table 5.1.   Feeding team members, areas of expertise, and team responsibilities

Team member*	Areas of expertise and team responsibilities
Speech-language pathologist (speech-language therapist)	Focuses on oral-motor development and stimulation, swallowing disorders, and adapted feeding devices and equipment
Occupational therapist	Focuses on sensory processing, oral-motor development and stimulation, positioning, self-feeding, and adapted feeding devices
Physical therapist (physiotherapist)	Helps identify movement disorders, positioning, adapted feeding devices, and equipment
Parent	Describes daily mealtimes, child's preferences, and feeding interactions
Caregiver	Describes daily mealtimes and feeding interactions
Developmental specialist	Provides knowledge of typical and atypical child development and implements developmental interventions
Dietitian	Addresses nutritional needs and intake and specialized diets
Social worker	Provides support, parent training, and access to resources
Behavior analyst	Conducts functional analysis and outlines behavioral strategies
Nurse	Monitors health conditions, medical conditions, and medical interventions
Pediatric gastroenterologist	Treats disorders of the gastrointestinal or digestive tract, including the esophagus, stomach, and small intestine
Pediatric neurologist	Diagnoses and treats nervous system disorders that affect the brain and muscles
Physiatrist	Diagnoses medical problems and provides input to treatment plan
Psychologist	Assesses feeding difficulties and observes feeding interactions
Radiologist	Interprets medical images to help develop treatment plans
Respiratory therapist	Evaluates and treats cardiopulmonary disorders

* Additional team members may be necessary depending on the child's feeding needs

The Individuals with Disabilities Improvement Act (IDEA) of 2004 (PL 108-446) addressed the importance of teaming and stated that Individualized Family Support Plans (IFSPs) for infants and toddlers with disabilities or developmental delays must include input from and collaboration among Early Intervention (EI) professionals such as developmental specialists (DSs), SLPs, physical therapists (PTs) and dietitians. In addition, several experts in the field have said that they also place value on teams and their positive impact on young children and their families (Campbell, Chiarello, Wilcox, & Milbourne, 2009; Rouse, Herrington, Assey, Baker, & Golden, 2002; Scherer & Kaiser, 2007). These authors emphasized communication, collaboration, and coordination among team members to reach desired outcomes. Campbell and Halbert (2002) reported on the opportunities for disconnect between team members and the implications of that disconnect for services. Especially in the area of feeding, it is critical to have all team members "on the same page" when designing feeding plans and determining their effectiveness (see Chapter 7).

In pediatric rehabilitation, Nijhuis et al. (2007) also advocated that team members communicate, engage in shared decision making and goal setting, and provide multiple avenues for parent and caregiver participation. Peña and Quinn (2003) pointed to the collaborative team process from an SLP perspective. Palisano (2006) offered a similar orientation when describing PT involvement in teams for children with cerebral palsy:

> The collaborative model of service delivery is based on the assumptions that effective service delivery for children with movement disorders…promotes outcomes that are meaningful to the child and family in daily life. The focus is on services that address child and family needs and priorities in settings where children live, learn, and play. (p. 1304)

Mutually agreed upon outcomes are critical for the success of any team, especially when the team is focused on feeding development. As indicated in Chapters 2, 3, and 4, a number of factors—including child preferences, parent and family preferences, community interactions, and community practices—come together around the issue of feeding. As such, the feeding team must fully embrace the contributions of all its members and recognize the context within which feeding services will be offered (Secrist-Mertz, Brotherson, Oakland, & Litchfield, 1997).

Chiarello et al. (2010) discussed the importance of coordination of team members when teaching new daily living and self-care skills to young children with cerebral palsy. The authors found that family priorities varied, but that team members working together was always necessary. From an occupational therapy viewpoint, Caretto, Topolski, Linkous, Lowman, and Murphy (2000) explained the role of these professionals in educating parents about infant care, including feeding in the context of the neonatal intensive care unit (NICU). Olsen, Richardson, Schmid, Ausman, and Dwyer (2005) provided similar recommendations for the participation of dietitians on NICU feeding teams, and Fung, Khong, To, Goh, and Wong (2004) provided recommendations regarding the need for pediatric neurologists on feeding teams working with children with a neurological disorder.

Throughout the early years, team members must share their specialized skills in ways that assist the child and all those who provide day-to-day care and services. For example, a behavior analyst can work with parents, caregivers, SLPs and others on the team to provide instructions on interventions to increase appropriate feeding behaviors (e.g., accept textured solids) while also decreasing inappropriate behaviors (e.g., spitting out food; Ledford & Gast, 2006; Matson & Fodstad, 2009; Piazza, Patel, Gulotta, Sevin, & Layer, 2003).

The following sections provide a brief overview of the team models (i.e., multidisciplinary, interdisciplinary, transdisciplinary) used in early childhood settings, along with the key components for effective and successful team functioning in order to attain desired child outcomes.

TEAM MODELS

Team members must work closely with children and their caregivers to ensure adequate nutritional intake and necessary skill development. Within this context, it is important to examine team models because each influences team member responsibilities and interactions (McGonigel, Woodruff, & Roszmann-Millican, 1994). Furthermore, the formation and orientation of a team reflects the combined values and experiences of its members and, as appropriate, the program or agency of which each is a part (e.g., Pre-kindergarten program; Tuckman, 1965). It is also important to remember that teams change and that new members must be instructed in team processes and procedures. The models described in the following sections represent three types of team structure and their respective points of view with regard to collaboration, communication, and coordination.

Multidisciplinary Teams

In multidisciplinary teams, professionals from different disciplines work independently for the most part. They sometimes share assessment tools and results and specialized strategies or techniques, but they implement their services separately. The multidisciplinary model often results in fragmentation and inconsistencies in the methods and means by which services are implemented across team members. Because autonomy is a central attribute of this model, multidisciplinary teams include only minimal coordination and often experience conflict over priorities. Each professional represents a distinct discipline and a primary focus of services. Feeding teams using this model lack common goals, often producing confusion for parents and caregivers as they try to follow disparate or conflicting recommendations without being considered full members of the team.

In addition, members of multidisciplinary teams make decisions individually, with little cross-discipline collaboration. The multidisciplinary model lacks communication because each team member works in isolation. Individual members form relationships with the child and the family, but limited team cohesiveness is achieved, especially because feeding occurs across multiple feeders and in multiple settings. Overall, this model is not conducive to coordinated services.

Consider the following example scenario. In a multidisciplinary feeding team, a toddler with cerebral palsy is seen individually by a DS, an OT, a PT, a SLP and a nutritionist. Team members have little formal interaction (e.g., team meetings) or informal interaction (e.g., phone calls, texts) with the other team members. Working with the mother, the SLP demonstrates a technique to assist lip closure during cup drinking. The technique is to be implemented with the child seated in his or her highchair. The child's mother describes the positioning to the PT who does not agree and shares frustration at not having been consulted about optimal positioning. The PT prefers the child be seated in a corner chair for mealtimes. This situation results in the SLP and PT offering the parent contradictory advice regarding positioning. Perhaps the nutritionist also offers the toddler's parent suggestions of calorie boosters to add to breakfast and dinner and ideas to increase the child's tolerance for textured foods, but doesn't share the information with the dietetic technician who visits once a week in the early morning. Figure 5.1 represents the configuration of a multidisciplinary team as a series of professionals each working with the child, but independently from each other.

Interdisciplinary Teams

Interdisciplinary teams have more formalized and ongoing channels of communication compared with multidisciplinary teams. Parents and professionals routinely share information and discuss progress. Communication typically occurs in scheduled meetings where professionals from different disciplines talk about shared cases. Parents are invited as well. Specific types of assessment are completed by individual team members, and the team meets in order to review results after they are compiled. The team evaluates the results, comes to a consensus, and develops the child's feeding plan.

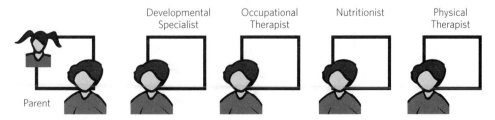

Figure 5.1. Multidisciplinary team

Research has found that professionals working with young children and their families prefer the interdisciplinary model to the multidisciplinary model; it is more inclusive of the parents and because each practitioner provides a viewpoint, helping to develop a holistic view of the child's development and progress (Homer, 2003; Horner, Bickerton, Hill, Parham, & Taylor, 2000; Körner, 2010; Simonsmeier & Rodríguez, 2007). In addition, an interdisciplinary model promotes greater awareness of discipline-specific strategies and assists with consistency across team members. This consistency is especially critical when addressing feeding difficulties. Körner (2010) advocated for existing multidisciplinary teams to move toward the interdisciplinary approach through training and evaluation of existing practices.

An additional benefit to the interdisciplinary model is that, with a greater focus on collaboration, a team leader emerges. Sometimes this leader emerges through input from the family or child, but often the professional who is providing the most direct services takes the lead. The team leader eases coordination among the team members and helps resolve conflicts. Miscommunication is reduced, and there is a greater emphasis on team development and cohesion. As described by Tucker (cf. 1965), an interdisciplinary team proceeds through four stages in its creation: forming, storming, norming, and performing. Leadership is especially critical during the initial three stages while team members forge a shared system of communication and a mutually agreed upon framework through which to address feeding difficulties—for example, as they select upon oral-motor exercises, determine whether enteral feeding (tube feeding) is necessary, and so forth.

Using an interdisciplinary model, the team assisting the toddler with cerebral palsy previously described would work together. The child would receive feeding-related services in a different manner with an interdisciplinary team. The DS, OT, PT, SLP and nutritionist would work together to address lip closure, positioning, and offering textured foods. The scenario involving the SLP and PT giving contradictory advice to the child's mother would be handled quite differently. The SLP and PT would meet and develop two options for the toddler's mother to use for lip positioning. Then the SLP would contact the remaining team members to advise them of the options and the PT's willingness to demonstrate their use. The DS would also ask the parent about her child's gains in feeding and other areas of development then bring this information, as well as the mother's recommendations, back to the team as they evaluate the existing feeding plan and prepare to update it. Figure 5.2 illustrates the structure of an interdisciplinary team.

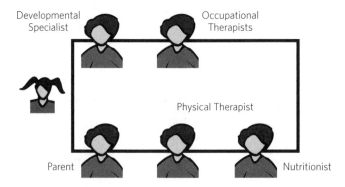

Figure 5.2. Interdisciplinary team

Transdisciplinary Teams

The transdisciplinary team model is characterized by collaboration and sharing of skills across disciplines. Once the professional is proficient in new skills outside her discipline, she is encouraged to implement them and continues to receive feedback and support. This practice is described in the literature as role release (McGonigel et al., 1994; Stayton & Bruder, 1999). With role release, a practitioner steps out of his or her primary professional role, and team members are able to implement strategies and techniques from another disciplines. For example, a DS would use a lip closure technique observed and practiced with the team SLP.

The authors describe six steps in the role-release process: role extension, role enrichment, role expansion, role exchange, role release, and role support (McGonigel et al., 1994). Throughout this process, there are successive opportunities for individual growth in each team member's discipline and for team-building activities to share and utilize discipline-specific information. The result is a unified approach to services.

In addition, parents and caregivers in transdisciplinary feeding teams are viewed as full team members. As members, they are encouraged to be involved in assessment, planning, implementation, and evaluation of feeding plans. All team members, to the extent possible, conduct assessments and implement team-determined feeding strategies together. This approach facilitates communication and shared decision-making, provides parents with greater access to other team members, and promotes consistency in carrying out a child's feeding plan.

The stages of team formation described by Tuckman (1965) are an integral part of this model. A mutually agreed upon framework guides the team and offers opportunities to reflect on child-specific feeding strategies and interventions. The transdisciplinary team model is guided by team consensus and "exchange of competencies between team members" (McWilliam, 2005, p. 129). Gisel et al., (2003) spoke to the need for transdisciplinary teams to treat feeding difficulties in children with cerebral palsy. The authors explained how professionals must work closely in order to provide support for the child's oral-motor skills, gross motor skills, and other associated areas of delay affecting oral intake.

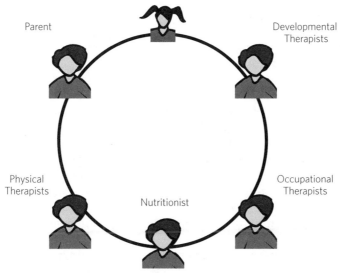

Figure 5.3. Transdisciplinary team

A unique component in the transdisciplinary model is the emergence of one professional who becomes the infant or toddler's primary service provider. The transdisciplinary team's primary provider is similar to the interdisciplinary team's leader, with the additional responsibility of ensuring opportunities for ongoing communication and professional development. This team member assists with co-ordinating services and promoting role release to meet a child's feeding needs. In a transdisciplinary model, the SLP in the previous scenario is the toddler's primary provider. The SLP works closely with the PT to learn positioning techniques and with the DS to learn play-based techniques for encouraging the child to accept textured foods. The SLP also draws on the mother's expertise about her child to confirm that team members' recommendations are consistent and can be integrat-ed into daily routines when team members are not present. Team members coor-dinate their schedules so at least two or three members attend feeding sessions. They also meet once a month to review the child's progress, share information and resources, and demonstrate new feeding techniques (see Figure 5.3 for a graphic representation of a transdisciplinary team).

FEATURES OF SUCCESSFUL TEAMS

The following sections discuss the key features of successful feeding teams and strat-egies to foster implementation of feeding plans and achieve key feeding outcomes.

Communication   An important feature of successful feeding teams is communication. All team members express themselves openly in order to facil-itate decision-making and provide coordinated services (Briggs, 1993; Wooster, Brady, Mitchell, Grizzle, & Barnes, 1998). Rouse, Herrington, Assey, Baker and Golden (2002) and Scherer and Kaiser (2007) specifically address the need for on-going communication among professionals and families with young children with gastrostomy tubes and cleft palate, respectively.

Communication is often lacking in multidisciplinary teams. It is present to varying degrees in interdisciplinary teams; and it is a vital part of transdisciplinary teams. The communication methods used by the team are critical to their success and must, to the extent possible, match each team member's preference. For exam-ple, case notes can be shared via e-mail after feeding sessions, and phone confer-ences or face-to-face meetings can be organized on a predetermined schedule (e.g., weekly, monthly, quarterly).

Communication is especially critical when team members change. Departing members must provide remaining and new team members with information about successful strategies. This is especially important when incoming team members have limited general experience or limited specific experience in the early childhood field (Campbell et al., 2009; Rapport et al., 2004).

Information sharing must stay within the feeding team to adhere with confi-dentiality requirements across disciplines (Kurjan, 2000). Each discipline follows regulations and procedures outlining access to reports and intervention plans. For feeding plans to be successfully implemented, there must be cross-discipline communication and resource sharing within the parameters set forth by each discipline.

An additional component of communication within a feeding team, no matter the model, is discussing the feeding plan with parents rather than informing parents after decisions have been made. Parents, family members, and caregivers are essential to all team configurations and must receive information and have their questions answered in a timely and clear manner, as well as be given opportunities to provide feedback to team members (Campbell & Halbert, 2002).

According to several researchers (Bruns & Thompson, 2010; Homer, 2003; King et al., 2009; Nijhuis et al., 2007; Peña & Quinn, 2003), in order for feeding teams to be successful, communication must have the following characteristics:

- Mutually determined expectations and procedures for informal and formal communication exchanges
- Ongoing and reciprocal communication
- Positive and easy-to-understand language with common (rather than discipline-specific) terminology
- A variety of communication methods to meet team-member preferences (e.g., face-to-face conversations, e-mail, texts)
- Method(s) to document and store communication among team members (e.g., paper files, secured web site)

Collaboration Friend and Cook (2009) defined collaboration as "a style for direct interaction between at least two co-equal parties voluntarily engaged in shared decision-making as they work toward a common goal" (p. 7). It is imperative that team members collaborate to develop, implement, and evaluate feeding plans. This collaboration must involve determining the necessary and most effective materials, strategies, and specialized interventions to address a range of feeding difficulties in infants, toddlers, and preschoolers. The feeding-related expertise and experiences of professionals, parents, other family members, and caregivers must be combined to identify strengths and formulate needs-based feeding plans.

The transdisciplinary team model is best suited to collaboration. As described in the scenario earlier in the chapter, role release requires a great deal of interaction so that team members can share expertise and provide feedback. One challenge in transdisciplinary teams is the possibility of professionals' unwillingness to cross discipline boundaries (McGonigel et al., 1994; Stayton & Bruder, 1999). This may be a particular concern surrounding feeding difficulties because professionals may need to step outside of what is familiar. For example, a PT may be asked to implement a feeding intervention prescribed by a SLP; if the PT is accustomed to providing adapted seating items rather than facilitating jaw control or cup drinking, the situation may be uncomfortable. Conversely, a SLP may feel uncomfortable asking a PT either to demonstrate use of a specialized positioning system or to position the child at the start of a feeding session. These are opportunities for learning across discipline boundaries. The professionals can discuss the strategies as well as share resources, such as handouts and videos. In this way, professional development is practical and meaningful and likely to lead to implementation of new strategies (Snyder & Wolfe, 2007). Team members must be open to learning new techniques to ensure optimal benefits for the children and families they serve. Because parents, family members, and caregivers often have insights and strategies to share with professionals, collaboration must extend to them as well (Bruns & Thompson, 2010; Palisano, 2006; Peña & Quinn, 2003; Secrist-Mertz et al., 1997).

An additional viewpoint on team collaboration was offered by DeMatteo, Matovich, and Hjartarson (2005). The authors described assisting children (birth to 15 years) with feeding and swallowing difficulties as follows, "the overall goal is to get children feeding or eating as quickly and as safely as possible, with the least hardship for the child and family. It is the responsibility of the clinician to use the best evidence to make decisions with the family to select the appropriate evaluations and interventions" (p. 154). This quote highlights the importance of informed decision making based on input from all team members and the importance of valuing the contributions of each team member. As illustrated by the interdisciplinary and transdisciplinary team models, team leadership is necessary for this to occur.

Collaboration also includes logistical considerations such as availability of resources, meeting times and locations, and informal opportunities to share information (Bell & Alper, 2007). Support from program or agency administration is an additional factor. Administrators must see the value in providing resources in order to improve team functioning, such as adjusting schedules so professionals can complete a feeding assessment together (see Chapter 6), approving funding for consultation, and working with the team leader to secure needed equipment (King et al., 2009). Resource allocation also extends to payment and/or reimbursement so team members can collaborate. For example, co-treatment is often not fully reimbursed because payment is based on one professional working with one child during a therapy session.

Coordination   Within all team models, there must be coordinated and consistent use of feeding strategies and specialized interventions (Lefton-Greif & Arvedson, 1997; Scherer & Kaiser, 2007). Gisel, Birnbaum and Schwartz (1998) recommended having all team members reach consensus with regard to the implementation of strategies and the evaluation of progress. For example, team members can meet with the child and caregivers and introduce new strategies together so that all professionals can observe and ask questions. If this is not feasible, the implementation of new strategies can be recorded, and the videos can be shared with all team members. In the previous example, the PT can be recorded trying a new piece of equipment to position the toddler during a home visit, and the video can be shown to the entire team at their next meeting. In addition, for monitoring progress, data sheets can be distributed among team members, and documentation methods can be reviewed (see Chapter 7). Team members must also identify when gains are not made and be able to make modifications to the feeding plan in order to further assist feeding development.

Coordination is also influenced by team members' schedules and changes to the team configuration (e.g., when a professional leaves the team and is replaced). A new team member must be oriented to the team's model, methods of communication and interaction, and decision-making process. Without a clear understanding of these components, the new team member is likely to encounter difficulties coordinating services with the other team members. In addition, more experienced team members must embrace the new team member and make necessary adjustments, especially if role release is involved. If the team leader leaves the team, the remaining professionals must decide who among them will take the leadership position. These varied situations have a direct impact on team coordination.

Coordination also can be adversely affected when one professional implements a strategy that is contrary to a strategy used by another team member. For instance, a DS might recommend that a young toddler with visual impairment use a weighted cup during all meals and snacks. If the dietitian encourages the child's mother to provide a bottle with Pediasure at breakfast and before bedtime to increase calorie intake, there is a conflict. The feeding team, as a whole, must come to consensus on the primary means of fluid intake to prevent such situations. Consensus can be reached through discussion, voting, or other means of dialogue about such issues. In the example (and in many situations), two methods are not necessarily mutually exclusive. In the example, a weighted cup and bottles of Pediasure might both be necessary to meet the child's nutritional needs; however, all team members, including the parent, must agree on the use.

Documentation   Documentation, whether pen-and-paper or electronic, is a crucial component for a successful feeding team. As described previously, if strategies are not implemented in a coordinated fashion, the child may show little or no progress. Anecdotal notes and data sheets, for example, can limit or eliminate uncertainty about a child's development in prioritized feeding skills and behaviors (see Chapter 7 for a description of documentation methods). Arvedson (2000) discussed the contributions of SLPs for children with suspected feeding difficulties in school settings. These professionals can observe the child during mealtime and share notes or checklist with other team members.

The importance of data collection is illustrated in the following example. During therapy sessions, a SLP notes increased tongue lateralization (moving side to side) and attempts at chewing semi-solids in a 2-year-old with Down syndrome. The child care provider indicates that the child pushes away solid foods. Finally, the OT rarely observes mealtimes during scheduled weekly visits, but offers the child oral stimulation exercises that encourage greater tongue movement. If all three professionals document the child's tongue movements and acceptance of semisolid foods, a clear picture of developmental gains and needs will emerge (see Chapter 7 for a discussion of data collection; see Appendix D for samples of data-collection forms). An additional consideration is the need for one or more agreed-upon data collection methods across team members. If each professional is using different types of documentation, it will be difficult to identify patterns and difficult to use the information to craft modifications and adaptations to existing interventions. The team model will likely dictate the degree of uniformity regarding documentation and data use (e.g., greater uniformity within a transdisciplinary team).

Training and Professional Development

Klein and Gilkerson (2000) indicated that professionals on a feeding team need to develop a knowledge base about feeding and about discipline-specific feeding strategies and interventions. The authors posited that an "important area for professional development is greater understanding of feeding issues" (p. 456). Communication and collaboration skills, along with mutually understood methods for facilitating coordinated feeding support and documentation are also needed as are effective team-participation skills (Körner, 2010; McWilliam, 2005; Stayton & Bruder, 1999).

Feeding teams need training opportunities to gain an understanding of feeding development and possible difficulties and an understanding of discipline-specific feeding expertise and strategies. Without some level of familiarity with cross-discipline strategies, collaboration and coordination can be negatively affected. For example, Power-duFur (2000) claimed that SLPs should not provide services to students with dysphagia (swallowing disorders) without gaining knowledge in this area. O'Donoghue and Dean-Claytor (2008) suggested that some SLPs are not aware of their lack of knowledge about dysphagia and could cause harm during therapy session. The authors asserted that "clinicians must understand when they are beyond their realm of clinical expertise and should seek appropriate consultations and referrals" (p. 196).

In a transdisciplinary team, training in strategies outside a team member's discipline is required. Informal and formal exchanges occur within the team. Workshops and similar activities provided by outside experts are also warranted. Additionally, feeding team members should seek continuing educational opportunities on topics outside of their field in order to improve their performance. For instance, a DS could attend a regional or state conference for SLPs or one focused on oral-motor development. Ideally, professional development should include hands-on activities and multiple opportunities for learning (Olsen et al., 2005; Wooster et al., 1998).

▧ ▧ ▧ TABLE TALK ▧ ▧ ▧

Gillian is a 3-year-old girl with pervasive developmental delay (PDD). She recently transitioned to a half-day Head Start program in the morning and her districts' half day prekindergarten (pre-K) program in the afternoon. Gillian receives all of her therapy services at the pre-K, including SLP and OT. Her mother, Jamie, also consults with a dietitian to help her daughter gain weight because Gillian has been at the 10th percentile for weight since she was 9 months old. Jamie's mother consults with Toni, a behavior analyst, to help address mealtime tantrums, especially at breakfast and lunch; the agreed upon strategy of praising Gillian when she remains at the table for at least 15 seconds works well, as does offering preferred foods after she tastes a nonpreferred or novel item.

Jamie gives Gillian breakfast at home (a cereal bar, a piece of nine-grain bread with grape jelly, and 4–6 ounces of apple juice) rather than have Head Start staff work with her for two meals. At lunch, Gillian generally accepts a few bites of each food and then yells, throws her plate, and leaves the table before the end of the meal. The lead Head Start teacher asks Jamie for suggestions, and Jamie shares several ideas that the behavior analyst has given her.

Unfortunately, the pre-K teacher has not asked for similar guidance for snack time. Jamie asked if the behavior analyst could visit the pre-K classroom, and the teacher agreed. However, scheduling a time that works with everyone's schedule has been difficult; 3 weeks have passed, and the observation has not yet occurred.

The pre-K teacher, Mrs. Garrett, called Jamie last week to schedule a meeting to discuss Gillian's disruptiveness in the classroom, specifically Gillian's snack-time behaviors and the fact that several of Gillian's peers are imitating her behavior. During the meeting, Jamie shares strategies from the behavior analyst and asks whether the pre-K teacher can use them. The teacher replies, "My aide and I have to manage 18 to 20 children. How do you expect us to follow this plan? There's just too much going on at snack time." Jamie leaves the meeting very upset and considers taking Gillian out of pre-K.

Discussion Questions

- Do you agree with Jamie and Toni's recommendations? Why or why not?
- How would you approach Mrs. Garrett about implementing the behavioral strategies that are used in Gillian's home and at Head Start?
- How could this situation be resolved by a transdisciplinary team?

6

Feeding-Related Screening and Assessment

What You'll Learn in This Chapter

This chapter provides

- A rationale for feeding assessment
- An overview of screening and assessment procedures and instruments
- Outcomes and next steps after a feeding assessment

■ ■ ■ FOOD FOR THOUGHT ■ ■ ■

"Ray, who is 45 months old, comes in from speech therapy. His friends are already at the snack table. Ray washes his hands and comes slowly to the snack table. 'Come over and sit by me,' says Ms. C., the pre-K aide. Ray sits down quietly and Ms. C. asks if he would like juice or goldfish crackers.

Ray shakes his head 'no.'

'Are you sure you don't want any tasty crackers?' Ray shakes his head.

Ms. C. says, 'That leaves more for me. How about some grapefruit juice?'

Ray looks at her and nods. Ms. C. pours the juice, and Ray takes a drink. He looks at the children at his table. He takes another drink, sets down his cup, and says, 'Goldfish please, Ms. C.'

She asks 'Are you sure you want goldfish?'

'Yes please.' Ray and Ms. C. sit together and eat crackers at the table.

Ms. C. notes Ray's behaviors in her observation notebook. At the beginning of the school year, he did not request items at snack and often ate by himself or did not participate. He also preferred soft foods and would refuse crunchy or hard foods. Ms. C. writes a note home to Ray's mom to let her know about his new skills."

Becca, Special Education Graduate Student and Pre-K Teacher

"Lizette, Vivian, and Melanie all drink and eat soy products instead of dairy. They have never been officially diagnosed with a dairy allergy, but their mother, grandmother, and great-grandmother all have the allergy, as do several other family members.

Lizette has more sensitivity to food than Vivian and Melanie. Lizette has had a blood allergy test done, but her mother has been told that it is not as accurate as a skin allergy test. One time, Lizette's mother ate a grilled cheese sandwich and cream of mushroom soup for dinner. That night after nursing, Lizette was extremely fussy. Even the nurses couldn't calm her down."

Laurie, Babysitter

As described in the story about Ray, observing a young child's mealtime interactions with adults, his food choices, and how he accepts fluids and eats foods with various textures provides important information to identify or confirm suspected feeding delays or difficulties. The information can also be used to develop interventions to improve a child's acceptance of foods and liquids, self-feeding skills, and related skills. Additional assessment approaches and methods are necessary to produce a complete representation of a young child's feeding development and possible difficulties, including allergies to specific food items. Borrowing from the literature on assessment of young children's social-emotional development, Carter, Briggs-Gowan, and Davis (2004) discussed in-depth assessment as the "gateway" to effective intervention and treatment.

WHAT THE LITERATURE SAYS

The American Academy of Pediatrics (2006) advocates screening for delays and disabilities, including those related to daily living activities such as feeding at several points during a child's early development. Screening is a brief testing procedure used to determine if a young child has reached key developmental milestones. If the child does not exhibit the typical skills, further assessment is indicated in the areas suspected to have a delay. There has also been a growing emphasis on examining young children's social-emotional and behavioral development (Carter et al., 2004; Conroy & Brown, 2004). The authors highlight the need to consider the context of children's lives, especially the environments in which they live. These environmental conditions can have direct effects on feeding and mealtimes. For example, a toddler who is cared for by caregivers with limited knowledge of child development may not be offered age-appropriate or adequate meal portions (see Chapter 4). This, in turn, can contribute to deficiencies in nutrition and inappropriate or disruptive mealtime behaviors such as throwing food or utensils.

A related area is utilizing mealtimes to examine parent–child interaction (Kelly & Barnard, 2000). Mealtimes offer opportunities to observe how a parent and young child respond to each other's cues, such as whether a mother stops feeding her infant when the infant turns his or her head away. There is also the need to gain knowledge about reciprocity during parent–child interactions. This is particularly critical when an infant or toddler is under-responsive to maternal cues (e.g., limited eye contact, less alert when awake) due to an underlying medical condition (e.g., cardiac defect) or disability (e.g., cerebral palsy, Down syndrome; Kelly & Barnard, 2000).

Early identification is also the focus of Early and Periodic Screening, Diagnosis, and Treatment (EPSDT) which is part of the United States Department of Health & Human Services. Through state networks of pediatricians and other health providers, this program targets low-income families with an emphasis on provision of health services for children. Identification of young children with disabilities or who are at risk for developmental delays, including delays that can have an impact on feeding, is discussed in the Individuals with Disabilities Education Improvement Act (IDEA) of 2004 (PL 108-446). This federal law stipulates that communities develop a screening system to identify children in need of special services through community outreach and related services. This is part of early intervention (EI) for infants and toddlers, as well as public school-based services for preschoolers. It is important to note that a similar emphasis on early identification is also evident in other regions, such as Canada, the United Kingdom, and Australia. In addition, the Diagnostic and Statistical Manual of Mental Disorders IV (DSM-IV-TR, American Psychiatric Association, 2000) recognizes feeding disorder of infancy or early childhood as "feeding disturbance manifested by persistent failure to eat adequately with significant failure to gain weight or significant loss of weight over at least 1 month...the onset is before age 6 years" (American Psychiatric Association, 2000, p. 108). In sum, screening and assessment is necessary to identify the presence and extent of feeding difficulties.

It is especially critical to screen a young child's nutritional status in order to identify deficiencies in vitamins and minerals necessary for growth and in order to determine whether the child's diet is meeting the recommended caloric intake. Charney (2008) posited the necessity of nutrition screening in child care settings. The author stressed the importance of the reliability (same results over time) and predictive value (results confirm findings of assessment) of screening results. As discussed in Chapter 1, feeding development follows a standard progression. Screening can identify "red flags" that indicate possible feeding difficulties. The red flags can be related to structural, physiological, behavioral, or nutritional causes, or they can be due to an underlying condition that causes delays or disabilities (e.g., cerebral palsy, Down syndrome). The feeding difficulties may also be short term or long term. Regardless of the origin of the problem, screening should be done to ascertain if a young child requires more in-depth assessment, including examination of oral-motor development, fine motor development, and feeding-related behaviors, such as age-appropriate self-feeding and interactions within feeding environments. Much can be learned when children are observed within feeding interactions, especially when a young child has a disability or is considered at risk for developmental delay. For example, feeding interactions are affected when an infant has a cleft palate. The child may have difficulty latching onto the breast, prolonged feedings, and excessive gagging (Kelly & Barnard, 2000; see Chapter 13). Medical examination of a child's digestive system is also recommended when feeding problems are suspected.

Leading authors in the feeding literature (Arvedson & Brodsky, 2002; Gisel, Birnbaum, & Schwartz, 1998; Manikam & Perman, 2000; Schwarz, Corredor, Fisher-Medina, Cohen, & Rabinowitz, 2001) advocate an in-depth assessment of a child's feeding skills in order to identify feeding strengths as well as the types and severity of feeding needs. This type of assessment collects information using a variety of methods and measures (e.g., observation, medical examination) and a variety of sources including parents and caregivers (Reilly, Wisbeach & Carr, 2000). Depending on the child's difficulties, other members of the feeding assessment team may include a gastroenterologist, nutritionist, behavioral psychologist, dietitian, occupational therapist (OT) and/or speech-language pathologist (SLP; Camp & Kalscheur, 1994; Lefton-Greif, 1994; Miller & Willging, 2003; Schuberth, 1994). For example, if a toddler has only eaten starchy foods, citrus fruits, and berries for the past 5 weeks, resulting in little weight gain and loose stools, assessment by a gastroenterologist can determine if a problem exists in the digestive system while his parent can check with his pediatrician to determine whether this behavior is age appropriate or indicative of a feeding problem. If a 4-year-old with cerebral palsy is having trouble with textured foods, for example gagging and choking most meals, an SLP can examine the child's skills through use of an assessment instrument that specifically addresses biting and chewing (see description of the Schedule for Oral-Motor Assessment). The resulting data can be used to develop a feeding plan—including a feeding schedule, procedures for food preparation, and positioning—to be implemented by the child's parent, caregivers, and clinicians (Morris & Klein, 2000; Olive, 2004; see Chapter 7 for information regarding feeding plans).

Burklow, Phelps, Schultz, McConnell, and Rudolph (1998) discuss the interplay of biological and behavioral aspects in the development and demonstration of feeding difficulties. Burklow et al., (1998) reviewed the feeding evaluations of 103 children with a disability or developmental delay (ages 4 months–17 years) and developed a coding system based on the following five categories: 1) structural abnormalities, 2) neurological conditions, 3) behavioral issues, 4) cardiac and respiratory problems, and 5) metabolic dysfunction. Diagnoses are based on examining assessment results within the five categories as well as identifying the underlying medical or health condition affecting feeding and mealtime behaviors. The authors emphasized that in order to determine the cause(s) and identify ways to address feeding difficulties, assessment must be thorough. An additional perspective was offered by Chatoor (2009) who discussed classification of feeding difficulties based on the infant's ability to self-regulate and on the quality of parent–child attachment. Chatoor and Khushlani (2006) discussed regulation issues affecting feeding for preschool-age children. All means of screening and assessment should be used to determine the breadth and depth of feeding difficulties.

SCREENING AND ASSESSMENT METHODS AND INSTRUMENTS

The following sections offer descriptions of a number of screening and assessment instruments commonly used with young children. The list is not meant to be exhaustive, but rather to provide an overview of the types and methods of feeding assessment. Most of the instruments are intended for use by early childhood special education (ECSE) professionals. Some require child observation or requesting that the child perform certain feeding skills. Others are completed by discipline-specific professionals, such as SLPs, with input from child care providers and ECSE professionals.

The instruments vary in length and method(s) for collection of information. It is noted when an instrument requires specialized training for conducting or evaluating the results. In addition, excluding the screening instruments and diagnostic tests, contact was made with instrument authors or researchers working with specific instruments in order to obtain copies of the instruments for review and to collect additional information about their use. If an author did not respond to the request, the instrument was not included in the chapter. The information presented here is not intended to recommend or endorse specific instruments or methods.

The following section provides an overview of screening procedures as well as procedures for obtaining a child's medical history, physical examination, and feeding history for additional background information. Use of a feeding diary, observation, and interview/parent report are also described. The second section focuses on rating scales, functional analysis, assessment "packages," and criterion-referenced and standardized assessment instruments. The final section offers an overview of diagnostic tests.

Screening

A number of authors have developed instruments to identify red flags that indicate feeding difficulties. Red flags may include extended feeding sessions, weak suck, excessive gagging, and food refusal (Swigert, 1998). These instruments are the initial step in determining the presence of a feeding problem. Individuals who work with young children on a daily basis are best suited to carry out this screening. Daily mealtimes offer ongoing opportunities to identify potential feeding difficulties.

Baroni and Sondel (1995) described the Nutrition and Feeding Risk Identification Tool (NFRIT). The NFRIT focuses on nutrition and feeding concerns for young children receiving early intervention (EI) services. This tool is completed by the parent(s) and includes input from the child's EI team. The Oral-Motor Feeding Rating Scale (OMFRS; Jelm, 1990) examines oral-motor movements and patterns. The scale is completed by a parent or professional through observation of a young child eating a meal. Data is collected concerning lip and cheek movement as well as tongue and jaw movement.

Several feeding-related items are included in the Ages & Stages Questionnaires®: Social-Emotional (ASQ:SE; Squires, Bricker, & Twombly, 2002). This screening instrument examines skills in areas including self-regulation, compliance, and daily living skills of 6- to 60-month-old young children. All eight ASQ:SE questionnaires include feeding-related items. Parents or caregivers rate each item as *most of the time, sometimes,* or *rarely or never*. A space marked "Check if this is a concern" accompanies each item. The NFRIT, OMFRS, and ASQ:SE identify young children in need of further feeding assessment.

Additional screening instruments have been developed for a specific program, agency, or region. A Look at Your Child's Nutrition (Gilliam & Laney, 2008) examines a child's appetite, feeding problems, allergies, and overall nutritional status. The Regional and Statewide Services for Students with Orthopedic Impairments (RSOI) in Oregon utilizes the Nutrition Screening–A Look at Diet and Health (Roberts, 2002). Parents complete items about their child's daily dietary intake, feeding concerns, and existing medical conditions.

The following six sections discuss a variety of methods to collect feeding information including medical history, feeding history, and observation. These methods may be informal or commercially available. A child care provider or ECSE professional should request that results be shared in order to provide input and be involved in making recommendations to address feeding needs and implementing strategies and specialized interventions (see Chapter 7).

Medical History

If screening results indicate a possible feeding problem, it is critical for a member of the feeding assessment team such as a pediatrician, gastroenterologist, or dietitian to collect the child's medical history, including a record of the child's height and weight gain since birth, medical procedures, and hospitalizations. The child's nutritional status—including a comparison of daily intake to growth and energy needs—should also be evaluated. This information offers insights into chronic problems such as slow or uneven weight-gain patterns, along with food selectivity and corresponding vitamin and nutrient deficiencies. In addition, the parent is asked about occurrences of gagging, vomiting, digestive system problems, and elimination issues including diarrhea and constipation. Instances of pneumonia, asthma, and other respiratory ailments should be documented and considered when collecting a child's medical history because a child's airway status can negatively affect food and liquid intake.

A thorough medical history can also begin to answer questions related to the affective aspects of eating and feeding-related interactions. Arvedson and Brodsky (2002) noted that 25%–40% of healthy toddlers demonstrate feeding problems, most of which are linked to developmental gains such as greater independence and control and most of which are manifested by eating small amounts or not sitting for a meal. When gathering a child's medical history, it is important to note how long relevant behaviors have been observed. Information should also be collected about delays in attainment of developmental milestones. The child's motor development should be evaluated because fine-motor and gross-motor delays are often manifested in problems with self-feeding and acceptance of textured foods or thin liquids (e.g., water, apple juice).

Physical Examination

A young child's physical appearance and oral-motor structures such as lips, tongue, and soft and hard palate should also be examined as part of a feeding assessment

(Lefton-Greif, 1994; Palmer, Drennan & Baba, 2000). This examination is typically completed by a pediatrician or nurse. An evaluation of physical appearance includes anthropometric measurements: height, weight, body mass index (BMI), body fat, and overall growth rate. BMI indicates amount of body fat based on a child's height and weight (Zemel, Riley & Stallings, 1997). BMI falls into one of the following categories: underweight, healthy weight, overweight, and obese. Respiration and heart rate should also be examined. An elevated heart rate, for example, can cause greater energy expenditure so that the suck–breathe–swallow sequence becomes difficult for an infant to maintain throughout a feeding. Arvedson and Brodsky (2002) and Lowery (2001) encouraged examination of feeding functions including degluititition (act of swallowing, which entails sucking and chewing), feeding (intake of food) and evidence of dysphagia. Results are used to determine the need for conducting additional, in-depth assessments to determine causation and treatment options.

According to Fraker and Walbert (2003) and Swigert (1998), physical examination for feeding assessment of an infant must include evaluation of the following reflexes:

- rooting (a touch to the cheeks or lips should cause the infant to turn toward the stimulus)
- suckling (front–back tongue movement when stimulus is placed in the mouth)
- sucking
- swallowing
- biting (pressure on the gums or rub left and right molar area)
- transverse tongue movement (tongue moves toward stimulation applied to the side of the tongue)
- gagging (touch to the back half of the tongue results in mouth opening)
- coughing

Responses that indicate possible feeding difficulties, such as tongue thrust and minimal lip closure, can be observed via this examination. These responses may signify lack of nonnutritive sucking. Nonnutritive sucking has been shown to assist infants with their suck–swallow–breathe pattern (Crist & Napier-Phillips, 2001; Derkay & Schechter, 1998; Miller & Willging, 2003).

Feeding History

Douglas (2000), Fraker and Walbert (2003), and Kedesdy and Budd (1998) recommended completing a feeding history as part of a feeding assessment. These authors all emphasized the valuable background information a feeding history provides about the child's attainment of feeding milestones such as initial response to solid foods, beginning cup use, feeding preferences, and short-term and long-term feeding concerns. Parents, caregivers, and ECSE professionals with knowledge of the child in these areas are the primary providers of this information. With regard to ESCE professionals, information should be gathered from present and former providers in order to prepare a complete representation of a young child's feeding development.

A feeding history gathers information about allergies and about medication(s) that may have an impact on feeding, such as appetite suppression from antihistamines and specific types of anti-seizure medications. A feeding history can also be used to learn about a child's meal and snack schedule, including average length of a meal, how much is eaten, and behaviors that interfere with eating. This information offers background on past as well as current feeding development and concerns.

A feeding history offers a holistic portrait of the child's feeding skills and areas of concern. Feeding histories inform further assessment by highlighting the types of additional information needed in order to develop appropriate strategies and interventions. In addition, it is critical to collaborate with the child's parent as well as other primary caregivers to gather a comprehensive feeding history. Kedesdy and Budd (1998) further advised that the types of information described here can be collected informally (e.g., notes, running records) or via completion of a formal, structured feeding history. Fraker and Walbert (2003) developed a formal feeding history that includes sections for the child's background information, medical information, feeding schedule, positioning, and breastfeeding versus bottle feeding. It also requests information about the child's favorite foods, liquid intake (including the type of cup used), and a list of concerns such as poor appetite, coughing, and avoiding meals. A referral guide is also included. The authors conclude that "early experiences should be documented as they can influence the sensory, emotional, and experiential aspects of current eating patterns" (p. 165).

Food Diary

A food diary is used to compile information about the food items and liquids a child accepts over a specified time period (e.g., 24 hours, 7 days; Johnson, Silverstein, Rosenbloom, Carter, & Cunningham, 1986). The resulting summary of the child's intake can be combined with other assessment results. For example, information about food ingredients, texture, and temperature can be included in a food diary to gather information on specific feeding concerns or to examine intake of a particular nutrient, such as iron. A food diary can also include location and duration of feedings and meals, seating (e.g., highchair, bean bag, mother's lap), response to presented foods and liquids, as well as the feeder and the amount and type of self-feeding.

Parents, caregivers, and professionals (including teachers, therapists, and aides directly involved in feeding activities and interactions with the child) document specific foods and liquids along with amounts that the child accepts at mealtimes and snacks (Yarnell, Fehily, Milbank, Sweetnam, & Walker, 1983). Adults with less frequent feeding interactions with the child can also provide information. A babysitter who watches the child once a week, as well as a grandparent who has the child for an overnight visit, can document a child's food and liquid intake. An important outcome of a food diary is intake information across individuals and settings. In addition, the feeding team can then review the resulting information to gain insight into the child's preferred foods and liquids as well as overall daily intake.

A food diary can be prepared in a checklist format or a more informal, open-ended format. Table 6.1 provides an example of a food diary based on a form developed for an early childhood classroom that serves preschoolers with autism. The form could be expanded to include space to document intake at snacks and dinner. Jacobi, Agras, Bryson, and Hammer (2003) utilized a more structured approach.

The authors created a standardized 24-hour calorie intake protocol. Parents of 135 preschool-age children completed the protocol to reflect their child's intake from a cooler that was delivered to their home. The cooler contained a variety of foods in age-appropriate portions (i.e., carbohydrates, 59.9%; proteins, 14.2%; fats, 25.9%). Results from the food diary indicated "their picky children as eating a limited variety of foods, accepting new foods less readily, requesting specific food preparation methods more often and expressing strong food dislikes" (p. 83). The information also offered the researchers information about ways to expose picky eaters to new foods. (Additional methods to assess picky eaters are presented in the following sections.)

Observation

Observation is a method of feeding assessment in which detailed information about mealtime behaviors and interactions are collected. Arvedson (2000) recommended observation as a means to examine a child's feeding relationship with primary caregivers (e.g., intake patterns, positioning). One such assessment instrument is the Toddler Snack Scale (TSS; Spegman & Houck, 2005). This instrument collects information about mother and toddler behaviors during a snack activity. Specifically, items assess mother–child engagement and negotiation of control and autonomy. After TSS items are scored, both members of the dyad are classified along a continuum: The mother is classified as *facilitative engaged, controlling engaged, superficial interaction,* or *controlling disengaged.* Toddlers are classified as *engaged assertive, intermittent engaged, compliant disengaged,* or *active disengaged* (Houck & Spegman, 1999).

Table 6.1. Food diary format with sample breakfast and lunch menu data

Monday	Tuesday	Wednesday	Thursday	Friday
BREAKFAST	**BREAKFAST**	**BREAKFAST**	**BREAKFAST**	**BREAKFAST**
✦Cheerios	✦Cheerios	✓oatmeal	✖breakfast burrito (2 bites)	✓blueberry muffin
✓apple pastry	✖sausage links (4 bites)	✦donut	✓orange juice	✓applesauce
✱apple juice (2 ounces)	✱apple juice (3 ounces)	✓orange juice	✱milk (1 ounce)	✱cranberry juice (2 ounces)
✓milk	✓milk	✱milk (1 ounce)		✓milk
LUNCH	**LUNCH**	**LUNCH**	**LUNCH**	**LUNCH**
✓sloppy joe with ✖bun	✓chicken patty with ✖bun (6 bites)	✓hot dog with ✖bun (6 bites)	✓turkey with gravy	✦chicken strips
✦corn	✓sweet potatoes	✖corn chips (10 bites)	✓mashed potatoes	✖macaroni & cheese (10 bites)
✓mixed fruit cocktail	✦banana slices	✓peas and carrots	✓green beans	✓green beans
✖sugar cookie (6 bites)	✦pudding	✓peach slices	✖dinner roll (8 bites)	✓mixed fruit cocktail
✓milk	✱milk (2 ounces)	✖chocolate chip cookie (5 bites)	✓pear slices	✓chocolate milk
		✱milk (2 ounces)	✱milk (2 ounces)	

Key:

✓ = refusal (pushed away, threw food item)

✦ = taste (accepts taste of food item)

✖ = ate portion of item (number of bites in parenthesis)

✱ = drank portion of item (number of ounces in parenthesis)

Observations should occur in the environments with which the child is most familiar and comfortable and where the child has most daily meals, such as in the home, child care, and community settings. Forms can be developed to document the child's physical actions and behaviors, as well as emotional reactions and responses. In addition, the number and types of inappropriate behaviors, such as food refusal and throwing food items, can also be recorded. The form can also include space to record the actions, reactions, behaviors, and emotional responses of the caregivers feeding and/or interacting with the child. In this way, patterns can be discerned indicating situations that encourage appropriate feeding behaviors in contrast with those that encourage mealtime challenges.

Fraker and Walbert (2003) described the need to observe signs of stress in infants, including burping, gagging, spitting up, arching, hiccups, and yawning. Swigert (1998) also recommended collecting observation of a young child's bite, chew, tongue movement, jaw control, and swallowing patterns. Morris and Klein (2000) developed the Mealtime Assessment Guide to assist with feeding observations. This guide includes six interrelated areas:

1) child's developmental skills,

2) mealtime relationship and interactions,

3) mealtime communication skills,

4) mealtime physical skills,

5) mealtime sensory skills, and

6) mealtime oral-motor skills (pp. 185–186).

The observer lists strengths and challenges in each area and compiles the data into a summary to use for intervention planning. Using observation of a feeding session, the Pediatric Scale (Perlin & Boner, 1994) records information about reflexes (e.g., rooting, gag, startle), facial responses, movements of the lips, tongue, mouth, and jaw along with coordination of suckling and sucking movements based on the child's age (0–3 to 24+ months).

The Holistic Feeding Observation Form (Lowman & Murphy, 1999) examines the following aspects of feeding for children with various disabilities: collaboration with the family, respiratory issues, oral-motor development, physical development/positioning, sensory development, communication, behavioral and socialization skills and feeding process, and implementation plan (pp. 231–233). The physical development/positioning section asks the observer to note the child's head and neck position; shoulder, trunk, hips, and pelvis stability; and knees, ankles, and feet position while eating and drinking. The authors emphasized the need to focus on area(s) the child's parents, caregivers, and professionals identify as concerns.

The Oral-motor/Eating/Speech Checklist is an observation tool used with children with autism (Flanagan, 2008). Items include observation of the food textures a child prefers and avoids. Information is also gathered through observation to describe of oral movements with liquids, semisolid foods from a spoon, soft solid foods (e.g., bread), and hard solid foods (e.g., pretzels).

Observation can also include specific oral-motor tasks. Mathisen, Worrall, Masel, Wall, and Shepherd (1999) used the Feeding Assessment Schedule (FAS; Johnson,

Handen, Mayer-Costa, & Sacco, 2008) in a study with infants with gastroesophageal reflux (GER). The FAS was also used to learn about the oral-motor development of infants with a form of spina bifida—a condition in which the backbone and spinal canal do not close before birth affecting muscle tone and overall motor abilities (Mathisen & Shepherd, 1997). The instrument is comprised of 10 subsets (e.g., lip, tongue, and jaw function; biting; food and saliva loss). Each is rated on performance and affective dimensions. For example, in the Swallowing subset, lip seal is assessed during swallowing, and the observer notes any increase in tension in the child's face and neck. The two components are scored independently. The FAS also includes presentation of four food textures (puréed, semisolids, solids, and liquids). Familiar spoons, bottles, and other feeding items can be brought from home. Sessions are videotaped for later viewing and scoring. The resulting profile offers information of the infant's oral-motor skills and areas of need. A similar observation instrument was described by Reilly, Skuse, Mathisen, and Wolke (1995), and Skuse, Stevenson, Reilly, and Mathisen (1995). The Schedule for Oral-Motor Assessment (SOMA; Reilly, Wolke, & Skuse, 2000) examines four categories of food textures (purée, semisolids, solids, cracker) and three methods of liquid intake (bottle, trainer cup, cup) for infants and toddlers 8–24 months of age. According to the scoring manual, the foci of the 15–20 minute observation are lip closure, tongue and jaw movements, swallowing, and quality of bite. Scoring is *Yes* (normal response) or *No* (abnormal response). Examples of abnormal responses include tongue thrusting, jaw clenching, and gagging (Reilly, Skuse, & Wolke, 2000). Research demonstrates the instrument's ability to identify young children with oral-motor problems. For example, Spender et al. (1996) used the SOMA in their study of young children (ages 11–34 months) with Down syndrome. The children demonstrated greater difficulty with textures compared with typically developing toddlers. Tongue protrusion and jaw control were also qualitatively different in the study participants.

Interview/Parent Report

An interview should be completed with the child's primary caregivers. In addition, information can be gathered through parent report. Parents can provide much insight into their child's eating habits during casual conversation such as at child care drop-off and pick-up. The child care provider, for example, can facilitate this feeding-related exchange by commenting on the child's food intake or demonstration of a new skill, by using general, open-ended questions to elicit information, and by probing to obtain more specific information and examples. An exchange may proceed as follows:

Ms. Parks (ECSE teacher): Jordyn enjoys eating breakfast when she arrives in the morning. She always finishes her plate and asks for more milk using her pictures. She also takes turns with her classmates to serve herself the breakfast items. Lately, she is not coming to the table for snack. She whines and resists when we try to bring her to the table.

Marsha (Jordyn's mother): That's interesting because we've noticed that she will eat an early dinner at home and refuse any food afterward. She's probably very hungry by the time she gets off the bus.

Ms. Parks: Yes, she eats two portions most days.

Marsha: Something her dad and I have noticed is that when we give her something to drink first she is more interested in a snack. She'll drink a little bit of water or diluted juice and then eat a few crackers.

Ms. Parks: That's helpful information. Tell me more about the foods Jordyn will eat for snack.

Marsha: All kinds of crackers, dried cereal, and sometimes raw vegetables.

Ms. Parks: We usually offer her granola bars and oatmeal cookies. My guess is when she sees us taking down the boxes to prepare for snack she checks out what we have. I think we'll have better success with crackers and such.

Mealtime routines and schedules that also should be examined within the context of an interview or parent report include mealtime and snack schedule, largest meal of the day, number of daily snacks, and whether the child is allowed to ask for food between meal and snack times. For infants, it is important to ask about the child's hunger and satiety cycle, alertness during feedings, and types and quantity of breast milk and formula consumed, as well as the use of on-demand or planned (e.g., every four hours) feeding. For example, a parent may report that her 8-month-old nurses four times a day, eats puréed fruits and vegetables at home, and is offered formula every 3 hours at the babysitter's house. A list of frequently requested foods, liquids, and snacks should be compiled for preschoolers. Seating during meals should also be discussed. Recorded details might include whether the child sits in a chair or booster at the table with other family members, in a separate highchair, or wherever he or she chooses (e.g., in the family room at the coffee table, on the floor of the dining room). The types of utensils, bottle or cup (including trainer cups with spouts and handles), and plates the child uses on a daily basis should also be discussed.

Babbitt, Hoch, and Coe (1994) advocated using interviews to collect information about environmental factors that can contribute to feeding difficulties (e.g., distractions in the dining room) and to learn about disruptive mealtime behaviors such as tantrums. Another tool for examining the feeding environment is the Behavior Focused Feeding Assessment (BFFA; Arvedson & Brodsky, 2002). This instrument collects information about individuals who feed the child, locations of snack and mealtimes, and schedule.

An additional tool for collecting information is the Routines-Based Interview (RBI; McWilliam & Casey, 2007; McWilliam, Casey, & Sims, 2009). The RBI gathers information about mealtime components including child engagement, opportunities for independence, and social relationships. Items ask about the family's rules at meals, handling of the transition to solid food, and opinions about the child feeding him- or herself independently. The administration instructions indicate that a home visitor—an individual who works with the family in their home and has the opportunity to observe daily routines—should collect the information. The Parent Mealtimes Questionnaire (Morris & Klein, 2000) collects information about the child's feeding history and parent concerns through use of open-ended questions about, for example, preferred formula for an infant, the transition to solid foods for a toddler, and favored food textures for a preschooler. There is an additional set of questions to complete if the child receives tube feedings. The Parent/Caregiver Questionnaire (Perlin & Boner, 1994) gathers similar information, including the time required for a typical meal and whether the parents had trouble introducing solid foods to the child. Information about utensils, bottle and cup type, and positioning are also requested from the child's parent or caregiver.

The Bright Futures in Practice program at Georgetown University designed the Nutrition Questionnaire for Infants (Story, Holt, & Sofka, 2002). The majority of its 12 items are open-ended questions, including one that asks parents to describe what a feeding with their baby is like. (This question also has a rating scale of *always pleasant, usually pleasant, sometimes pleasant,* and *never pleasant.*) Another item on the questionnaire asks if parents are concerned or have questions about feeding their baby. The Nutrition Questionnaire for Children (Story, Holt, & Sofka, 2002) is composed of 14 items, including items that ask about the number of meals and snacks and amount of juice consumed by the child daily and that ask whether the family had difficulty obtaining enough food or funds with which to buy food over the previous month. The intent of both questionnaires is to gather background information, screen for red flags, and assess developmental risk. The program also provides parent training materials related to feeding, nutritional health, and overall health and development. For more information, see Story, Holt, and Sofka (2002).

Swigert (1998) offers two interview forms. The Initial Feeding Evaluation is for infants 4 months and younger; the Interview Form for Children with Feeding Problems focuses on infants, toddlers, and preschoolers who are over 4 months old. The forms are intended to be completed by a clinician with caregiver input. Both versions include items about the child's medical, birth, developmental, and feeding histories. The last section includes questions about consistency, liquids, textures of foods, and favorite foods. The Initial Feeding Evaluation also contains items requiring examination of the infant's lips, jaw, tongue, cheeks, palate, and gums as well as observing nonnutritive and nutritive sucking behaviors. Information is also collected concerning feeding related distress such as sweating, tonal change, gasping, coughing, and choking. For older infants and young children up to 5 years of age, information is gathered about food texture (smooth, semi-chunky, and chunky baby food; mashed table food; and regular table food), spoon use (remove food, attempt to self feed), cup use, and biting and chewing skills. The form also has space to note adaptations and assistance, such as providing jaw support, thickening juice, and using an Easy Grip Spoon.

An additional facet of interviewing a young child's parent is collecting information about family concerns. Specifically, background information can guide the assessment process by raising awareness of unique family circumstances that may have an impact on feeding (e.g., primary caregiver, living conditions). While the need for this type of information has not been extensively described in the feeding assessment literature, families with children with disabilities indicate that this information should be considered. For example, prominent authors have emphasized learning about family priorities for individual members and the family unit (Bailey, Hebbeler, Scarborough, Spiker, & Mallik, 2004; Harry, 2008a). The interview method of collecting information is also referred to as "ethnographic interviewing" (Westby, 1990). Ethnographic interviewing calls attention to the family's context in

Table 6.2. Overview of information-collection forms to evaluate feeding development

Information-collection format	Purpose	Example
Medical history	Background information about illness, health conditions, and so forth that may adversely impact feeding	Developed by physician and reviewed by feeding team
Physical examination	Medical professional collects anthropometric measurements, respiration and heart rate, and feeding structures	Developed by physician and reviewed by feeding team
Feeding history	Collect information about feeding milestones, intake, allergies, etc.	Feeding History Form (Fraker & Walbert, 2003)
Food diary	Summary of the child's intake including portion size, location of meals and snacks, and specific presentation information (e.g., temperature, texture)	Description of a 24 hour calorie intake protocol (Jacobi, Agras, Bryson, & Hammer, 2003)
Observation	Compile information about child's mealtime behaviors and interactions, emotional responses, and inappropriate behaviors	Mealtime Assessment Guide (Morris & Klein, 2000)
Interview/parent report	Gather information about mealtime routines, food preferences, and environmental factors affecting feeding (e.g., location, noise level)	The Parent/Caregiver Questionnaire (Perlin & Boner, 1994)

order to inform planning that takes into consideration identified values, beliefs, and resources.

Table 6.2 provides an overview of the assessment methods described in this section.

Appendix B, on the CD-ROM, provides the Feeding Protocol assessment instrument used to collect both family background information and examples of specific feeding concerns and needs. It has an interview format and can be used in its entirety or in sections as warranted by the child's level of feeding development and possible difficulties. The Feeding Protocol is intended as one component of a comprehensive feeding assessment to be completed with input from parents, caregivers, and ECSE professionals. It should not be the sole data collection instrument.

The following sections describe rating scales available commercially. These instruments focus on parent or caregiver input relating to one or more facets of feeding development and concerns. Information is also provided about functional analysis, criterion-referenced assessment instruments, and standardized instruments (see Table 6.3).

Checklists and Rating Scales

This section provides an overview of ratings scales addressing a number of facets of feeding, including parent attitudes about feeding, parent–child interactions during feeding, feeding development and issues (e.g., chewing patterns, daily intake), and disability-specific feeding behaviors. A description of several assessment instruments in each category is provided in the Appendix at the end of the chapter. Feeding assessment "packages" (multiple assessments developed by a single program or organization) are also presented.

As discussed in Chapters 2 and 3, parent attitudes inform feeding practices and parent perceptions of their child's feeding skills and needs. Instruments such as the Comprehensive Feeding Practices Questionnaire (CFPQ; Musher-Eizenman, & Hol-

Table 6.3. Overview of feeding-related assessment tools

Type of feeding-related evaluation tool	Purpose	Example
Checklists and rating scales		
Parent attitudes	Collect parent perceptions about child's feeding behaviors, skills, and needs	Comprehensive Feeding Practices Questionnaire (Musher-Eizenman & Holub, 2007)
Parent–child interactions	Compile observations and ratings of parent–child interactions as a view into the parent–child relationship	Toddler Snack Scale (Spegman & Houck, 2005)
Feeding development and issues	Examines feeding development and identifies indicators of feeding delays and problems	Early Feeding Skills Assessment (Thoyre, 2010)
Disability-specific feeding behaviors	Gathers information for young children with disabilities that impact feeding, such as autism and cerebral palsy	Brief Autism Mealtime Behavior Inventory (Lukens & Linscheid, 2008)
Assessment "packages"	Assembles feeding assessment information using materials developed by a professional group or community program	Nursing Child Assessment Feeding Scale (part of Nursing Child Assessment Satellite Training; Sumner & Speitz, 1994)
	Uses behavioral strategies to identify antecedents, behaviors, and consequences related to feeding difficulties	Behavioral Feeding Assessment (Kedesky & Budd, 1998)
Criterion-referenced assessment	Collects data multiple times to evaluate the child's demonstrated and emerging skills and feeding needs relative to the child's overall functioning level	Assessment, Evaluation, and Programming System for Infants and Children (AEPS®), Second Edition (Bricker, 2002)
Standardized assessment	Uses standardized procedures, scoring, and interpretation to compare child's feeding skills with same age peers	Vineland Adaptive Behavior Scales (Sparrow, Balla, & Cicchetti, 1984)

ub, 2007) examine factors related to parent perceptions of feeding including eating patterns. The Feeding Demands Questionnaire (Faith, Storey, Kral, & Pietrobelli, 2008) examines parents' emotional responses to their child's eating, and it explores their perceptions related to the types of foods their child likes and dislikes. Parent–child interactions during feeding frame a number of additional feeding assessments. For example, Spegman and Houck's (2005) Toddler Snack Scale (TSS), administered during a snack activity, examines mother and toddler behaviors, focusing on engagement and negotiation of control and autonomy. Scores indicate the overall type of interactions between the dyad such as mothers categorized as *controlling engaged* who parent toddlers classified as *compliant disengaged*.

Two additional areas explored by checklists and rating scales are feeding development and disability-specific feeding behaviors. The Developmental Pre-Feeding Checklist (Morris & Klein, 2000) examines feeding development from 1–24 months. For example, the 9-month section lists the swallowing of semisolid food and the movement of the jaw during chewing, along with behavioral descriptions. Parents rate each skill as *present-spontaneous, present with facilitation*, or not present. This instrument is also available in a format with skill grouping such as feeding position, sucking liquids from the cup, and lip movements in chewing. The Brief Autism Mealtime Behavior Inventory (BAMBI; Lukens & Linscheid,

2008) is composed of 18 items focusing on mealtime behavior of children with autism. Items investigate food preferences (e.g., crunchy or sweet foods), flexibility (e.g., same food items, seating arrangement, manner in which food is served), and disruptive behavior during mealtimes (e.g., crying, aggression toward self or adult). Frequency information is also collected along a continuum of *never/rarely* to *almost every meal*. Refer to the Appendix for additional assessment instruments in each of these areas and sample items.

Feeding Assessment Packages   A number of professionals, groups, and community programs have developed feeding assessment materials. For example, the *Nursing Child Assessment* Satellite Training (NCAST) program utilizes the Nursing Child Assessment Feeding Scale (NCAFS; Sumner & Speitz, 1994). The NCAFS is an observational checklist that examines parent–child interaction during feeding activities. Dyads are videotaped and NCAST-trained individuals view the videotape and score items as *present* or *absent* based on behavioral criteria. The Feeding Scale contains 76 items and includes parent/caregiver subscales (Sensitivity to Child's Cues, Responses to Distress, Fostering Social-Emotional Growth and Fostering Cognitive Growth) and child-related subscales (Clarity of Cues and Responsiveness to the Caregiver). Parent/caregiver items address whether the parent/caregiver comments on hunger signals from the child before feeding and whether the caregiver interacts with the child while the child is feeding. Child-related items ask about the child's gaze during feeding and responsiveness to feeding attempts (for further information see Hodges, Houck, & Kindermann, 2009). Specialized training is required to score NCAFS items (Huber, 1991; Kelly & Barnard, 2000).

The RSOI in Oregon provides a variety of feeding assessment materials (Roberts, 2002), including an Observation of Feeding in School form. Space is available to note the child's positioning, alertness, responses to textured food items, and consistency of liquids. A detailed Oral-Motor Evaluation form can be completed by a nurse or SLP. In addition, the Risk Factors Indicating Possible Swallowing Dysfunction checklist includes 26 items to evaluate the presence of dysphagia. Results are used to plan interventions that address the child's feeding difficulties including improving chewing skills and adding thickeners to liquids. (The RSOI Nutrition Screening form is described earlier in this chapter.)

An additional method of collecting feeding assessment data is through completion of a functional analysis. This is a type of behavioral assessment is commonly utilized with children with developmental delays (Girolami & Scotti, 2001).

Functional Analysis   Functional analyses of mealtime behavior allow information collection to determine the reason for inappropriate behavior (Babbitt, Hoch, & Coe, 1994; Fischer & Silverman, 2007; Girolami & Scotti, 2001; Piazza et al., 2003a). Piazza and Addison (2007) describe the importance of identifying the function of the child's inappropriate mealtime behaviors. Information is collected via an antecedent, behavior, consequence (ABC) structure: antecedent (what occurs prior to the behavior), behavior (e.g., duration of tantrums and frequency of gagging), and consequences (what occurs after the behavior). Environmental and physiological conditions that may affect behavior (e.g., hunger, illness, medication) are also considered. The Behavioral Feeding Assessment (Kedesdy & Budd,

1998) offers a means to collect this information. Often, multiple individuals collect functional analysis data that is then pooled to identify behavioral patterns (Piazza et al., 2003a). Authors also emphasized parent involvement throughout this process (Najdowski, Wallace, Doney, & Ghezzi, 2003). Most important, parent input often offers a different viewpoint about noted antecedents and consequences surrounding feeding difficulties. Altogether, results of a functional analysis help to establish the reinforcers that support a child with autism or other developmental delay or disability in acquiring and maintaining appropriate feeding behaviors.

The following two sections highlight the use of criterion-referenced assessment systems and standardized assessment instruments. Criterion-referenced assessment focuses on a child's skill development and feeding needs over time. Standardized assessment instruments have a set of procedures that must be followed for testing, scoring, and interpreting results. In addition, the child's results are compared with a large sample of same-age children to determine the presence of developmental delay or disability.

Criterion-Referenced Assessment

Criterion-referenced assessment focuses on a child's growth over time. Data is collected multiple times, and development is evaluated relative to the child's demonstrated skills, emerging skills, and feeding needs. The Infant/Toddler Sensory Profile (Dunn, 2002) includes a section related to feeding. This instrument helps evaluate young children (7–36 months) with sensory processing disorders. Caregivers rate the infant or toddler on a 5-point Likert scale (*almost always, frequently, occasionally, seldom,* and *almost never*).

Most criterion-referenced systems couple assessment and intervention targets for children ages birth through 5 years. The Hawaii Early Learning Profile (HELP) provides an assessment for children birth through 3 years (Furuno et al., 1988) as well as an assessment for children ages 3–6 years (Teaford, Wheat, & Baker, 2010). HELP includes items examining a young child's feeding skills. The Assessment, Evaluation, and Programming System for Infants and Children (AEPS®), Second Edition (Bricker, 2002) also contains items examining a young child's feeding development, including items about food texture and variety and use of utensils.

The AEPS and HELP utilize an assessment, instruction, and evaluation cycle. Assessment results inform daily instruction. The final component includes ongoing monitoring and formal evaluation. Progress in feeding-specific skills and behaviors can be documented and used to inform instructional decisions.

Standardized Assessment

Standardized assessments possess extensive reliability (consistency of results over time) and validity data (instrument items sufficiently address the topic or topics under study). Items are administered following a scripted protocol with materials that are part of the kit (e.g., 1" blocks for stacking). Training is also necessary for examiners. Finally, results from a standardized instrument are necessary for eligibility under the Individuals with Disabilities Education Improvement Act (IDEA) of 2004 (PL 108-446) for infants, toddlers, and preschoolers with disabilities or developmental delays to receive services.

The Battelle Developmental Inventory–Second Edition (BDI-2; Newborg, 2004) is a standardized instrument for use with infants and for children up to age 7 years, 11 months). It examines developmental milestones in five domains (Adaptive, Personal–social, Communication, Motor, and Cognitive). Eating is included in the Self-Care section of the Adaptive Domain. Items examine acceptance of puréed foods, semisolid foods, solid foods, and utensil use. Age ranges are provided reflecting their emergence (e.g., 8–11 months discusses bite-sized of food." Either the child is asked to demonstrate the item, the child is observed during a mealtime or snack activity, or a parent or caregiver is interviewed. Responses are scored as follows: 2 (*meets item criteria*), 1 (*attempted item but did not meet all item criteria*) or 0 (*incorrect response, no response, or no opportunity to respond*). The instrument includes adaptations such as how to offer manipulatives and other items to a child with a visual impairment. The BDI-2 also includes a screening instrument.

The Vineland Adaptive Behavior Scales–Second Edition (Vineland-II; Sparrow, Cicchetti, & Balla, 2005) focuses on daily functioning in the domains of Communication, Daily Living Skills, Socialization, Motor Skills, and (as an option) Maladaptive Behavior Index of children and adults with and without disabilities. Feeding items are included in the Daily Living Skills domain. For a young child, a parent is asked about eating, drinking, and use of tableware (e.g., eats soft food, sucks or chews on crackers, holds bottle unassisted, sucks from straw, feeds self with spoon). Information can be collected using the Parent/Caregiver Rating Form, Teacher Rating Form (ages 3–21 years), Survey Interview Form, and an Expanded Interview Form. Items are rated using the following scale: 2 (*usually or habitually performed without help or reminders*), 1 (*performed sometimes or partially without help or reminders*), 0 (*never performed without help or reminders*), N (*no opportunity*) and DK (*don't know*). Results can be used to determine qualification for specialized programs, development of treatment plans, and (when used numerous times) to report progress (Sparrow et al., 2005).

DIAGNOSTIC TESTS

A variety of diagnostic tests are available to determine the basis of many anatomically-based feeding difficulties (Arvedson & Brodsky, 2002; Lefton-Greif, 1994; Lowery, 2001; Marquis & Pressman, 1995; Newman, Keckley, Petersen, & Hamner, 2001; Sheppard, 1995; Wolf & Glass, 1992). For example, Miller and Willging (2003) recommend use of flexible endoscopic evaluation of swallowing (FEES) to identify pediatric dysphagia. The descriptions provided in the following sections are an overview of diagnostic tests primarily focused on allergy testing, swallowing difficulties, and the identification of gastroesophageal reflux (GER). In-depth information is available in Morris and Klein (2000) and from medical professionals trained in these specialty areas.

Allergy Testing

Woods (2003) stated that

> early, accurate diagnoses of childhood food allergy…will allow for the initiation of the
> key elements necessary for the care of the food-allergic patient, including education

about avoidance diets and the development of emergency care plans for the treatment of allergic reactions. (p. 1637)

The primary types of food allergies affecting young children are allergies to milk, nuts (specific types or all types), and eggs. Some young children demonstrate mild symptoms; others experience anaphylactic shock (i.e., an immediate or almost immediate response including swelling, stomach pain, dizziness, and difficulty breathing). Høst et al. (2003) identified the primary indications for allergy testing for young children as vomiting, diarrhea, colic, and wheezing. The authors further noted that children under the age of 4 years with food allergy "almost always show symptoms from two or more organ systems concomitantly" (p. 562).

There are three approaches to testing for food allergies (see Høst et al., 2003). Sicherer (2002) advocated controlled elimination of suspected foods from the child's diet. The author further recommended reintroduction of a small amount of these foods to confirm the allergic response. Woods (2003) noted that some food allergies can be outgrown by the time a child reaches 5 years of age (e.g., soy, wheat). Another option is allergy testing conducted by an allergist or dermatologist (i.e., a doctor specializing in skin conditions). Skin pricks with suspected allergens are made on the forearm or back (Eigenmann & Sampson, 1998). A positive result including redness or a raised welt indicates an allergic reaction and is visible upon examination. Finally, allergen specific immunoglobulin E (IgE) antibody is the universal marker for allergy testing. The radioallergosorbent (RAST) or serum test includes a blood-draw that is examined in a laboratory for specific IgE antibodies. Elevated results usually indicate an allergy (Tan, Sher, Good, & Bahna, 2001).

The following diagnostic tests focus on one or more components of swallowing.

Videofluoroscopic Swallowing Study   A videofluoroscopic swallowing study (VFSS), also termed a modified barium or cookie swallow, is a video X-ray imaging study focusing on examination of the child's oral structures to analyze swallowing as well as passage of liquids and food boluses into the esophagus and stomach (Benson & Lefton-Greif, 1994; Darrow & Harley, 1998; Derkay & Schechter, 1998; Morris & Klein, 2000; Siktberg & Bantz, 1999). It is recommended for young children at risk for aspiration and/or suspected of having GER (e.g., young children with cerebral palsy). A VFSS is most often administered in a specialized examination room in a clinic or hospital.

Swigert (1998) described several ways to prepare barium for a VFSS. Liquid barium can be added to formula or fruit juice or can be thickened with commercial thickener or rice cereal (it must pass through a nipple). Barium paste can be mixed with puréed fruit or vegetable. Or barium powder or paste can be added to chewable foods such as cookies. In addition, it is important to provide familiar items such as the child's spoon and preferred formula or favorite snack item to help make the child comfortable during the procedure (Morris & Klein, 2000). It is also recommended that the radiologist and SLP conducting the VFSS work with the child's parent or guardian to keep the child calm and engaged. The parent can also assist the child to be comfortable in an infant carrier or seating system that accommodates a larger child, such as a Tumbleform seat.

The radiologist or SLP reviews the VFSS images during and after the procedure to identify if and how often aspiration occurred. The advantage of observing
the child's swallowing mechanism as it occurs is the provision of a visual image
of aspiration that can be further examined and interpreted within the context of
the VFSS session (e.g., the child's facial expression at the time of aspiration can be
observed). It is also important to note coughing and choking during the VFSS because these responses can indicate that liquid or a food bolus has passed into one
or both of the child's lungs. There is a caution that a VFSS may not detected GER
at the time of the procedure (Derkay & Schechter, 1998; Palmer, Drennan, & Baba,
2000). Therefore, a VFSS may need to be repeated to verify the presence or absence
of a problem with the esophagus or stomach.

Flexible Endoscopic Evaluation of Swallowing   An alternative to VFSS is
a flexible endoscopic evaluation of swallowing (FEES). This procedure assesses
the structure of the airway through insertion of a thin, flexible fiberoptic scope
attached to a camera. After application of topical anesthesia, the scope is passed
through each nostril to the pharynx (Morris & Klein, 2000). This is a brief, in-office
procedure that is performed in a more familiar setting than the examination room
for a VFSS, possibly facilitating a child's cooperation during the procedure. Additional advantages are that the FEES procedure does not require introduction of
barium and that the necessary equipment is portable.

Preferred liquids and food items should be offered. The child is given a variety of food consistencies containing green food dye to assist visual review of the
images of the throat and larynx during swallowing. The child may be asked to
tuck his chin, for example, to evaluate changes during a specific phase of swallowing or of the swallowing mechanism. A FEES also provides information about how
the child manages secretions or identifies if secretions, liquids, or foods are aspirated. A FEES is usually performed by an otolaryngologist (ear, nose, and throat
doctor) and SLP. Rees (2006) stated that results of a FEES procedure can accurately
diagnose aspiration. The FEES can also be utilized as a complement to a VFSS.

Upper Gastrointestinal Series   Similar to a VFSS, an upper gastrointestinal (GI) series is a radiologic study that evaluates the anatomy and function of the
esophagus, stomach, and intestines; specifically, the first part of the small intestine
or duodenum. The procedure is used to identify structural malformations including tracheoesophageal fistulas (TEF; a condition in which the esophagus does not
extend to the stomach but attaches to the windpipe) and obstructions along the GI
tract (Darrow & Harley, 1998). If a fistula is diagnosed, further oral feedings are
discontinued until it is surgically repaired.

An upper GI series entails both fluoroscopic and x-ray exposure, so repeated
use is not recommended. Furthermore, this procedure needs to be completed on
an empty stomach, so intake must be limited for 4–8 hours prior to the procedure.
An upper GI series is completed in approximately 5 minutes. The resulting X-rays
are examined for appearance of the structures and possible malformations in the
gastrointestinal system.

pH Probe   An additional method of collecting feeding assessment information is use of a pH probe. This procedure requires insertion of a sensor through the nose to the farthest part of the esophagus to monitor the presence of acid from the stomach coming up into the esophagus (Marquis & Pressman, 1995; Morris & Klein, 2000; Newman et al., 2001). An x-ray is taken after the probe's insertion to verify that it is in the correct location. A sensor is also placed on the child's back to help collect information about acid level. Both sensors provide information directly to a recording device. GER episodes can be accurately and specifically documented with a pH probe. Recorded data provides a reflux score which is compared with reflux scores of same-age children who have undergone the procedure.

A hospital stay is required to complete this test. The sensor monitors the acid level in the esophagus for a period of 18–24 hours. Heart rate and oxygen level can also be monitored if necessary, such as for a young child with respiratory concerns. The parent remaining with the child is also asked to write down the child's activities including eating, walking, sleeping, and so forth in order to provide the professional who interprets the results with a complete picture of the time period. It is recommended that a child has no foods or liquids except for water, apple juice, or breast milk for approximately 4 hours before the procedure. There is also a need to discontinue anti-GER medications (e.g., Maalox, Tagamet, Zantac) for 2 days prior to a pH probe. This procedure may not detect acid episodes after meals, which can limit the usefulness of the results (Newman et al., 2001).

Gastroesophageal Scintigraphy   Gastroesophageal scintigraphy can be used to detect the presence of reflux from the stomach into the esophagus, and it can also be used to evaluate esophageal function and stomach emptying. A radioisotope (a radioactive material ingested or injected into the body) is added to formula or solid food to facilitate observation of food passage. Measurements of reflux are collected over 60 minutes in 30- to 60-second intervals while child is in the supine position (lying on the back). As with the pH probe, results are compared with data from same-age children to determine if a GER problem exists. Swigert (1998) asserted that a gastroesophageal scintigraphy is as effective as an upper GI series or 24-hour pH probe. Results may include false positive readings due to the positioning necessary for the procedure.

Ultrasound Imaging   A less invasive means of examining the digestive tract is ultrasound imaging (Morris & Klein, 2000). Ingestion of a radioactive material is not necessary, and the child's parent can hold the child or be close by during this procedure. The equipment is less alarming in appearance than, for example, a VFSS, so the child is likely to be less apprehensive about the procedure. Positioning is also less of an issue because movement will not adversely affect the images.

A hand-held wand is moved over areas of the body where gel has been spread. The ultrasound machine processes the information from the wand and produces images on a gray scale. There are distinctive images of skin, muscle and fluid for example. The machinery can also be used to label specific images. A technician, radiologist, or other medical professional with the necessary training can interpret the images and share findings and recommendations.

Table 6.4. Overview of diagnostic tests

Type of diagnostic test	Purpose	Considerations
Allergy testing	Identifies specific allergens in child's diet	Skin prick test can cause discomfort
Videofluoroscopic swallowing study (VFSS)	Examines passage of liquids and food boluses with a focus on the pharyngeal swallow stage or when food moves from the oral cavity to the entrance of the esophagus	Inpatient clinic or hospital procedure requiring the use of barium; may not detect all instances of aspiration; procedure may need to be repeated for accurate diagnosis
Flexible endoscopic evaluation of swallowing (FEES)	Detects presence of pediatric dysphagia	Uses a topical anesthetic; often used as a complement to a VFSS
Upper gastrointestinal (GI) series	Evaluates the anatomy and function of the esophagus, stomach, and intestines	Repeated use is not recommended for young children; procedure must be completed on an empty stomach
pH probe	Requires insertion of a sensor through the nose to collect data about reflux episodes	May need to immobilize child's hands so probe is not removed; procedure lasts 18–24 hours; procedure often requires a hospital stay
Gastroesophageal scintigraphy	Identifies presence of reflux from the stomach into the esophagus	Similar to an upper GI series and pH probe; use of radioisotope; may have false positive results
Ultrasound imaging	Produces images of the digestive tract	Less invasive procedure; useful to examine anatomy of digestive tract

An overview of the purpose and specific considerations of the diagnostic tests described here are presented in Table 6.4.

OUTCOMES OF FEEDING ASSESSMENT

There are a number of outcomes related to feeding assessment results. First, is the identification of specific feeding challenges, such as disruptive mealtime behaviors, food allergies, and GER. In addition, information gathered from the various assessments offers a holistic representation of a child's feeding strengths, emerging strengths, and needs that can be used to inform intervention planning (Arvedson & Brodsky, 2002; Chatoor, 2009; Fischer & Silverman, 2007; Olive, 2004; see Chapter 7). In other words, completion of a variety of feeding assessment instruments ensures a comprehensive representation of a young child's mealtime skills and behaviors. Finally, feeding assessment data provides a means to address a young child's overall nutritional status, developmental feeding skills, and patterns of parent–child interactions during feeding opportunities. The information is also a starting point to monitor progress in specific areas of feeding development (see Chapter 7).

Although beyond the scope of this chapter, Schwarz, McCarthy, and Ton (2006) described a "treatment alternatives algorithm" for children with developmental disabilities encompassing many of the approaches presented in this chapter (p. 214). The authors provided a decision tree to guide assessment of feeding difficulties. The treatment plan is developed based on determination of the cause of the feeding problem and its presentation. For example, if aspiration is identified after completion of a feeding history and diagnostic test such as FEES, treatment recommendations can include dietary supplements, use of anti-GER medication, and possible gastrostomy tube placement (see Chapter 14 for a complete discussion of tube feeding).

Chapters in Section III discuss a range of feeding complications and strategies as well as specialized interventions to address them. Ongoing assessment is necessary to determine progress and necessary modifications to resolve feeding difficulties.

■ ■ ■ TABLE TALK ■ ■ ■

"Feeding evaluations are complex. It's not just about discovering the answers to simple questions like, 'What foods or liquids does your child eat/drink?' It's also about the more subtle and complex influences that the child's environment, behavior, body awareness, and oral control have on the feeding experience; as well as considering the integration of the sensory and oral-motor systems as they work in coordination one with the other.

To begin an evaluation, you have to start by collecting a complex case history of the child, including pregnancy, birth, early feeding experiences, and health/medical issues that have influenced the child's development to this point. But, it doesn't stop there. You also have to consider the environmental and behavioral components of the feeding experience, as well as the structure and function of the body and mouth.

As an evaluator, you have to become an investigator...seeking answers to complex questions regarding the child and his or her feeding experience as a complete package. If you are evaluating a young boy, for example, you must ask: 'Can this child touch his hands to his mouth? Can he tolerate foods/nipples/fingers in his mouth, or have his oral experiences been so negative that he gags at the sight of food or its containers? Can he tolerate the smell of food and/or liquid? Does he have enough strength and coordination to adequately remove food or liquid from a spoon, bottle, or cup or to manipulate and chew the foods presented? Does he react negatively to feeding experiences with anyone who attempts to feed him or only to certain people and/or in certain environments?'"
Lesley, SLP

Discussion Questions

■ What is your response to Lesley's perspective on feeding assessment?

■ What types of feeding assessment instruments best address the behavioral and environmental components of a feeding disorder?

APPENDIX

Rating Scales

Parent Attributes

Name and author(s)	Number of items, assessment type and rating scale descriptors/labels	Brief description
Comprehensive Feeding Practices Questionnaire (CFPQ) Musher-Eizenman and Holub	49 item rating scale Frequency: Never, Rarely, Sometimes, Mostly, Always Agreement: Disagree, Slightly disagree, Neutral, Slightly agree, Agree	Examines parent attitudes related to feeding including child control, encourage balance and variety, involvement, monitoring and teaching about nutrition, eating patterns and restrictions for weight control
Feeding Demands Questionnaire Faith, Story, Kral, and Pietrobelli	8 item rating scale Agreement: Disagree strongly, Disagree moderately, Disagree slightly, Neither agree or disagree, Agree slightly, Agree moderately, Agree strongly	Examines overall food intake along with the degree to which mothers pressure their children to accept specific types of foods
Maternal Rating of Infant Behavior Mathisen, Worrall, Masel, Wall, and Shepherd	19 item rating scale Frequency: Most, Many, Some, Occasional, Rare	Examines maternal or caregiver perceptions concerning infant feeding behavior. Items involve aspects of anxiety, enjoyment, difficulties and special feeding concerns
Pediatric Assessment Scale for Severe Feeding Problems Crist, Dobbelsteyn, Brousseau, and Napier-Phillips	15 item rating scale Frequency: Always, Sometimes, Never (10 items) Parent checks remaining five items child will accept and swallow without difficulty including cold foods, pureed foods and mixed textures	Examines feeding issues related to oral and tube feeding, food preferences including texture and temperature and swallowing skills
Stanford Feeding Questionnaire Jacobi, Agras, Bryson, and Hammer	70 item rating scale Frequency: Never, Rarely, Sometimes, Often, Always	Examines areas related to picky eating, including child's intake over a typical day, history of weaning (breast and bottle) and general eating behaviors such as eating in front of the television and assisting in food preparation

Parent–Child Interaction

Feeding Interaction Schedule Described in Spender, Stein, Dennis, Reilly, Percy, and Cave	Timed observation, parent statements and rating scale items (five and nine point scales, not described)	Examines parent–child interactions during feeding including parent's emotional tone and child's response to food presentations such as acceptance or rejection
Feeding Scale Chatoor, Getson, Menvielle, Brasseaux, O'Donnell, Rivera, and Mrazek	Two observations two weeks apart to complete 46 item rating scale Four point rating scale (not described)	Examines dyadic reciprocity, dyadic conflict, talk and distraction, struggle for control and maternal non-contingency

Feeding Development/Issues

Behavioral Pediatrics Feeding Assessment Scale Crist and Napier-Phillips	35 item rating scale Frequency: Never, Rarely, Sometimes, Often, Always	Examines child-specific eating behaviors and parents' feelings and strategies for managing feeding problems.
The Children's Eating Behavior Inventory Archer, Rosenbaum, and Steiner	40 item rating scale Frequency: Never, Seldom, Sometime, Often, Always Yes/No responses for problem identification	Examines frequency of eating behaviors, feeding preferences, parent control and identification of mealtime problem behaviors
The Child Eating Behavior Inventory (Oregon Research Institute) Described in Lewinsohn, Denoma, Gau, Joiner Striegel-Moore, Bear, and Lamoureux	89 item rating scale Yes/No responses	Examines pickiness, food refusal, struggle for control and positive parental behaviors
Developmental Pre-Feeding Checklist Morris and Klein	Checklist with ratings (complete items based on child's age) Choices: Present-Spontaneous, Present with Facilitation, Not Present	Examines feeding skills chronologically from 1–24 months or grouped by feeding skill area such as sucking liquids from a cup

The Early Feeding Skills Assessment Thoyre	36 item rating scale Various: Yes/No; Never, Occasionally, Often; All, Most, Some, None	Examines responses of preterm infants in readiness to feed, oral feeding skills and oral feeding tolerance. A baseline level of oxygen saturation as well as respiratory and heart rate are collected. Length of feeding session and positioning are also documented. Supports provided by the feeder are also noted, such as repositioned infant and support to jaw.
Food Neophobia Scale Pliner and Hobden	10 rating scale items and tasting session (e.g., guacamole, rice crackers) Agreement: Strongly disagree to agree strongly on a seven point scale	Examines child's responses to novel foods or eating situations

Disability-Specific Feeding Behaviors

The Brief Autism Mealtime Behavior Inventory Lukens and Linscheid	18 rating scale items Frequency: Never/Rarely to Almost every meal	Examines mealtime behavior of children with autism, including food preferences, flexibility and disruptive behavior
Feeding Assessment Survey Johnson	10 item rating scale Frequency: Never, Sometimes, Often, Very frequently	Examines mealtime behaviors of children with autism

7

Planning and Monitoring Feeding Progress

What You'll Learn in This Chapter

This chapter provides

- A description of the process to develop feeding plans in conjunction with Individualized Family Support Plans and Individualized Education Plans
- An explanation of monitoring and its importance for young children with feeding difficulties
- An overview of the use of anecdotal records, observations, and data-based approaches to monitoring progress

■ ■ ■ FOOD FOR THOUGHT ■ ■ ■

"Stacia is 50 months old. She sits down at the snack table with the other preschoolers while we are having graham crackers and milk. I offer each child the items.

Stacia says, 'Yes please,' to both items. She takes her graham cracker and breaks it into four pieces. She takes one graham cracker piece and sets it in her milk cup. She looks at me then back down. She picks up the graham cracker out of the milk and eats it. She takes her second graham cracker piece and puts it in her milk cup.

She takes it out and eats it. She says, 'Mike has three left.'

I ask 'How many do you have?'

She looks down at her pieces. She smiles and breaks each piece in half. 'One, two, three, four!' She takes a piece and smiles."

Becca, Prekindergarten Teacher

"After months only eating very few table foods Phillip, who is 19 months old, is now beginning to try vegetables and certain fruits. Toddler room teachers say he is doing better but still not great at eating. He'll try a variety of things, and sometimes he surprises them by eating two or more helpings of foods he likes."

Eva, Child Care Provider

"During mealtimes I have noticed that my 29-month-old nephew Jerrell is working on grasping foods in order to feed himself. He doesn't quite know how to pick up food using a pincer grasp and tends to place his hand flat down on top of foods, balling them up and then trying to place them in his mouth. He usually drops the majority of the food once he opens his hands."

Latosha, Aunt

These quotes illustrate the importance of planning feeding goals and monitoring their attainment. Whether a toddler is meeting a feeding milestone or a child with delays is demonstrating a new skill, designing appropriate plans and capturing information for review by the feeding team is crucial to the child's progress. Documenting progress identifies which strategies and specialized interventions need to be adjusted to aid in continued improvement in mealtime skills and behaviors.

WHAT THE LITERATURE SAYS

Effective planning and progress monitoring are critical for young children, especially those with delays or disabilities (Carta, Greenwood, Walker, & Buzhardt, 2010; Grisham-Brown & Pretti-Frontczak, 2003; Guralnick & Conlon, 2007). For young children with disabilities, the Individuals with Disabilities Education Improvement Act (IDEA) of 2004 (PL 108-446) stipulates the parameters for determining eligibility for services; it also stipulates parameters for planning and monitoring developmental gains in infants and toddlers and instructional goals for preschool-aged children. The Individualized Family Support Plan (IFSP) and Individualized Education Plan (IEP) are the planning documents. Each is developed by a team that includes professionals and the child's parents, and both documents prescribe timelines and procedures for their implementation.

Much of the literature focuses on the development, implementation, and evaluation of IFSPs and IEPs (Grisham-Brown & Hemmeter, 1998; Grisham-Brown, Pretti-Frontczak, Hemmeter, & Ridgley, 2002; Jung, 2007; Rosenkoetter & Squires, 2000). IFSPs focus on infants and toddlers who currently receive specialized services/supports due to diagnosed disabilities or developmental delays or infants and toddlers who are at risk for delays. IEPs are for preschoolers receiving services in public schools and related settings, such as Head Start. IFSPs and IEPs are briefly described in the following sections, along with specific planning components that include feeding development.

Individualized Family Support Plans

Like the feeding team (discussed in Chapter 5), the IFSP team includes parents and caregivers. All team members work together to create outcome statements based on the child's current levels of development and the family's priorities (Jung & Grisham-Brown, 2006). Outcome statements highlight the expected results for both the child and the family, including a 6-month plan that outlines what needs to occur to achieve each outcome and the professionals who will provide the necessary supports, materials, and so forth. The document also specifies who will monitor progress and the methods used to determine the child's developmental gains. For many infants and toddlers, IFSPs are implemented in the child's natural environment, which can be in the home as well as community settings. Jung (2007) promotes integrating activities and strategies in IFSP outcome statements into daily routines such as dressing, mealtimes, and play activities. This naturally embeds instruction into daily activities and routines (Pretti-Frontczak & Bricker, 2004). Box 7.1 provides examples of feeding-related IFSP outcome statements for Josie and Sammy.

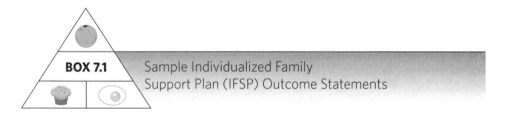

BOX 7.1 Sample Individualized Family Support Plan (IFSP) Outcome Statements

Josie was born at 30 weeks gestation. She experienced respiratory difficulties throughout her 7 weeks in the neonatal intensive care unit, requiring gavage feeding and eventual placement of a gastrostomy feeding tube. She is now 15 months old. Josie receives most of her nutrition through tube feedings. Her feeding team has agreed that it is appropriate to begin oral stimulation and to offer tastes of baby food at this time.

IFSP Outcome statement: We want Josie to accept tastes of baby foods.

• After receiving training from the speech-language pathologist, Josie's mom and grandmother will provide facial massage to Josie's cheeks and jaw before tasting sessions.

• Before each bolus feed during the day, Josie's mom and grandmother will offer Josie tastes of baby food (beginning with fruits and evaluating for vegetables in 2 months).

• Depending on her alertness, Josie will be positioned either in an infant seat or in the arms of her mother or grandmother.

• Food will be offered using the tip of a pacifier at all times (evaluate for spoon feeding in three months).

Sammy is 10 months old. He was born with cleft lip and palate. His lip was operated on when he was 3 months old. Surgery to correct the cleft palate is scheduled 2 weeks after his first birthday. He enjoys feeding activities and has not had any problems with intake. Sammy exhibits delays in fine motor skills which are also being addressed on his IFSP.

(continued)

Box 7.1.   *(continued)*

IFSP Outcome statement: We want Sammy to eat at least half of his daily foods by mouth.

- Sammy's parents, home child care provider, and speech-language pathologist will work with him and document his daily intake. Consult with physical therapist once a month for positioning.
- Sammy will be positioned in an adapted highchair or Rifton corner seat.
- An infant coated spoon and Haberman feeder will be used.

The IFSP is reviewed every 6 months. It can be reviewed sooner if the child meets some or all documented outcomes or there is a significant change in medical, health, or developmental status (e.g., post-surgery, "burst" of developmental gains).

Individualized Education Plan

Preschoolers receiving services under IDEA have IEPs. It is important to note that IEPs are only implemented in a school setting or other program that receives federal funding such as Head Start. Annual IEP goals and short-term objectives (STOs) are not applied to the home setting. There may be coordination between the home and school settings, such as using a successful strategy in both places, but the responsibility lies with the school-based team. In contrast, for the majority of infants and toddlers, IFSP outcomes are carried out solely in the home setting by their families, caregivers, and IFSP team members.

For preschoolers with disabilities, the IEP focuses on annual goals and benchmarks. Recent changes to IDEA recommend a 3-year IEP with annual reviews of benchmarks tied to state standards. STOs must be developed for students (age 3 to 21 years) with significant delays. STOs can also be included in the IEP at the discretion of the IEP team. STOs are tied to annual goals and are reviewed and updated annually. The examples provided here emphasize annual goals and STOs addressing feeding.

The IEP includes current levels of functioning based on assessment results (see Chapter 6 for descriptions of feeding assessments), types of services (e.g., speech-language therapy and counseling) and placement information (e.g., pre-kindergarten classroom half day and early childhood special education classroom half day). Annual goals are also included. These are general statements focusing on increasing, improving, and developing skills. Annual goals typically focus on educational content areas (e.g., reading and science) and behavior change (e.g., increased social interaction). However, for 3- to 5-year-olds, annual goals can also address developmental needs, including fine motor skills and feeding.

When developing annual goals, it is helpful to include a brief rationale for the skills selected for instruction. For example, the statement "Ronnie will increase self-feeding skills" is further explained by "in order to prepare for kindergarten." The rationale explains "why" the goal is important. In this case, Ronnie will need to be an independent feeder in kindergarten. More specifically, he will need to open containers (e.g., milk carton) and use a spoon and fork.

STOs assist team members to implement IEP annual goals by providing specific, observable, and measurable steps to reach annual goals through several linked STOs for each annual goal (Bateman & Herr, 2006). Each STO must include an active verb such as complete, imitate, or share. Active verbs promote specificity and enable teachers to observe and identify incremental skill development. The behavior can be further described by including whether adults and/or peers are involved. An additional benefit of STO specificity for the feeding team is that data is more easily collected when STOs can be readily observed by a child's teachers and therapists. With specific STOs, skill development is incremental and progress can be better monitored.

There are additional components in STOs that support their implementation and monitoring. STOs should include one or more conditions describing the amount and/or type of assistance the child should receive (e.g., hand-over-hand, verbal reminder, model) as well as specialized materials. In the case of feeding-related STOs, materials can include a specific feeding chair, spoon, or cup that must be available at every meal and snack opportunity. Praise can also be part of an STO condition. Finally, the IEP team decides on criteria to indicate how well or how often the child must perform the skill (e.g., 5 of 5 times daily or with 100% accuracy). As a result, specific conditions, behaviors, and criteria in STOs are developed to be achievable and meaningful to the child.

It is imperative to develop STOs that can be integrated into the child's daily activities and routines (Grisham-Brown & Hemmeter, 1998; Grisham-Brown et al., 2002). An objective focusing on tasting new foods can be implemented during mealtimes, snack, cooking activities and, as appropriate, community outings. If, on the other hand, the skill relates to fine motor development, such as increased independent feeding, it is necessary to identify activities during the child's day that provide opportunities for skill acquisition and practice. Finger feeding requires a pincer grasp, as does handling small objects during sensory play. A variety of manipulatives such as small knobs on puzzle pieces also include this skill. In all, these opportunities encourage rapid learning and generalization of skills and behaviors. In the monitoring progress section that follows, the methods provided are ones that are easy to implement within the context of a child's daily life, whether in a home, school, or community setting, which helps make IFSP outcomes and IEP goals and STOs simple to monitor.

Some young children may require a more specialized plan than outcomes in the IFSP or IEP goals and objectives. For example, Piazza et al. (2003b) describe a series of interventions used to treat food refusal in three young children. The procedures were provided while the children were "admitted to an intensive pediatric feeding disorders day treatment program" (p. 365). A behavior therapist headed the team and worked with parents and professionals at the facility to develop, implement, and monitor each child's feeding plan. A similar approach was used to treat one child's refusal to accept fluids (Patel, Piazza, Kelly, Ochsner, & Santana, 2001), to decrease three children's packing behavior (holding accepted food in the mouth without chewing or swallowing), and to increase another child's acceptance of textured foods (Patel, Piazza, Layer, Coleman, & Swartzwelder, 2005; Piazza et al., 2003b). After completion of a day in-patient program or discharge from a full-time residential program, the interventions must be employed in the home and community settings to ensure continued progress. The specialized team will, in most cases, remain involved through contacts with parents and follow-up procedures as necessary (e.g., provision of specialized equipment or supplements, review of behavioral strategies such as fading and extinction).

Box 7.2 offers examples of feeding-related IEP annual goals and STOs for Josie and Sammy.

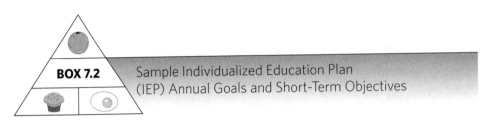

Josie is now 40 months old. She continues to be fed through a gastrostomy tube. There have been some advances with oral feeding, but during and for several weeks after a respiratory illness or hospitalization Josie refuses to eat anything by mouth. She has also experienced a number of episodes of aspiration after drinking thickened liquids. After clearance from her pediatrician and pulmonologist, her early childhood special education teacher, classroom aid, and speech-language pathologist have agreed to try a number of methods to encourage Josie's oral intake.

IEP annual goal: Josie will increase tolerance of oral stimulation activities in order to prepare for oral feedings.

IEP short-term objectives:

- Given Tumbleform feeding seat in semi-upright position, a Textured Grabber and physical assistance, Josie will grasp the Textured Grabber to make contact with her cheeks or lips for at least 30 seconds during three out of three daily opportunities for 5 out of 5 days.
- Given Tumbleform feeding seat in semi-upright position, a Chewy Tube and praise, Josie will tolerate the Chewy Tube placed inside her mouth and rubbed against her top and bottom teeth for at least 15 seconds during two of three daily opportunities for 5 out of 5 days.
- Given Tumbleform feeding seat in fully upright position, Josie will use her tongue to taste puréed fruits placed on her lips during two of three daily opportunities for 4 out of 5 days.

Sammy's cleft palate surgery went well. During his toddler years he was able to eat and drink age-appropriate items but needed assistance to hold cups and required use of adapted spoons for snack and mealtimes.

Sammy began attending a half-day prekindergarten classroom 2 months ago. He is doing very well developmentally, especially in the areas of language and social skills. He continues to lag behind his peers in fine motor development which is interfering with a number of self-feeding skills. His feeding team (same members as his IEP team) addressed these areas on his IEP.

IEP annual goal: Sammy will improve self-feeding skills in order to prepare for kindergarten.

IEP short-term objectives:

- Given a small-sized angled spoon and scoop dish and praise, Sammy will feed himself at least 75% of semisolid foods, such as pudding, five out of five opportunities per week.
- Given a small-sized angled spoon and scoop dish, Sammy will feed himself at least 50% of solid foods such as meat pieces and mixed vegetables at least four out of five opportunities per week.
- Given a Sip-Tip cup and verbal cues, Sammy will grasp Sip-Tip cup with both hands and drink at least 4 ounces of liquid at lunchtime each day for a minimum of 1 week.

OVERVIEW OF INSTRUCTIONAL APPROACHES

Infants, toddlers, and preschoolers require an array of instructional approaches to achieve IFSP outcomes and IEP goals and STOs. Many published approaches are naturalistic, which refers to their integration into the child's daily activities and routines and across settings. This integration is referred to as embedding. Additional materials or equipment are typically not necessary. Furthermore, these activity-based approaches support generalization of skills targeted on an IFSP or an IEP (Pretti-Frontczak & Bricker, 2004; Sandall & Schwartz, 2008).

The term generalization refers to the application of an acquired skill or demonstration of an acquired behavior in contexts and with individuals that were not part of the original learning environment. In other words, new skills learned in one situation are used in new situations. For example, a preschooler learns how to put on a shirt and pants. With repeated opportunities and feedback, the child will exhibit this skill with various types of shirts and pants (e.g., with and without elastic waist) and in new situations (e.g., at home and at grandmother's house). Similar results can occur with eating and drinking skills, such as when a child self-feeds or cleans up following a meal in multiple settings.

There is a range of naturalistic supports to facilitate learning. A young child can be given visual representations (e.g., photos, line drawings) of materials and activities; parents, caregivers, professionals, and peers can model the skill or behavior; a task analysis can be completed to break down teaching a skill or activity into its component steps; a nonpreferred activity or task can be paired with a preferred one (e.g., complete a puzzle and then have five minutes of computer time); and choices can be provided (e.g., book to be read by caregiver or color crayon for art activity; Jung, 2007; Sandall & Schwartz, 2008).

It is important to note that all of these approaches can be used to encourage feeding development (Bruns & Thompson, 2010). For example, if a preschooler is reluctant to eat vegetables due to food selectivity or texture aversion, a choice can be offered: "Would you like to taste the carrots or green beans first?" This can be paired with a taste of a preferred food after the child accepts the taste of a carrot or green beans. Child engagement in activities and routines is critical to skill development, as noted in McWilliam and Casey (2007) and VanDerHeyden, Snyder, Smith, Sevin, and Longwell (2005); these authors provided strategies similar to the ones previously described to foster engagement (e.g., environmental arrangement, embedding).

The environment also plays a role in skill development. Numerous authors emphasize the importance of examining physical space and social dimensions (e.g., child-to-provider ratio, supervision during small group activities; Bruns & Mogharreban, 2008; Carta & Kong, 2009; Davis & Fox, 1999; Mogharreban & Bruns, 2009; Sandall & Schwartz, 2008). Lighting, temperature, and access to materials are examples of environmental considerations that can affect attainment of IFSP outcomes and IEP goals and STOs. Attention must be paid to the characteristics of the settings in which the child participates. Whether the activity is an art activity or self-feeding, the physical space and social dimensions must be reviewed by the IFSP or IEP and modified accordingly. For example, a toddler with noise sensitivities may need to eat breakfast in a separate room from peers at a child care center because the sounds of parents and children arriving and materials being put away may interfere with the child's intake. However, the child should be encouraged and systematically taught to tolerate the noise level as much as possible. The child may be encouraged to remain at the table in 30-second increments, eventually learning to tolerate the noise and eat in the child care room and other settings as well as participate in family-style meals (Davis & Fox, 1999).

In addition to the approaches previously described, feeding-related IFSP outcomes and IEP goals and STOs can also be addressed using more formal (less naturalistic) methods such as adapted feeding utensils and positioning systems. Section III provides a variety of strategies and specialized interventions, including bottles and cups available to assist young children with anatomical differences (e.g., cleft palate) and seating considerations for infants, toddlers, and preschoolers with neurological disorders such as cerebral palsy. Depending on the child's feeding strengths and difficulties, these approaches can be combined with naturalistic methods to promote specific areas of feeding development.

MONITORING PROGRESS

Planning for feeding development and monitoring progress must be carried out by the child's feeding team. Each member will have implementation and data collection responsibilities.

Most of the published work on feeding difficulties highlights the range of problems and possible solutions (Bachmeyer et al., 2009; Cooper-Brown et al., 2008; Douglas, 2000; Samson-Fang, Butler, & O'Donnell, 2003; Schwarz, 2003) rather than providing in-depth discussion of methods to monitor progress in feeding skills and behaviors. Luiselli (2000), however, did provide such a discussion. Several techniques were used with a 3-year-old child to increase his intake and to teach self-feeding. Professionals taught the child's parents how to collect and document information regarding his feeding behaviors and intake, and data was collected during each treatment session in the home. In addition, "Criterion changes were instituted based on a review of the mealtime data" (p. 353); specifically, as the child made progress, the number of required eating responses to receive reinforcement increased. (This child was allowed to play with preferred toys only after he met criterion for intake.) Bachmeyer et al. (2009) and Piazza, et al. (2003a) illustrated other behavioral methods used in progress monitoring. Improvements were noted for the children in their studies, with documented increases in appropriate mealtime behaviors.

An assumption should not be made that most child care providers, parents, and other caregivers have the background in behavioral interventions and data collection to successfully complete procedures such as the ones previously described. Training in child development and early childhood curriculum methods does not typically include this content. It also cannot be assumed that other members of a child's feeding team, such a speech-language pathologist (SLP) or dietitian is trained in behavioral theory. Nevertheless, there are a number of easy-to-implement methods to track feeding progress. An overview is provided here with more detailed information and examples later in the chapter.

Because data are recorded, changes in feeding skills and behavior are measured and observed. Depending on how information is collected and analyzed, obvious as well as less obvious changes can be noted and used to develop and/or revise a child's feeding plan. Furthermore, especially for young children with disabilities, it is important to record all changes, whether large or relatively minute (in feeding and other areas of development). For example, a toddler with a feeding disorder accepting a new texture is a milestone. An infant with gastroesophageal reflux (GER) accepting three rather than two ounces of a new formula is also noteworthy. Finally, a preschooler demonstrating the ability to complete an 8-step mealtime clean-up task is significant.

Monitoring progress also addresses another component of growth. While behavior change is observable and specific, social change is also important. Kazdin (1977) emphasized the relationship between behavioral change and increases in socially acceptable behavior. This is especially significant for families with young children with disabilities and feeding difficulties. When children have the ability to eat age-appropriate foods, parents can more easily prepare meals, and children can more easily participate in family and community events (e.g., holiday dinner at grandparent's house, pot luck at church). In this way, progress has several beneficial outcomes for the child and for individuals who are involved in the child's day-to-day feeding activities.

Categories of Progress

Before describing methods of progress monitoring, it is critical to first define the four categories of progress that data can indicate: steady progress, slow progress, variable progress, and no progress (Alberto & Troutman, 2008; Cooper et al., 2007). Steady progress is demonstrated over time as the child gains targeted skills in a continuous manner. Slow progress is when a child shows improvement in a feeding-related skill but at a slower rate than expected. This may be evidenced in a toddler with Down syndrome acquiring self-feeding skills. Developmental milestones will be reached, but at a slower rate (Kumin & Bahr, 1999).

Variable progress occurs when advances in a skill area are not consistent—for example rapid growth for a period followed by no change for a number of weeks. An example would be when an older infant accepts tastes of puréed vegetables

Table 7.1. Types of progress and examples

Type of progress	Definition	Examples
Steady	Child demonstrates gains toward targeted skills in a continuous manner	Child increases formula intake from 2 ounces to 3 ounces to 4 ounces at regular intervals Child feeds himself or herself from a spoon with less and less spillage
Slow	Child shows improvement at a slower rate than expected	Child increases formula intake from 2 ounces to 2½ ounces to 3 ounces per feeding Child feeds herself from spoon but with a great deal of spillage even with adult assistance Child accepts textured foods such as puréed peaches and is hesitant to eat soft peach slices
Variable	Child makes gains but in an inconsistent manner	Child increases formula intake from 2 ounces to 3 ounces to 2½ ounces to 4½ ounces per feeding Child feeds herself from spoon with varying amounts of spillage Child accepts textured foods such as puréed peaches and peach slices at some meals but refuses them at others
No progress	Child exhibits no change over a defined time period	Child does not increase formula intake; remains at 2 ounces for 1 month Child feeds herself from a spoon with a great deal of spillage (more than half) for 2 months Child only accepts puréed foods

for several days and then refuses both familiar and unfamiliar offerings. Variable progress is also seen in older children—for example when a preschooler demonstrates gains over the first 10 days drinking from an open cup but then, the following week, requests a favorite Sippy cup and refuses to use the open cup.

The fourth category—no progress—describes periods of time during which a child stops making progress (e.g., 2 weeks, 1 month). This circumstance warrants immediate review of strategies and specialized interventions. Corresponding changes to the feeding plan will likely be required. Table 7.1 provides examples of the four types of progress.

Finally, there is the possibility that previously acquired skills will be lost. Such losses can occur with a specific skill or overall. Depending on the individual child, loss of acquired feeding skills may be due to factors such as illness, alterations in medication, and change in one or more aspects of the mealtime routine.

Dimensions of Behavior

There are several dimensions of behavior change that can be used to document progress (Alberto & Troutman, 2008; Cooper et al., 2007; Lingo, Barton-Arwood, & Jolivette, 2011). For example, frequency (or rate of response) can be calculated. If a new food is offered 10 times and the child tastes it twice, the frequency would be 2 of 10 times. Frequency can also be calculated as a percentage (20%).

Feeding-related skills can be broken down into steps in a process referred to as task analysis. This method provides highly detailed information about a child's progress. For example, when a child is learning to self-feed, the component skills can be listed, and a rating—present, emerging, or not present—can be given for each component. Over time, the data indicates progress and identifies areas requiring additional intervention (e.g., a child is able to lower the spoon into the bowl and scoop food onto the spoon but spills most of the food before it reaches his or her mouth).

Finally, trials to criterion measure the number of times required for a child to reach a predetermined criterion (standard or rule for evaluation). One infant may need 5 trials to reach criterion (e.g., drinking 5 or more ounces without vomiting), while another child needs 12 trials before meeting the same criterion. The criterion can be linked with an amount of food or liquid, a specific feeding-related skill, or another targeted area from the child's feeding plan. A child can also work on several criterions simultaneously unless the skills are developmental and must be acquired sequentially (e.g., accepting semisolid foods prior to accepting solid foods).

Additional Monitoring Methods for Children with Disabilities

When working with young children with disabilities or developmental delays, there are additional monitoring methods. As described in Chapter 6, criterion-referenced assessments such as the Assessment, Evaluation, and Programming System for Infants and Children (AEPS®), Second Edition (Bricker, 2002) and the Hawaii Early Learning Profile (HELP; Furuno et al., 1988) include feeding-related items that can be tracked over time. The AEPS Child Observation Data Recording Forms and Child Progress Record includes space to update the child's skill level and provide descriptive information about progress. Another assessment, the Individual Growth and Development Indicators (IGDI) includes tools that focus on infants and toddlers in the areas of communication, cognitive problem solving, movement, social skills, and parent–child interaction (Carta et al., 2010). These areas all contribute to the development of feeding skills such as self-feeding. (See Table 12.1 for examples of gross motor and communication skills.) Data for IGDIs are collected in a play context, which facilitates monitoring progress because the child's behaviors are spontaneous and occur within daily activities and routines.

Guiding Questions

Before selecting the data-collection method or methods, several questions must be answered by the child's feeding team: (a) What? (b) Who? (c) When? and (d) Where? (Lingo et al., 2011).

What? First, the feeding behavior or skill to be monitored must be selected. With agreement from all members of the feeding team, several IFSP feeding outcomes or IEP STOs can be addressed simultaneously. However, it is often best to begin by focusing on one or two interrelated behaviors or skills rather than multiple areas. When a child has difficulties accepting textured foods as well as self-feeding, for example, the feeding team needs to prioritize and ensure coordination (see Chapter 5). If self-feeding is selected based on parent preference and team consensus, team members must then decide the specific skills to target as well as needed materials and equipment (e.g., angled spoon, feeding chair with shoulder and hip supports).

Who? Next, a decision must be made regarding who will gather the monitoring data. Depending on the age of the child and the settings where he participates, a number of people may be selected to gather data. Parents, caregivers, teachers, and other members of the child's team will probably each be considered as possible data collectors. Often, the professionals who are with the child at mealtimes (e.g., SLPs or caregivers) are the obvious choices for data collectors. Training should be provided as needed.

When? Decisions about the time of day (during which activities and routines) feeding data will be collected are also necessary. These times can be limited or expansive. For example, the targeted feeding skills may be observed only during morning snack, or they may be observed every time the child takes food or fluid during the day.

Where? Finally, the location for monitoring must be agreed upon by team members. Again, this can be very limited—"only at home," for example, or "only at child care." Or it can be expansive—"everywhere the child takes food or fluids." See Table 7.2 for a summary of guiding questions for data collection.

Frequency of Data Review

The frequency with which the resulting data will be reviewed must be decided (Alberto & Troutman, 2008; Cooper et al., 2007). As described previously in this chapter, progress can be steady, slow, or variable. Examining the data at predetermined intervals is necessary to see patterns of progress and to make necessary adjustments. For example, if data indicate that Josie (see Box 7.1) is showing steady progress with

Table 7.2.   Guiding questions for progress monitoring

Question	What must be identified to develop a progress monitoring plan
What?	Specific feeding behaviors (e.g., remaining at table for three minutes) or skills (e.g., self feed finger foods) as described in IFSP, IEP, or specialized feeding plan
Who?	Parents, caregivers, child care provider, pre-K teacher, Head Start teacher, clinician, or other professional or combination determined by feeding team
When?	Number of opportunities or times that a behavior will be monitored and data will be collected during a feeding session, mealtime, or throughout daily activities and routines at home, child care center, public school setting, and so forth
Where?	Location or setting where child participates in feeding activities and data will be collected; may include home, child care center, public school classroom and/or in the community

accepting tastes of fruits after 2 weeks, the feeding team may decide to move forward with offering tastes of vegetables. If she shows no progress with vegetables after 1 week, the team may decide to return to fruits for several days before trying vegetables again. Or the team may decide to offer both types of baby foods and take data on the number of tastes of each type that Josie accepts. Possible frequencies for evaluating data include daily, every 5 days, weekly, or twice a month. However, it is critical not to wait too long, especially if the child is not moving forward in the targeted outcome, one or more STOs, or any component of a specialized feeding plan. In some cases, progress may not occur or a loss of previously acquired skills may take place. Collecting monitoring data also identifies these circumstances and can assist the feeding team to make changes to a child's feeding plan, such as adjusting portion size or identifying the need for adapted seating. The following sections present several methods with examples of specific techniques to collect and examine feeding data—the "how" of data collection and experimental design.

Anecdotal Records

Anecdotal records are written observations. They can vary along several dimensions. They can be brief or detailed, and they can be open-ended or follow a predetermined format. A predetermined format might be as simple as half sheet of paper with space for the child's name, the data collector's name, the date, and the time, along with space to write phrases and/or sentences about what is occurring in the context of the targeted behavior, routine, or interaction (Lincoln & Guba, 1985; see Figure 7.1 for an example). It is important to note that all types of anecdotal records focus on behaviors and interactions within the child's environment(s).

One of the difficulties with anecdotal records is that caregivers should write these records just as the skills are demonstrated or shortly afterward. Using index cards or similar note paper can help team members complete anecdotal records as behaviors happen, or brief reminders can be written on index cards, digitally recorded, or saved on some other type of electronic device for later elaboration. An additional consideration with anecdotal records is the need to capture the anecdotes with specific and objective terminology. Much like IEP STOs, anecdotal records should include "no impressions or perceptions." Anecdotal records should be written and collected from feeding team members and other caregivers who interact with the child during mealtimes. Together, anecdotal records taken by all members of the feeding team provide a holistic view of naturally occurring feeding opportunities and skill development.

Figure 7.1.   Sample anecdotal record form

Child's name: __Lily R.__

Person completing anecdotal record: __Jenna (Classroom teacher)__

Date: __May 4, 2011__   Time: __Time: 11:45am – 12:15pm__

Location: __Child care center__   Peers: __Bobby L., Sammy M.__

Anecdotal Record #1:
Lily took eight bites of the hot dog. She smiled and made open mouth sounds after each bite. She also

smiled and clapped while taking bites of a sugar cookie. Lily also pointed to the milk contained three

times during the meal and drank each time the container was given to her. As previously documented,

she pushed refused the mixed vegetables and attempted to throw the peaches. She did watch Bobby

take bites of his peaches.

Date: __May 5, 2011__   Time: __11:45am – 12:15pm__

Location: __Child care center__   Peers: __Bobby L., Sammy M.__

Anecdotal Record #2:
Lily did not eat very much today. The only food she accepted from her lunch was eight bites of

a dinner roll. She repeatedly pushed away the plate with turkey with gravy and closed her mouth when

mashed potatoes were presented. She also threw the bowl with the pumpkin pie and said "no." Lily's

speech and language pathologist observed the meal and encouraged Lily to try each food. She also

offered her tastes of vanilla pudding since that is one of Lily's preferred foods. Lily took a few bites and

then closed her mouth and turned her body and face away.

Food Diary

As described in Chapter 6, a food diary provides a summary of a child's intake. The feeding team determines the number and format of the entries. A diary can focus on one feeding opportunity each day, or it can consider all mealtimes. Food texture and temperature also can be tracked. Location and duration of meals, positioning and seating, and the amount of food accepted from a feeder or by self-feeding can also be included. The format can be informal, such as jottings in a notebook, or more formal (see Table 6.1 and Figure 7.2).

The pivotal component is aligning the information collected in the food diary with the child's relevant IFSP outcomes, IEP STOs, and/or the goals on the child's specialized feeding plan. As indicated in Boxes 7.1 and 7.2, the targeted areas of skill development affect the information that is documented in a child's food diary.

Observational Recording

Similar to anecdotal records, observational recordings can be used to collect data about a child's feeding behaviors and skills. The difference between anecdotal re-

Figure 7.2.   Sample Completed Food Diary

Child's Name: Lily R.

Dates: May 2–6, 2011

Location of meal: Child care center
(Select one: home, child care center, public school classroom, community, other)

Meal: Lunch
(Select one: breakfast, morning snack, lunch, afternoon snack, dinner, bedtime snack)

Monday	Tuesday	Wednesday	Thursday	Friday
♪ sloppy joe ✖ sloppy joe bun (6 bites) ✦ corn ✓ mixed fruit ✖ sugar cookie (6 bites) ♪ milk	✖ chicken patty (4 bites) → chicken patty bun (12 bites) ♪ sweet potatoes ✦ banana → ! pudding (15 spoonfuls) ✳ milk (3 ounces)	✓ hot dog ✖ hot dog bun (8 bites) ♪ corn chips ♪ mixed vegetables ✓ peaches ✖ sugar cookie (5 bites) ✳ milk (4 ounces)	✓ baked turkey ✓ gravy ♪ mashed potatoes ♪ green beans ✖ dinner roll (8 bites) ✓ pumpkin pie → milk (6 ounces)	✦ chicken strips → ! macaroni & cheese (15 bites) ♪ green beans ✓ mixed fruit ♪ chocolate milk

Key:
✓ = rejected (child pushes or throws away item)
♪ = refused (child does not touch, lick, mouth, or taste item)
✦ = tasted (child licks, mouths, or sucks on item or brings food from utensil to mouth)
✖ = ate portion of food item (number of bites)
✳ = drank portion of item (number of ounces)
→ = finished eating / drinking item (approximate amount)
! = requested (child asks for more)

cords and observational recording is that observational recording is more formal in structure and exclusively data-driven, with little descriptive documentation. However, anecdotal records can be collected to supplement observational recordings (Alberto & Troutman, 2008; Cooper et al., 2007). Several general types of data can be collected to monitor progress. Counting the frequency of a behavior (how often it occurs) or the duration of a behavior (how long it lasts) are two examples that can be gathered alone or in combination. A brief description of event, duration, and momentary time sampling is offered in the section that follows. These examples are included because they represent commonly used methods of observational recording. Additional methods may be recommended by the child's feeding team. Often, a behavior analyst will take the lead on this aspect of progress monitoring because behavior analysts have specialized training in this area.

Event Recording   In order to determine the number of times a child engages in a specific eating-related behavior or demonstrates a specific feeding skill within a predetermined period of time (the behavior's frequency; e.g., twice in 15 minutes), data should be collected in the form of event recording. This method is preferred for brief, discrete behaviors and skills that are easily observed. Explained in another way, each instance of the behavior or skill must be clearly and consistently identified across all team members who are collecting data. Each time an infant munches on a cracker, for example, is counted as an event and represented by a tally mark. In addition, as described previously in the section on STO development, the more specific and observable the behavior or skill, the easier it will be to observe and count. In addition, event recording is preferred when collecting information across several days, weeks, and so forth.

Duration Recording   When the feeding team is interested in determining the amount of time between the beginning and the end of a specific behavior, skill, or skill sequence, duration recording should be used. For example, a toddler is having difficulty drinking from a Nosey cup (a cup that does not require the child to bend his or her neck or tilt his or her head). The child care provider receives training to document a duration recording by beginning to count by seconds each time the child brings the Nosey cup to his or her mouth until the child returns the cup to the table. (For a skill such as this, the child care provider may also be instructed to document the number of ounces the child drinks each time he or she brings the cup to his or her mouth, which can be captured in a food diary.) The drawbacks of this method are that it requires continuous observation on the part of the adult who is recording the data and that the specific behavior may not take place during the designated time resulting in "0" being marked on the data sheet for nonoccurrence.

Time Sampling   The final method focuses on recording when a behavior occurs (or if it does not occur) during a specified time period. The time period can be very brief (e.g., 10 seconds or 1 minute) or it can be the duration of a meal-time. For example, a 10–minute snack session can be divided into 10 observation intervals (each of which would last 1 minute) to gauge whether a child remains in a booster seat (momentary time sampling). The corresponding data sheet would have 10 cells or boxes. The feeding team determines whether the observer watches the child for the entire minute (whole interval) or one portion (a partial interval; e.g., the first 15 seconds). At the end of each minute, the adult observes the child and marks an "X" if the behavior occurred or the skill was observed and a "0" for nonoccurrence. When using whole-interval time sampling for longer periods of time, the observer is required to remain with or nearby the child. This may be difficult to achieve in some home and early childhood settings.

Level of Assistance   Tracking the level of assistance a child required for a feeding-related skill is an additional component of progress-monitoring data. Assistance types include physical assistance, modeling, verbal cues (reminders), and no assistance (independent performance of the task). Data sheets that track level of assistance should include the subskills necessary for the target skill to be achieved. In other words, they should break down the steps for the target skill. (See the description of task analysis in the Instructional Approaches section of this chapter). It may also be necessary to collect event or duration recording data for the subskills.

Data sheets are developed to match a child's specific feeding needs. Examples of data sheets designed to collect specific types of data are shown as follows: Figure 7.3, Event Recording; Figure 7.4, Duration Recording; Figure 7.5, Time Sampling; and Figure 7.6, Level of Assistance. It is important to note that more than one behavior or skill can be documented on one data sheet. The team is responsible for ensuring that the data is collected as required for multiple feeding behaviors and skills. Depending on the method selected and the child's actions, data may be collected multiple times during one mealtime (or other designated data-collection time) only once, or not at all (nonoccurrence). To aid in progress monitoring, it is helpful to include a comments section on data-collection sheets to capture additional information (e.g., child's mood, environmental distractions, first demonstration of a skill).

The feeding team must work together to determine the most efficient and meaningful form of data collection for progress monitoring (Cooper et al., 2007; VanDerHeyden et al., 2005). It is also important to decide on the least intrusive

Figure 7.3.   Sample Format for Event Recording Data Sheet.

Child's Name: Lily R.   **Observer:** Jenna (classroom teacher)

Specific behavior/skill: Brings finger food to mouth, takes a bite, and chews for 5 seconds

Date	Time	Total number of occurrences per date											
May 2, 2011	Start: 11:30am End: 11:50am	Y	Y	Y	Y	Y	Y	Y	Y	Y	Y	Y	Y
May 3, 2011	Start: 11:30am End: 11:50am	Y	Y	Y	Y								
May 4, 2011	Start: 11:30am End: 11:50am	Y	Y	Y	Y	Y	Y	Y	Y				
May 5, 2011	Start: 11:30am End: 11:50am	Y Y	Y Y	Y	Y	Y	Y	Y	Y	Y	Y	Y	
May 6, 2011	Start: 11:30am End: 11:50am	N											

Y = tally mark for occurrence; N = tally mark for nonoccurrence

Comments: Lily R. will feed herself bread (hot dog bun on Wednesday and dinner roll on Thursday) and sugar cookies (Monday and Wednesday). She is resistant to other finger foods when prompted (e.g., "Lily, try what is on your plate"). On Friday, she refused chicken strips but fed herself 3 ounces of macaroni and cheese using a spoon. On Tuesday, she brought a chicken patty to her mouth, bit it, and chewed it four times.

Figure 7.4.   Sample Format for Duration Recording Data Sheet.

Child's Name: Bobby L.   **Observer:** Bettie (classroom aide)

Specific behavior/skill: Brings Nosey cup to his mouth, drinks, and returns cup to the table

Date	Time begin	Time end	Duration of behavior
May 16, 2011	11:45:10	11:45:38	28 seconds
May 16, 2011	11:49:22	11:49:40	18 seconds
May 16, 2011	11:52:05	11:52:12	7 seconds
May 16, 2011	11:55:50	11:56: 17	22 seconds
May 16, 2011	12:02:12	12:02:32	20 seconds

Comments: Bobby L. used his Nosey cup five times during lunch. He was given his favorite drink (chocolate milk). The instance when he brought the cup to his mouth and returned it to the table in 7 seconds was due to the child being distracted by a plate falling to the floor at the table next to him. He was asked to pick up the cup immediately after but waited several minutes.

Figure 7.5.   Sample Format for Time Sampling Data Sheet.

Child's Name: Chase V.   **Observer:** Tina (classroom teacher)

Specific behavior/skill: Remain in seat during snack

Interval 1 10:00–10:01	Interval 2 10:01–10:02	Interval 3 10:02–10:03	Interval 4 10:03–10:04	Interval 5 10:04–10:05
X 10:00:00	X 10:01:00	X 10:02:00	0 10:03:00	0 10:04:00
X 10:00:15	X 10:01:15	X 10:02:15	0 10:03:15	0 10:04:15
X 10:00:30	X 10:01:30	X 10:02:30	0 10:03:30	X 10:04:30
X 10:00:45	X 10:01:45	X 10:02:45	0 10:03:45	X 10:04:45
X 10:01:00	X 10:02:00	0 10:03:00	0 10:04:00	X 10:05:00

X = ; O =

Comments: Chase was engaged continuously in eating a snack for approximately the 3 minutes. He fed himself bite-size crackers and took a few sips of cranberry juice. At 10:02:50, he said "No." He stood up from his chair and left the table at 10:03:00. He walked to the cubbies and said "Go home." I brought him back to the table and helped him sit down at 10:04:30, so he could continue his snack.

Figure 7.6.   Sample Format for Level of Assistance Data Sheet.

Child's Name: Sammy M.   **Observer:** Ricky (Classroom aide)

Specific skill: Grasp cup with both hands and drink at least 4-ounces of liquid at lunchtime

Date	Sub-skills	Level of assistance
May 9, 2011	1. Reach for cup with both hands	V
	2. Grasp cup with both hands and bring to mouth	V
	3. Open mouth for liquid	I
	4. Keep mouth open and both hands on cup	I
	5. Move cup away from mouth with both hands	M
	6. Return cup to table and release	I
May 10, 2011	1. Reach for cup with both hands	V
	2. Grasp cup with both hands and bring to mouth	V
	3. Open mouth for liquid	I
	4. Keep mouth open and both hands on cup	V, M
	5. Move cup away from mouth with both hands	V, M
	6. Return cup to table and release	I
May 11, 2011	1. Reach for cup with both hands	V
	2. Grasp cup with both hands and bring to mouth	M
	3. Open mouth for liquid	I
	4. Keep mouth open and both hands on cup	I
	5. Move cup away from mouth with both hands	P
	6. Return cup to table and release	P

I = Independent, V = Verbal cue (reminder), M = Model, P = Physical assistance

Comments: Sammy was able to independently demonstrate at least two subskills daily. I use the verbal cue, "What do you do next?" He is successful with moving to the next step of the skill. Sammy required physical assistance on May 11th due to not feeling well. His mother sent a note that he complained of a stomachache at dinner the previous night and wanted her to feed him.

method so that the child's behaviors are as natural as possible. For example, it is preferred that the feeding team member who works with the child also record necessary information (e.g., complete the entry in food diary, take duration recordings) rather than including an additional person solely for this purpose. If a child needs a more specialized feeding plan (Patel et al., 2001; Patel et al., 2005), multiple team members may need to participate in this aspect of data monitoring. As previously indicated, the team must also establish a schedule for reviewing progress-monitoring data and take appropriate action based on the results. Recommendations from individual members of the child's feeding team should be sought throughout this process for all IFSP outcomes, IEP STOs, and goals from specialized feeding plans. Adjustments are part of the process and offer opportunities to further tailor the feeding plan to the child's feeding strengths, emerging skills, and needs.

■ ■ ■ TABLE TALK ■ ■ ■

Mr. and Mrs. Franklin had been very concerned about their son's feeding. When Emerson was almost 3 years old, he ate only finger foods such as chicken nuggets, cheese cubes, and pretzels. Emerson would push food away when it was presented on a spoon. Many times, he also screamed and hit himself around the face and said "No spoon!!" Mrs. Franklin became very distressed each time this occurred, which could be several times a day.

Emerson would sit at the table at mealtimes but only drink juice or milk. He tried some pasta off his mother's plate on several occasions, but otherwise he sat with his parents without eating.

Mrs. Franklin worked as an SLP. She asked her colleague, Jamie, a specialist in oral-motor disorders, for advice. Jamie gave Mrs. Franklin some oral stimulation ideas such as cheek massage and using Chewelry. These interventions did not produce appreciable change, so Jamie called in Barry, a behavior analyst. He offered several techniques to encourage Emerson to hold a spoon and bring it to his mouth. For example, Barry would offer Emerson the spoon to hold in one hand and a piece of cheese to hold in the other. He counted how many seconds Emerson would hold the spoon before dropping or throwing it. A second technique he suggested was to track how long Emerson would hold a spoon with a piece of chicken nugget on it. Barry encouraged Emerson's parents to model bringing a spoon to their mouths and note if their son attempted to do the same. Finally, Barry asked Mrs. Franklin to write down anecdotal notes of Emerson's feeding activities two to three times a week, describing what he ate, his behavior, and her feelings about progress or lack thereof.

Discussion Questions

■   Do you agree with Jamie and Barry's recommendations?

■   How would you take data on the techniques Barry suggested?

■   How would you approach progress monitoring in this situation?

Strategies and Specialized Interventions

INTRODUCTION

> *"Feeding delays frequently occur concomitant with a host of developmental disabilities or ongoing health conditions…General features of feeding interventions…include beginning at the child's current skill level and advancing intervention based on child performance, communication about performance with regular caregivers and monitoring the child's health status throughout the process."*

(Kedesdy & Budd, 1998, p. 311)

Section III offers in-depth information and resources on general feeding strategies and specialized interventions for a variety of feeding difficulties. Chapter 8 provides an overview of general feeding considerations for young children in individual and group settings, including meeting nutritional guidelines, promoting healthy eating habits, choosing formulas and foods, and positioning. For group settings, there is a discussion on involvement of young children in food preparation and family-style meals.

Chapters 9 through 14 present an array of strategies as well as specialized feeding interventions designed to address the needs of young children with specific feeding difficulties associated with at risk conditions, disabilities, and anatomical differences.

Chapter 9 discusses the unique needs of young children who are at risk for feeding difficulties due to prematurity and young children who have been diagnosed with organic or nonorganic failure to thrive. Negative feeding experiences can adversely affect development in this area. Key developmental considerations for feeding success are described.

Chapter 10 reviews sensory-based feeding issues, including sensory processing problems and feeding issues specifically related to young children with sensory integration disorders and autism. Behavioral strategies and environmental modifications are described.

Chapter 11 discusses young in children with oral-motor difficulties including dysphagia, aspiration, and gastroesophageal reflux. Pica (eating nonedible items) is also discussed. Strategies and specialized interventions focusing on oral-motor exercises, adjusting food items, and fluids to increase intake and positive interactions during mealtimes are discussed. Medication to treat oral-motor difficulties is briefly described.

Chapter 12 discusses the needs of infants, toddlers, and preschoolers with neurological disorders. Young children with cerebral palsy often experience feeding difficulties; appropriate positioning, and specialized supplements, and calorie boosters are discussed.

Chapter 13 explores specialized interventions for young children with cleft lip and palate and specialized interventions developed for infants, toddlers, and preschoolers with difficulties with tongue and jaw control. Surgery to repair clefts is discussed, along with recommendations for fluid intake and food presentation prior to and after surgeries.

Chapter 14 examines tube feeding, including reasons for tube placement, different types of enteral systems, and stoma (i.e., site of the tube) care. Recommendations for oral stimulation and intake are also discussed within the parameters of safety and the likelihood of continuing or beginning oral feeding.

Each chapter in Section III offers "Feeding Nuggets," brief listings of resources including books, DVDs, and web sites focusing on chapter topics.

8

General Strategies for Feeding Young Children

What You'll Learn in This Chapter

This chapter provides

- A discussion of nutritional guidelines for young children
- General considerations related to young children who are picky eaters or have food sensitivities and allergies
- Recommendations for positioning to enhance feeding experiences
- Examples of individualized and group strategies in home and group settings

---

■ ■ ■ FOOD FOR THOUGHT ■ ■ ■

"The first time my husband, Gary, met my extended family, he noticed the little ones weren't eating their veggies. He convinced two of them that green beans were good because peas were hiding inside the shell and after you ate the peas, you had grass to dip in the catsup/dressing. It was quite humorous watching them break open the bean, pull out the 'peas,' and dip the shells. One of the kids even did an ant on a log version... fill the shell with catsup & place the peas on top. But for some reason, this trick never works for our boys."

Elisa, Parent

"Trevian began child care at 8 weeks. He would eat 4 ounces every 3 hours. When his bottle was finished, he would get upset. He could be calmed using a pacifier but would get hungry again before 3 hours. His bottles were increased to 6 ounces. Later, his ounce intake was increased from 6 ounces to 7 ounces. He is now 4 months old and eats rice cereal (about 2 ounces) once a day along with his 7-ounce bottles every 3 hours. "

Lesley, Child Care Provider

"To try to get Holly, to eat more throughout the day when she was 7 months old, she was given rice cereal mixed with a fruit or veggie. Due to phlegm issues, eating cereal was difficult for her and she would often gag and choke on cereal. When she was 10 months old, she began eating breads and drinking breast milk from a Sippy cup, and she quickly advanced to all table food. We saw a change in Holly's behavior. She does very well with table foods now."

Lesley, Child Care Provider

"Jessica is 14 months old. I wash her hands and then sit her in her chair. I place a bib around her neck. She feeds herself completely. She uses her hands mostly, but she holds the fork in her hand. Sometimes she will hand me her fork so that I can get a piece of food on it and then she will feed herself with the utensil. She sips from her Sippy cup efficiently. When she sets the cup back down though, sometimes she sets it into her food bowl."

Evie, Child Care Provider

"The Child Development Laboratories (CDL) participates in the Child and Adult Care Food Program through the Department of Education. They serve nutritious meals based on their guidelines. CDL makes sure that meals have low levels of salt, sugar, and fat. CDL teaches the children that their food is for eating and not playing with. CDL serves all of their meals family style. The children are encouraged to serve themselves and then pass the food to their neighbor. The children do not have to eat every food served. The children are never forced to eat any type of food.

If the children are having problems serving themselves, the hand-over-hand method is practiced.

The staff are encouraged to talk about how they are enjoying their own food, and children are allowed to try foods when they are ready to try them. All staff that are in the classroom during a meal are expected to sit and eat with the children. It is a social time for the children, and staff are expected to engage in conversations. Staff are also expected to eat at least one spoonful of every food served unless they have an allergy or religious belief that conflicts with eating a particular food. Staff are discouraged from insisting that the children use 'please' or 'thank you' but they should use it themselves. Children are encouraged to use signs or words to express that they would like more food. Signs for 'more' and 'finished' are taught in the infant room and carried on to the toddler room. If children spill during the meal, they are required to help clean up their own mess."

Kacie, Graduate Assistant at CDL and Early Childhood Special Education Graduate Student

"At 54 months, Baxter sits down at the snack table at pre-K. We are having mixed fruit from a can.

I ask him if he would like fruit. He says 'Yes, please.' I continue to move around the table.

'I need a spoon,' Baxter yells as I continue to scoop out fruit.

'Baxter, we have not all been served yet so no one has a spoon yet,' I explain. He looks around the table. I finish serving and pass out spoons. Baxter picks up his spoon and begins to eat. He eats the pears, peaches, and cherries. He leaves the grapes.

'More please,' he says pushing his bowl toward me.

'Baxter, you need to finish what you have before you can have more fruit.'

'But I don't like those ones,' he says pointing at the grapes.

'If you want more fruit, you need to eat what you have first.' I look back over to Baxter and his bowl is now empty.

'More fruit please!' he says with a smile.

I get my spoon to serve him and say, 'You ate all your grapes, Baxter. Now you can have more fruit!'

I serve him the fruit, and he finishes the bowl and asks to be excused."

Ashley, pre-K Teacher

"We serve breakfast and lunch family style to 20 children (13 girls, 7 boys) between the ages of 3 and 5 years. The children get their own dishes, utensils, and milk/juice. They learn to set the place setting, serve themselves, open and pour milk, and clean up after themselves. Some children come to school knowing manners and how to use utensils, and we teach the others."

Kara, Head Start teacher

The previous examples provide an overview of feeding situations and strategies to address feeding problems. Young children progress through key milestones (e.g., beginning solid foods, drinking from an open-mouth cup) resulting in age-appropriate, independent feeding. There are also gains in overall development as evidenced by Kara and Ashley's experiences. While many children meet feeding milestones effortlessly, some infants, toddlers, and preschoolers may require the use of specific strategies to facilitate this form of development.

As discussed in Chapter 1, feeding milestones are attained in a predictable manner by most young children. Some children, however, encounter difficulties that negatively affect eating activities. Morris and Klein (2000) suggested a variety of ways to encourage independence during mealtimes. They suggest promoting choice making, respecting children's preferences, and participation in meal preparation. The authors also emphasize problem solving to arrive at favorable feeding solutions. For example, instead of battling with a toddler over food choices, a parent or caregiver can enlist the child's input. The sensory components of food items and fluids (e.g., textures and temperatures) should be explored, and adjustments made based on the child's responses (see Chapter 10). Trachtenberg (2007) and others (cf. American Academy of Pediatrics Committee on Nutrition, 2008; Birch, 1999; Birch, 2008) also stressed the importance of forming healthy food habits during the early childhood years. The following sections provide recommendations and strategies to promote such habits early in a child's life.

MEETING NUTRITIONAL GUIDELINES

Nutrition is recognized as a critical part of development (Britten, Marcoe, Yamini, & Davis, 2006; Marcoe, 2001). The United States Department of Agriculture (USDA) developed recommendations in the form of a pyramid depicting the daily requirements of the main food groups for optimal growth. In 2010, the pyramid was updated to a plate design, emphasizing more fruits, vegetables, and whole grains. (For more information, visit the USDA web site: http://www.choosemyplate.gov/.) New guidelines also emphasize meeting young children's nutritional needs by offering a variety of foods, emphasizing water as a primary beverage, and using salt in moderation in foods prepared at home, child care, and other settings, as well as checking sodium levels in prepackaged and restaurant foods.

Developing Healthy Eating Patterns

Infants present a unique stage in feeding development, with much of the focus on increasing intake and introducing solid foods at appropriate times. Parent and caregiver ability to understand an infant's cues is very important. Mentro, Steward, and Garvin (2002) focused on interpreting an infant's visual, communicative, and motor responses as indicating readiness to feed (e.g., movement of arms and legs when bottle is presented, babbling when finger foods are offered). Satter (1986, 1990) also emphasized the feeding relationship and indicated that parents and caregivers should offer opportunities for exploration and at the same time set limits regarding food activities. Nicklaus (2009) indicated that early feeding experiences, especially for infants who are breastfed, should offer a variety of taste experiences. The first 12 months of a child's life acquaint him or her with food experiences that lay the groundwork for future feeding development.

Variety   The rapidly growing and changing bodies of young children require a varied diet. Meals and snacks must provide a combination of healthy and favored options. In addition, guidelines indicate that at least one of a child's preferred foods should be included at every meal to improve intake. Young children should receive appropriate serving sizes of foods from all food groups (grains, vegetables, fruits, dairy, proteins, and fats). Children also need more frequent and smaller portions compared with older children and adults. In general, 2–3-year old children should receive approximately 1000 calories a day, and 4–5-year old children should receive 1400 calories a day (Britten et al., 2006). A child's activity level also factors into daily caloric needs; more active children may require more calories than less active children.

Recent research has found that basic nutritional recommendations for very young children are not always met. In the Feeding Infants and Toddler Study (FITS), Fox, Pac, Devaney, and Jankowski (2004) reviewed data from a random national sample of approximately 3,000 children ages 4–24 months. Of this group, 20–30% did not regularly consume vegetables or fruits. In fact, by 18 months, French fries were identified as the most commonly eaten vegetable. In addition, more than half of the sample's toddlers ages 19–24 months ate dessert or candy on a frequent basis. The authors emphasized the need for parents and caregivers to offer healthy choices, such as cheese, yogurt, and whole grain cereal in place of the desserts and candy. In a later examination of infant feeding practices, Siega-Riz et al. (2010) found that, compared with infants in previous studies, fewer infants were consuming infant cereal. Furthermore, infants in their study had a lower than expected intake of fruits and vegetables. There was a positive finding regarding toddlers: compared with toddlers in earlier studies, toddlers in their sample showed a decreased intake of desserts or candy, sweetened beverages, and salty snacks (Siega-Riz et al., 2010).

These findings emphasize the need for young children to be presented with a variety of vegetables and fruits daily. Green, leafy vegetables are particularly important, as are a variety of fruits, including berries and apples. Early exposure assists with the development of lifelong healthy eating habits (Briefel, Reidy, Karwe, Jankowski, & Hendricks, 2004; Eliassen, 2011; Parlakian & Lerner, 2007). Supplements should only be used when necessary; children should receive their calories and nutrients from foods. (Additional information regarding supplement use is provided in a later section of this chapter.)

Self-Regulation of Food Intake

An infant's feeding patterns for meals and snacks are established prior to his or her first birthday (Skinner, Ziegler, Pac, & Devaney, 2004). The infant is an active agent in this process, learning to regulate hunger and satiation as well as developing a taste for the variety of foods provided. Preferences are also formed. For example one child may prefer carrots and squash rather than green beans at meals or a specific cereal rather than crackers for snack. Skinner et al. (2004) reported that older infants and toddlers eat up to seven times a day with most eating three meals and two snacks. Breakfast was found to be highest in nutritional value for calcium and iron. Eighty percent of toddlers received an afternoon snack consisting of one or more of the following: milk, water, cookies, crackers, chips, and fruit drinks. Skinner et al. (2004) also recommended deferring the introduction of and limiting exposure to low-nutrient, high-calorie foods. They recommended snack foods such as cut-up fruit, raw vegetables, strips of cooked meats, and whole-grain crackers with toppings such as jam, cream cheese, or peanut butter (low-fat options are best).

Briefel et al. (2004) supported the previously described suggestions, indicating that children should be explicitly taught to recognize hunger and satiety cues. For example, parents and caregivers can explain to young children that it is acceptable to not finish a meal if their stomach feels full and to ask for a second helping only if they feel hungry. In other words, children should be taught to "listen" to their bodies, such as when their stomach "growls" or when they feel tired. It is also important for children to understand that if they are not aware, an appetite for a favorite food may take precedence over satiety signals, causing overeating and discomfort. Body awareness and healthy eating habits can help prevent childhood obesity. Parent and caregiver support in limiting unhealthy foods and in modeling appropriate food choices is critical to these efforts (Bluford, Sherry, & Scanlon, 2007; Epstein, Myers, Raynor, & Saelens, 1998; Faith, Scanlon, Birch, Francis, & Sherry, 2004).

Birch and Fisher (1998) indicated that children as young as 3 years have the ability to regulate their food intake (see Chapter 1). A variable that influenced this was the feeding practices of parents and caregivers. The authors described how parent controls on food, for example, may result in the child seeking high-fat foods rather than healthier options. When parents limit children's access to foods, it can adversely affect the child's understanding of hunger and satiety, leading to less self-control around food. Establishing healthy eating patterns requires age-appropriate feeding practices and expectations. Johnson (2002) recommended that parents "offer foods at appropriate times by matching them to the child's stage of development; act as role models for appropriate eating behaviors; and learn to set appropriate limits for their children's eating behaviors" (p. S93). The author focused on advice for parents, but the same advice could be given to caregivers and professionals working with preschoolers.

STRATEGIES FOR PROMOTING FEEDING SUCCESS

During the preschool years, nutritional requirements and an ongoing need to develop healthy eating habits continue to be primary feeding concerns (Birch & Fisher, 1998; Johnson, 2000; Skinner et al., 1999). However, many young children tend to be picky eaters, and food sensitivities and allergies affect food preparation and intake.

Finally, optimal positioning must be considered. Instead of allowing a toddler to walk around with food, for example, the child should be encouraged to sit in a chair that is an appropriate size, such as a booster seat (with or without a tray). Mealtime positioning must also support each child so she is comfortable and able to be as independent as possible.

Strategies for Picky Eaters

In a study examining eating patterns of 118 toddlers, Carruth et al. (1998) found that

> a limited number of food exposures and trials to determine the toddler's food likes and dislikes are probably insufficient to anticipate that toddlers will learn to accept a wide variety of foods. If insufficient exposure results in…rejections, parents may consider this problematic eating behavior. (p. 185)

The authors further emphasized that limited opportunities with novel foods does not necessarily produce a picky eater. Picky eating is largely related to a developmental phase focusing on independence and autonomy and is often coupled with the emergence of neophobia (fear or unwillingness to try new things). A toddler with strong preferences for familiar and preferred foods is, in fact, exhibiting age-appropriate behavior. Idiosyncrasies, such as only eating one type of cereal for breakfast, requiring that a sandwich be cut a certain way, or using a specific cup for juice but not for milk are developmentally appropriate responses. These behaviors are typically short term, and even while they are ongoing, it is important for caregivers and parents to continue offering new foods to establish healthy eating patterns (Jana & Shu, 2008; Mascola, Bryson, & Agras, 2010). Modeling is also very important. Healthy eating patterns are encouraged and reinforced by parents, caregivers, and other adults who model a varied diet without forcing or cajoling the child to try new foods.

Carruth, Ziegler, Gordon, and Barr (2004) focused on the optimal number of food presentations to counteract picky eating. The sample of 3,022 infants and toddlers required at least 10–12 experiences before determining the item was disliked. When a child turns away or pushes a food item away, it should be removed. This response by a parent, caregiver, or other provider lets a young child know that she is valued. The new item should continue to be offered; the child will explore or accept it when developmentally ready (Carruth et al., 1998; Carruth et al., 2004;

Fox et al., 2004; Nicklaus, 2009). Mascola et al. (2010) noted that in their sample, approximately 20% of children ages 2–11 years demonstrated picky eating habits. Problems arose with children who displayed this behavior for longer than 2 years, resulting in the need for specially prepared meals and some behavioral concerns (e.g., tantruming when favored food was not readily given or was not available). Taken together, these findings indicate the importance of repeated presentations within the context of an individual child's developmental progress.

Morris and Klein (2000) noted that

> children's decisions to eat a new food are based primarily on their sensory perceptions of the food. If they don't like the way it looks, smells or feels when they touch it, they may refuse to have anything to do with it. (p. 11)

This observation should be kept in mind during the neophobic phase. Some degree of apprehension around new foods is to be expected in toddlers. If the child continues to limit intake as an older toddler, a feeding assessment should be conducted to rule out specific feeding disorders. (See Chapter 6 for more information about feeding assessment; see Chapter 10 for feeding strategies for children exhibiting more problematic picky eating, such as children with a sensory processing disorder or an ASD.) Box 8.1 provides a variety of strategies for use with picky eaters; the strategies can be used individually or in combination.

Food presentation includes the way food is assembled (Johnson, 2002; Nicklaus, 2009). For example, many young children do not like casseroles and stews

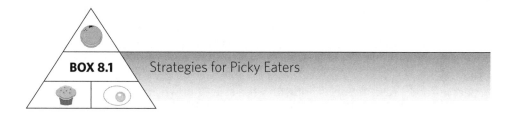

BOX 8.1 Strategies for Picky Eaters

- Offer nutritious foods for snack and mealtimes throughout the day, especially if the child refuses foods from a certain food group; find substitutes as necessary
- Pair new food with a familiar or preferred food item
- Model trying new foods or foods that child does not readily eat
- Provide choices, but not too many
- Affirm child's choices rather than bargain or negotiate
- Use creative food presentation to gain child's attention
- Provide praise for exploration and/or acceptance of a new food item
- Offer small portions for tastes rather than a serving size
- Offer dips and spices for bland foods
- Encourage child to assist in meal preparation and offer tastes of ingredients
- Allow the child to help shop for ingredients
- Promote experiences with different foods by color, shape, or texture
- Match child's preferences for feeding method and food choices when possible, such as offering a food that is usually eaten with a spoon as a finger food

because of the mixture of ingredients. When ingredients (e.g., pieces of stew meat, boiled or baked potatoes, carrots) are presented singly, young children may be more likely to consume the foods. This need for familiarity may extend to a favored plate or cup—items which can be taken to a restaurant or relative's home with the result that the child eats more and healthier foods.

Attractive food presentation, whether in portion or display, can increase intake of healthy foods (Parlakian & Lerner, 2007). Portion size has been investigated as it relates to food presentation. Looney and Raynor (2011) examined the affects of portion size with a sample of preschoolers. Apple sauce and chocolate pudding were offered in small or large portion sizes. Children selected the large portion regardless of the food item. McConahy, Smiciklas-Wright, Mitchell, and Picciano (2004) further discussed the importance of age-appropriate portion sizes, indicating that parents, caregivers, and other adults working with young children should offer guidance on the frequency of eating as well as the amounts and types of foods consumed. Cooke (2007) indicated that parents and caregivers should offer toddlers and preschoolers a variety of foods to ensure that they meet their caloric needs and to broaden food acceptance. (For more information, see the General Considerations and Individual and Group Strategies sections later in this chapter.) Furthermore, dietary patterns that increase the likelihood of favorable lifelong habits are developed in early childhood.

Young children tend to eat small portions such as half a slice of deli meat and a tablespoon of blueberries. This encourages completion of a snack or meal. Conversely, a large portion has the potential to discourage the child from eating (or even tasting) the food item. In one study described in Chapter 1, serving children a double sized portion of carrots actually enhanced the amount of carrots eaten. However, a triple serving size led to eating fewer carrots (Spill, Birch, Roz, & Rolls, 2010).

Food presentation is an important consideration when it comes to offering young children novel foods, familiar foods, and preferred foods. It can also be used to encourage intake of healthy foods that are not preferred. One important aspect of food presentation is adjusting the size of bowls, plates, and utensils to correspond with the child's size and fine motor skills. There are a variety of commercially available cups that offer a progression in size and flow-rate. For example, one brand offers a 4-ounce cup with an adjustment valve and spout top and 8-ounce and 9-ounce cups that have straws and adjust to an open presentation.

There are myriad ways of presenting foods to encourage young children to consume them. Presentation should be visually appealing and draw on familiar topics. For example, "bagel snakes" (mini bagel halves filled with tuna or chicken salad and connected end to end), "ants on a log" (celery filled with peanut butter or cream cheese with raisins on top), "smiley face sandwiches" (with raisins for eyes and nose and a fruit slice for mouth) and "traffic light" fruit skewers (combination of apple, mango, honey dew and cantaloupe pieces with yogurt dip) are examples of child-friendly ways to offer nutritious foods. Toddlers and preschoolers can also be provided with ingredients such as whole grain crackers, cheese slices, sliced olives, and baby carrots and instructed to prepare their own creations. Parents and caregivers can also offer smoothies and shakes in an array of colors using blenderized fresh fruit, yogurt, and milk. Smoothies can also include vegetables such as sweet potatoes, spinach, and avocados.

Compared with the typical trajectory in feeding development, the eating patterns of many young children with disabilities are markedly different. For example, parents of children with autism spectrum disorder (ASD) often provide accounts of their children's limited and/or selective intake compared to preschoolers without an ASD. Children with ASD often consume insufficient amounts of vitamins A and E, calcium, and fiber, and many parents of children with ASD describe a generalized resistance to tasting new foods (Lockner, Crowe, & Skipper, 2011). Provost, Crowe, Osburn, McClain, and Skipper (2010) reported that mothers with 3–6 year olds with ASD described their children as picky eaters. Specifically, they reported their children resisted tasting new foods and often threw or dumped food items. Typically developing young children may exhibit the same or similar behaviors, but the behavior usually does not become an established habit. (See Chapter 10 for more information about feeding development for young children with ASD.)

Food Sensitivities and Allergies

Food sensitivities and allergies are most often related to peanuts, milk, eggs, tree nuts (including almonds and cashews), soy, and wheat. Children might also experience problems with citrus foods and green vegetables, such as broccoli. Food sensitivities, also known as food intolerance, indicate that the food should be reduced or eliminated from the child's diet (Wood, 2003). Some foods that cause sensitivity can be slowly reintroduced while the severity of the child's symptoms is documented in order to help determine whether the child's tolerance has increased. It is also beneficial to work with a dietitian and/or a pediatrician to make decisions about which foods to keep and which foods to reduce or remove from a child's diet. Food sensitivities are individual; siblings (even twins), for example, may exhibit very different responses to the same food item, with one experiencing great discomfort and the other tolerating the food well.

With food allergies that trigger an immune-system response—such as sneezing, runny nose, coughing, difficulty breathing or wheezing, itchy skin and/or eyes, hives or rash, swelling, stomach cramps, nausea and diarrhea—more decisive action must be taken (Høst et al., 2003). Some reactions are so severe that an injection of epinephrine (EpiPen) is necessary to prevent death. Some allergies are outgrown by the time a child is 5 years old, while other allergies remain throughout childhood and beyond (Wood, 2003).

It is important to identify foods that can substitute for the items the child cannot consume. The substitute should provide nutrients the child would otherwise get from the typical food and, at the same time, reduce the likelihood of adverse reactions (Keet et al., 2009; Stahl & Rans, 2011). For example, a child who has difficulty with cow's milk can be offered almond milk, rice milk, or soy milk. These substitutions provide many of the nutrients the child would otherwise get from cow's milk without causing an adverse reaction. If a child has difficulty digesting citrus fruits, other types of fruits should be offered, along with supplemental vitamin C in some cases. Parents and caregivers must thoroughly read food labels and be familiar with terminology indicating the presence of possible allergens. For some children, only foods prepared at home may be safe to eat—regardless of participation in child care, Head Start, and/or other settings.

Classrooms must eliminate all traces of allergens. This requires support from program administrators as well as cooperation from other families with a child at the setting (e.g., not sending in treats containing one or more allergy-causing ingredient/s). All caregivers—including relatives, babysitters, and other adults who interact with the child at mealtimes—must be made aware of food sensitivities and allergies and the appropriate actions to take if or when a child has an allergic reaction. Peers can also be taught about food allergies so they understand their classmate's experience and needs.

Springston et al. (2010) explored experiences of over 1,000 caregivers of children with food allergies. The consistent finding was distress related to day-to-day limitations caused by the allergy. This response was strongest when multiple food allergies were present. In addition, Flammarion et al. (2011) described a correlation between weight and height for young children with food allergies. The sample of children with food allergies showed lower weight and shorter height compared with same-age peers without food allergies. Children with more than two food allergies were the smallest. These findings indicate the varied presentation of food allergies and illustrate the necessary accommodations to meet the mealtime needs of children affected by them.

Positioning

Comfortable positioning for both the child and feeder is an integral component in successful feeding. For an infant who is nursing or bottle fed, there are several positions or holds. For example, parents and caregivers can utilize the cradle hold or football hold. Infants can also be placed in a side-lying position or supported on a pillow. A description of these common holds is offered in Table 8.1. It is up to the feeder and infant dyad to determine the most successful hold. In addition, as the infant grows and displays more voluntary movement (e.g., supports head, sits independently), feeding positioning will need to be modified.

An older infant or toddler typically uses a highchair at the family table or at the child care table for mealtimes. Beginning at approximately 18 months of age, a booster seat can be used. Booster seats are portable and easier to keep clean than most highchairs. They also permit the child to sit directly at the table because they attach to chairs. This provides a number of benefits, including easier access for the child and greater participation in mealtime activities (e.g., passing bowls of food). Many booster seats can also be placed on the floor and have a tray that can be used to hold food and drink items. Most preschoolers can sit on an adult-sized chair with little or no additional support. Child care centers, Head Start, and prekindergarten classrooms are equipped with adjustable tables and child-sized chairs.

Table 8.1. Common infant positions for nursing or bottle feeding

	Description
Cradle hold	Cradle the infant's head in the fold of the arm holding infant and provide support to the infant's bottom. Position infant on his back or slightly turned to one side to provide eye and body contact with the feeder. Alternate sides so the infant uses neck and shoulder muscles on both sides.
Crossover hold	Place the arm around the back of the infant, supporting the infant's head, neck, and shoulder. Be sure the hand is placed at the base of infant's head with thumb and index finger at infant's ear level. As in the cradle hold, facilitate eye and body contact.
Sidelying hold	Place child in sidelying position with head and shoulders elevated (semi-upright). Lower arm is used to cradle infant's back and bottom. Can use a rolled-up receiving blanket so the infant is close to the feeder and provided with necessary support to maintain the position.
Football hold	Place a small pillow or nursing pillow under the infant. Cradle the infant by placing a hand under the head to support the neck. Bring infant close to feeder. Infant's legs and feet should be tucked under the feeder's arm.

Regardless of the type of seating, there are several requirements for safe and successful mealtimes. Children must be able to keep their head and neck at midline (in line with belly button and facing forward), their shoulders pushed back, and their torso centered. Hips and bottom need to be flush with the back of the seat, and feet need to be flat on the floor or other support. For young children who require additional assistance to meet these requirements, Chapter 12 provides examples of positioning techniques and specialized feeding chairs. It is important to note that the feeder also needs to be comfortable during feeding activities (Morris & Klein, 2000). The feeder should have comfortable seating. Also, when feeding an infant, the feeder (at least initially) can determine the preferred hold. After learning the infant's preferences related to nursing or bottle feeding positions, the feeder can use other holds.

INDIVIDUALIZED STRATEGIES FOR PROMOTING FEEDING SUCCESS

In addition to the general considerations described previously, some young children require individualized strategies to encourage feeding development. Among these are specialized formulas; adapted utensils, cups, and plates; calorie boosters and supplements; and thickening products. Each is briefly described in the following sections.

Specialized Formulas

Infant formulas are easily digested by most newborns and older infants, but some infants require specialized formula for reasons such as protein sensitivities and/ or allergies, gastroesphageal reflux (GER), gastrointestinal problems, and conditions related to prematurity. Other infants need a high-calorie mixture to promote growth. Soy-based, lactose-free, and predigested formulas are available. Most of these formulas are produced by companies (e.g., Carnation, Mead Johnson and Ross) that also make nonspecialized formula. It is important to note that the Special Supplemental Nutrition Program for Women, Infants, and Children (WIC) authorizes payment for some specialized formulas. The program receives federal funding through the Food and Nutrition Service of the Department of Agriculture. Table 8.2 provides information related to several types of specialized formulas.

Table 8.2.   Examples of specialized formulas

Specialized formula	Reason(s) for use
Enfamil EnfaCare Lipil, Similac Neosure	Specialized formulation for premature infants
Isomil, Prosobee Lipil, Good Start Supreme Soy	Soy-based formulas for easier digestion
Similac with Iron, Similac Advance with Iron, Enfamil with Iron	Provide additional iron
Enfamil Lipil	Provide additional fats (lipids)
Enfamily Lactofree, Similac Lactose Free Advance, Neocate	Soy-based formulas for infants with cow's milk allergy or milk protein intolerance
Alimentum, Gentlease, Nutramigen, Pregestimil	Hypoallergenic formula options to reduce gas and colic symptoms due to protein, carbohydrate, and/or fat sensitivity or intolerance
Neocate	Developed for infants with multiple protein intolerance
Peptamin Junior	For infants with gastrointestinal dysfunction

It is also important to note that regardless of the type of specialized formula required, its preparation must follow product instructions. For example, the exact amount of powdered formula must be mixed with the exact amount of water. When measuring powdered formula, level scoops (versus heaping scoops) of formula should be used. It is also important to remember that concentrated formula is intended to be diluted with water (in proper proportions as indicated) and never offered "as is." Adherence to these guidelines for both standard and specialized formulas ensures that an infant receives the appropriate amount of fluids for growth.

Adapted Utensils, Cups, Plates and Bowls

Mealtime utensils—as well as cups, plates, and bowls—are available in many styles and shapes. The key considerations are the child's age and fine motor skills. For example, a 21-month-old may need a spoon with a larger bowl or longer handle in order to successfully bring food to his or her mouth. A young preschooler can benefit from a plate with an inner lip to reduce spillage. Note that both of these examples focus on understanding which aspect of feeding needs to be supported and finding the appropriate item to address that need. A related focus is on promoting independence. For example, an adapted cup can actually limit a child's ability to drink independently if the cup is too heavy or too large for small hands. Parents and caregivers may need to test a number of feeding items to identify the type that is most suitable. Advice from a speech-language pathologist (SLP) or occupational therapist (OT) may also be necessary. These professionals can provide suggestions about items, such as appropriate sized scoop bowls, angled spoons, and specialized grips on spoons, forks, and cups.

There are many options for adapted feeding items such as Maroon spoons, which have a larger bowl to hold food and a longer handle for easier grasping. There are also Flexi-cut cups to facilitate chin tuck during drinking. Many such products are available from commercial retailers such as One Step Ahead. Other items must be ordered through specialty catalogs such as Beyond Play.

Calorie Boosters and Supplements

Some children's diets may need to include calorie boosters or supplements. These may be short-term or long-term additions to the child's diet, depending on the reason they are needed, the child's weight gain, and the child's overall nutritional status (Morris & Klein, 2000). Recommended calorie boosters often include heavy or whipping cream, butter, avocado, sour cream, cheeses (grated, shredded, or cubed), plain yogurt, powdered milk, wheat germ, and yogurt or ice cream smoothies. While adding calories, many of these items also provide more than recommended amounts of fat. Low-fat or nonfat alternatives include margarine, jams and jellies, wheat germ, brown sugar, and nonfat dry milk powder. The specific combination will vary based on the child's dietary needs, the availability of items, and parent and caregiver preferences. There are also infants, toddlers, and preschoolers who require these foods due to gastrointestinal conditions such as gastroesophageal reflux (GER). The use of calorie boosters for this group is often more long term and determined by input from the team of professionals working with the child.

Most infant diets include sufficient amounts of necessary nutrients without additional supplementation. However, multivitamins may provide necessary vitamins and minerals that certain young children, especially picky eaters, are lacking. For several reasons, it is important for parents to consult with a medical professional, such as a dietician or pediatrician, before beginning multivitamin supplementation. There are recommendations and restrictions regarding multivitamin use, and some multivitamin supplements may provide more than the recommended amount of one or more key nutrients, which can negatively affect absorption and other digestive processes (Briefel, Hanson, Fox, Novak, & Ziegler, 2006). In addition, a medical professional will determine the correct dosage and manner of presentation (e.g. liquid, chewable).

Children must understand that the multivitamin or a supplement is meant to provide a specific vitamin or nutrient; it is not intended as candy or a "treat," even if the taste is sweet and it is in the shape of a favorite cartoon character. Otherwise, a young child may ask for more and not understand why the request is refused or may try to access more vitamins without assistance from an adult. Many multivitamins (because of high amounts of A, D, E, K, and iron) can be toxic if more than the correct dosage is ingested. Supplements should be stored in a location only accessible to adults in order to prevent the child from taking extra doses. Multivitamin supplement use should be reviewed as the child grows, and multivitamins and other supplements should not replace a well-balanced diet. In addition, if a child is on medication for an unrelated issue (e.g., airborne allergies), possible drug interactions must be considered. Products such as Pediasure, Ensure (liquid and pudding), and Nutren Junior offer ready-to-serve options. Dietitians have specialized knowledge concerning nutrition and calorie intake and can provide information related to appropriate calorie boosters and supplements that are appropriate for a young child's needs.

Thickening Products

Some young children may require that food items and/or fluids be thickened before they can be consumed. There are several consistencies that are described by the foods they resemble: nectar, honey, or pudding. Apple sauce, puréed foods (e.g., carrots), and gelatin powder are examples of thickening products that can be added to foods, depending on a child's needs.

Many young children who do not need this much viscosity (thickness) will still require some thickening agent with specific food items and/or fluids to reach a desired consistency. This problem is most common with soups or other "thin" foods. Mayonnaise, yogurt (plain or flavored), and sour cream can be used for this purpose. Adding thickener to some juices may also be recommended.

Commercially available thickeners include Thick-it, SimplyThick and Thicken Up. Thick-it, for example, contains modified cornstarch and maltodextrin (a type of easily digestible carbohydrate derived from corn and used in dry foods, dairy products, and beverages). The thickener is added to hot or cold beverages as well as food items and dissolves within 30 seconds. Thickeners do not change the appearance or taste of the item to which they are added.

A number of foods with thicker consistencies can help young children transition from purées to more textured foods: oatmeal, mashed potatoes, mashed sweet potatoes, avocados, and refried beans, for example. Choose foods based primarily on the child's preferences. An additional point to bear in mind is that the need for thickening products will most likely be short-term. (The needs of young children who require long-term use of thickeners are described in Chapters 11 and 12.)

GROUP STRATEGIES

The preceding sections described nutritional guidelines for young children and discussed general considerations for successful feeding experiences. Individual strategies were also presented. This section focuses on group strategies to promote a variety of feeding and developmental skills.

Food Preparation

An essential part of a snack time or mealtime is preparation. Involving children in the food preparation process allows them to explore the properties of ingredients (e.g., the fact that butter melts when heated, the differences between raw and cooked foods), to follow sequences in recipes, and to learn about safety when handling foods and equipment such as can openers and pots. However, the most significant outcome is that a child's self-esteem is increased by becoming an active participant in food preparation, rather than remaining a passive recipient of adult-prepared foods. This type of active involvement can also result in the child having a greater interest in trying new or unfamiliar foods (Johnson, 2002).

When young children participate in the kitchen, adults may have to work harder for supervision and clean-up than they would have worked without "help." Yet, as indicated previously, the outcomes are valuable. Food preparation must be matched to a child's age level and developmental skills. For example, a 2-year-old can bring the ingredients to the adult and help stir them together, but a 4-year-old can add ingredients, stir ingredients, and transfer muffin mix from a bowl to a cupcake pan. Variations among individual children will be evident. Parents, caregivers, and other providers with knowledge of the specific child can determine which food preparation tasks are appropriate. The following information provides an overview of the range of preparation tasks as well as examples of developmental outcomes:

- Preparing a grocery list can introduce new vocabulary and promote literacy and numeracy skills.

- Going to the store to purchase food items can improve motor development. For example, fine motor skills are necessary for writing grocery lists, and gross motor skills are necessary for walking around the store, removing items from shelves, and unpacking items after arriving home.

- Preparing classroom snacks improves social skills such as turn-taking and following a sequence; serving snacks improves one-to-one correspondence skills.

- Preparing a meal for a classroom celebration involves large- and small-group interactions and children's ability to following directions. It can also provide opportunities to discuss foods from different cultural groups and holiday traditions.

There are a number of food preparation activities that can be adjusted for toddlers and preschoolers. Very young children can help with rinsing fruits and vegetables, cutting soft fruits with a dull knife, and making sandwiches. Related activities such as throwing away refuse, and setting and clearing the table, are additional meal-related tasks that can be undertaken by young children. It is important for children to begin making a contribution using their own effort early in life (Eliassen, 2011). Positive experiences provide the foundation for ongoing involvement in food preparation as the child grows older and can take on greater responsibilities.

Family-Style Meals

As described in Chapter 4, mealtimes are a critical part of family identity and a means to learn about family traditions. In addition, young children often eat one or more daily meals outside of the home in settings including child care, prekindergarten, and similar programs. Therefore, it is critical to provide a positive feeding environment in group settings.

Family-style meals provide opportunities for young children to eat together, and also work on turn-taking and other social-emotional skills. Toddlers and preschoolers can take part in food preparation (described previously), and they have the opportunity to observe peer and adult behavior during mealtimes (Parlakian & Lerner, 2007). It is imperative that child care providers and other adults in group settings participate in all aspects of mealtimes. Young children learn by observation, so adults have much to offer by modeling appropriate mealtime behaviors.

Setting the table, turn-taking to pass food and drinks, conversing during the meal, and cleaning up after the meal are opportunities provided by family-style meals. Elisassen (2011) noted that the most advantageous aspects of including young children in family-style meals could be offering familiar, preferred, and novel foods within a supportive environment. There are also myriad ways of incorporating the individual strategies described in this chapter.

Skill Development Opportunities   Participation in food preparation and family-style meals affords opportunities to target children's skill development in multiple areas. The use of activity-based intervention (ABI; Pretti-Frontczak & Bricker, 2004) provides young children with multiple opportunities to acquire and use new skills. Using the ABI framework, daily routines and activities are a means to encourage development (see Chapter 7 for more information about ABI). Meal and snack times fall into the category of routines in that they occur at approximately the same time each day and follow a similar sequence of actions. Regardless of the specific skill that is being addressed (e.g., accepting textured foods, moving from a spout to an open mouth cup), a range of other skills are also addressed. For example, while working on accepting textured foods, a child would likely also be sitting in an appropriate position to access the textured foods (gross motor), asking for more (expressive language), and following a sequence of steps to put items away when the meal is completed (cognitive/problem solving). Most young children enjoy exploring and learning about their food. Toddlers, especially, tend to poke and touch food items. Preschoolers may continue this exploration as well as take a more active role in food selection. Mealtime routines can also be expanded to include developmental activities such as hand washing and tooth brushing.

Morris and Klein (2000) discuss the array of skills inherent in self-feeding: communication, language, and social interaction skills (e.g., mealtime manners and conversation), along with fine-motor skills. It is critical that parents, caregivers, and professionals provide meaningful and, as necessary, structured opportunities for young children to learn and practice these developmental skills during mealtimes and other feeding-related activities, such as grocery shopping and meal preparation.

Feeding skill development aligns with critical developmental periods for young children. Feeding activities provide many chances to see development in action, such as the first time an infant holds her bottle, or a preschooler pours herself juice without spilling. These skills are celebrated by parents, caregivers, and others who interact with the child as they represent the achievement of important milestones.

There is also a correspondence between developmental milestones and changes in eating behaviors. For example, young toddlers who have just learned to walk often do not remain seated to eat for more than several minutes. This is to be expected due to the nature of their new walking skill. Walking requires practice. With their newfound independence comes an apparent desire for nonstop exploration, and they are generally less likely to stop to eat an entire meal or snack. To encourage children of this age to participate in mealtimes at home and in community settings, it is important to offer preferred foods, have children assist in food preparation, and provide fun food presentations. Toddlers do not have long attention spans, so it is also important to keep meals simple and short.

As described previously, all facets of food preparation offer skill development. During meal preparation, children have opportunities to practice literacy skills, such as reading sight words on food packages and following recipes. Mealtimes supply preschoolers with opportunities to practice new number concepts. They practice one-to-one correspondence while setting the table, and they practice counting while providing specific portions, such as three meatballs. In addition to eating healthy foods, preschoolers sharing a meal are learning about distributing food items, utensils, and so forth. There are also learning opportunities in the social, emotional and language areas during mealtime interactions. Like other activities that offer important learning opportunities, feeding activities require planning to produce successful outcomes.

ABI's emphasis on naturally occurring and meaningful opportunities fits with feeding in EC settings because a considerable amount of time is spent on feeding. In fact, young children may have up to two meals and several snacks each day in an environment outside of their home. In addition, ABI is a powerful tool for examining other classroom activities and routines to identify occasions to include or add feeding-related skills (Pretti-Frontczak & Bricker, 2004). Feeding-related skills can be incorporated into other parts of the school day (not just mealtimes and snack times), and feeding skills often extend to other critical learning areas. For example, snack items can be discussed during morning meeting, cookbooks can be included in the literacy area, and a store or restaurant can be created or expanded in the dramatic play area. In addition, centers and teacher-directed activities should be examined for opportunities to include feeding-related materials such as food items (actual or pretend), utensils, and empty boxes and containers to facilitate learning across developmental areas.

SUMMARY

The general strategies described here offer a set of considerations for addressing feeding-related skill development and learning across domains, including ways to provide successful feeding experiences to picky eaters and young children with food sensitivities and allergies. The individual and group strategies reflect a variety of ways to introduce novel foods, and they focus on addressing the current, individual needs of each child in various areas of feeding development, such as food acceptance, utensil use, and self-feeding. Keeping in mind the uniqueness of each child's preferences and development will help the child develop and maintain better eating skills.

Table Talk

Jill works in the preschool room at My Kids Child Care Center. This is her second year at the center. The room has 18 children between 3 and 4½ years of age. Most of the children have attended the center since they were infants.

This year, Jill's group includes three children new to the center. Addilyn, who is 40 months old, is allergic to eggs and wheat. She can have a taste of foods containing these items, but will have a rash and runny nose if she eats more. Jimmy and Jacob are 42-month-old twins, and both are picky eaters. Neither boy eats any vegetables. Jacob drinks milk, while Jimmy prefers diluted juice or water. Both boys eat a variety of breakfast foods but typically do not try the meats and grains offered at lunch time. In addition, Jimmy only sits for 2 to 3 minutes before leaving the table to eat in the book area.

The preschool room has a cooking activity each week. The children either make a snack or prepare a food item to celebrate a child's birthday or an upcoming holiday. Children work together to prepare the ingredients and follow recipes. They work on turn-taking skills, and they learn new vocabulary words related to the ingredients, measurements, and so forth. All snacks and meals are eaten family style with the children seated at kidney-shaped tables. There is one adult for every two tables. Expectations are that children serve themselves and converse during mealtimes.

Jill needs to review upcoming cooking activities to ensure Addilyn can participate in their preparation and taste or eat the results. She also prepared a letter to send home to parents alerting them not to send in foods containing the items that trigger Addilyn's allergies. Jill isn't sure how to work with Jimmy and Jacob. Typically, by the time the children reach the preschool room, picky eating habits are not an issue and children are accustomed to family-style meals. She plans to talk with the toddler room teacher about ways to encourage the twins to explore other types of foods. Until then, she continues to offer both boys the group's regular food items at breakfast, lunch, and snacks.

Discussion Questions

- What additional steps should Jill take to address Addilyn's allergies?
- What suggestions do you have for Jill to try with Jimmy and Jacob to expand their intake?
- How would you approach family-style eating at My Kids Child Care Center?

FEEDING NUGGETS

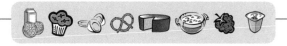

Books

Feeding Your Child For Lifelong Health by Susan Roberts and Melvin B. Heyman (1999)

The Yale Guide To Children's Nutrition by Milosevic William Tamborlane and Joseph Warshaw (1997)

The Baby Food Bible: A Complete Guide To Feeding Your Child From Infancy On by Eileen Behan (2008)

Web Sites

Healthy Meals Resource System:
http://healthymeals.nal.usda.gov

For activities related to allergies:
http://www.fankids.org/

For more information about the USDA's feeding recommendations:
http://www.choosemyplate.gov/

For more information about picky eaters:
www.parenting.com http://www.mypyramid.gov/preschoolers/HealthyHabits/
PickyEaters/makefoodfun.html

For additional information about epinephrine administration and possible side
effects: http://www.ncbi.nlm.nih.gov/pubmedhealth/PMH0000211/
http://www.epipen.com/how-to-use-epipen

For more information about Special Supplemental Nutrition Program for *Women,*
Infants, and Children (WIC):
http://www.fns.usda.gov/wic/
http://www.chtc.org/dl/handouts/20050301/20050301-1.pdf

For more information about adapted utensils and other items:
http://www.onestepahead.com
http://beyondplay.com

For more information about the importance of children helping with food
preparation:
http://teamnutrition.usda.gov/Resources/Nibbles/Nibbles_Newsletter_31.pdf
http://www.mypyramid.gov/preschoolers/HealthyHabits/PickyEaters/
kitchenactivities.html

9

Young Children At Risk for Feeding Difficulties

What You'll Learn in This Chapter

This chapter provides

- An overview of feeding difficulties related to prematurity
- An overview of failure to thrive
- Strategies and specialized interventions to address these issues with examples to illustrate them

■ ■ ■ Food for Thought ■ ■ ■

"Juan was born 3 weeks premature and weighed 5 pounds, 7 ounces. He was on oxygen the first day and had a feeding tube. When the NICU staff took him off the oxygen, they tried to feed him a bottle with breast milk and he couldn't suck on the nipple. They brought him to me to see if he could breastfeed, but he couldn't latch on and suck. He was on a feeding tube with fluids and breast milk for 10 days. A speech therapist came to work on his mouth formations and tried to get his tongue moving to suck milk from the bottle. We used little preemie nipples that were easy to put in his mouth to begin bottle feeding. He preferred hard nipples so when I tried to breastfeed, I had to use a nipple cover. He took milk at home from the one brand of bottles best because they had harder nipples. He only drank 2 ounces at a time and would eat all day long and sleep throughout. Now (at 29 months), he likes the hard, nipple-like hole in the Playtex Sippy cups the best. He wouldn't use soft nipples on bottles or cups."

Evelyn, Parent

"The girls were in the Level 2 Nursery of the NICU for all 10 days they were in the hospital. They were born at 35 weeks. At week 30, I went into preterm labor and spent 5 weeks in the hospital. The girls received breast milk and Neosure. The hospital has a very aggressive feeding regimen for preemies to get their bodies working in the real world as fast as possible. Around day 5 or 6, Josie decided she no longer wanted to drink from a bottle so she was tube fed for 48 hours then went back to the bottle. She did not lose weight during this episode. The doctors said this is fairly normal and to think nothing of it because she went back to bottle feeding. They drank breast milk by bottle from birth until 12 weeks. Then they drank formula. They were on Neosure for weight gain for the first 6 months and then transferred to regular formula because of their awesome weight gain. While breastfeeding/pumping we still added Neosure for the extra calories. Breast milk has 20 calories per ounce and the doctors wanted the babies to get 24 calories. When we started introducing textures, they were okay, not anymore troubled by the texture than any infant eating something new.

Now they eat like typical toddlers—MESSY! They can drink from regular cups, Sippy cups, straws, and sports bottles. They can manipulate their forks and spoons. They even bus their own dishes to the floor in front of the kitchen sink because they cannot reach the sink."

Amanda, Parent

As these scenarios show, many of the typical feeding decisions that a parent makes after a child is born (especially those related to caloric needs) become more complicated when an infant is born early. The more professionals know about special feeding issues with young children born prematurely and about feeding issues related to children with organic or nonorganic failure to thrive, the better they can work with these populations.

PREMATURE INFANTS

An infant is premature if born before 37 weeks of gestation. (An average full-term newborn is born between 38 and 41 weeks of gestation.) Premature infants are categorized into three groups: 1) low birth weight (LBW; under 1,500 grams); 2) very low birth weight (VLBW; under 1,000 grams), or 3) extremely low birth weight (ELBW; less that 800 grams). Good nutrition in infancy is essential for typical growth and optimal development. However, babies born prematurely can have challenges getting adequate nutrition because of their unique nutritional needs, and it is common for premature infants to have feeding disorders. To eat successfully, infants need to have a coordinated suck–swallow–breathe pattern. This skill is under-developed or absent in infants born before 34 weeks of gestation (Bullock,

Woolridge, & Baum, 1990; Dailey Hall, 2001). An inability to coordinate sucking, swallowing, and breathing can lead to lower levels of oxygen in the blood, slowing of the infant's heart rate during feeding, aspiration of milk (breathing it into the lungs), and even cessation of breathing (Tenhaaf, 2008). Feeding disorders are very common among premature infants because they often have weak muscle tone (hypotonia), weak oral movements, and lack of stamina for feedings and other activities—and because they may be irritable, difficult to awaken for feedings, and disorganized behaviorally (Dailey Hall, 2001).

Gastrointestinal Function and Development of the Fetus

At 10 weeks gestation, an infant's gut is formed and rotates into the abdominal cavity. The fetus can swallow amniotic fluid by around 16 weeks gestation, and by 24 weeks, there is some gastrointestinal movement. Actual peristalsis, or muscle contractions in the digestive tract that move food, begin around 29–30 weeks gestation. A fetus develops coordinated sucking and swallowing by 32–34 weeks gestation. By the time the infant is ready to be born, he or she can swallow amniotic fluid which "includes carbohydrates, proteins, fats, electrolytes, immunoglobulin and growth factors" (UCSF Children's Hospital, 2004). An infant born prematurely doesn't have time to develop these crucial processes and skills. Subsequent feeding issues can affect weight gain (Dailey Hall, 2001), later cognitive and developmental outcomes (Daley & Kennedy, 2000), and the foundation of the parent–child relationship (Sheppard & Fletcher, 2007). Because of these concerns, "it is of critical importance to ensure that the early feeding experiences of premature infants are both safe and efficient" (Tenhaaf, 2008. p. 1).

Problems Related to Prematurity

Infants born prematurely are very small, but may have a relatively large head compared to their body size. They have little hair, and their skin may be very thin and pink or red. They have trouble maintaining their body temperature because they have so little fat. They often look perfectly formed, and for the most part, this is true externally. Internally, their organs are formed, but not mature enough to function correctly. Possible problems associated with prematurity are as follows:

- Immature lungs, brain, immune function, and bowel function
- The inability to suck and swallow
- Elevated risk of necrotizing enterocolitis (NEC; a condition in which parts of the bowel die)
- Illnesses that may interfere with adequate enteral feeding, such as respiratory distress syndrome (RDS; difficulty in breathing; occurs in infants with immature lungs) or patent ductus arteriosus (a heart problem in which the vessel between two major arteries does not close)
- Complications due to medical interventions that rule out oral feeding such as umbilical vessel catheters or exchange transfusions (UCSF Children's Hospital at UCSF Medical Center, 2004)

Generally, the lungs of premature infants do not function, which is a critical problem and one of the primary concerns when an infant is born early. Lungs mature in utero at about 34–37 weeks gestation, when the alveoli begin to produce surfactant that reduces surface tension in the lungs so that the air sacs can expand at birth and the infant can breathe. Most premature infants outgrow lung functioning problems in the first few months.

Another complication due to premature birth is immaturity of the brain, which can lead to apnea (forgetting to breathe), bleeding (hemorrhage), or permanent injury to the brain. The immaturity of the brain may also lead to problems with the sucking and swallowing reflexes necessary for feeding.

The premature infant is also at risk for infections due to poor immunity. Infections can put the infant at serious risk and can lead to sepsis (infection in the bloodstream), or necrotizing enterocolitis (inflammatory disease of the intestines caused by feedings that don't pass through the intestine well).

Another issue affecting premature infants (especially those who are critically ill) is extrauterine growth restriction in which premature infants develop severe nutritional deficits in the first weeks after birth and are under weight and height when they go home (Clark et al., 2003). Extrauterine growth restriction is a critical issue related to malnutrition in preterm infants, and more research is necessary to determine the best approach to treatment. Some of the treatments being studied are early feeding, protein requirements, supplementing formula with breast milk (or breast milk with formula), and nutritional support. In addition, the causes of necrotizing enterocolitis and the overall health consequences of extrauterine growth restriction are being studied (Clark et al., 2003).

Nutrition for the Preterm Infant   The nutritional needs of premature infants and their ability to meet nutritional needs by taking in food are different from that of a full-term newborn. A comparison with the uterine environment is important when evaluating appropriate foods for premature infants. A full-term infant swallows amniotic fluid, so foods chosen for the premature infant should be as similar as possible to this fluid. Two foods provided for premature infants that are chemically similar to amniotic fluid are breast milk and formulas designed specifically for premature infants. Premature infants who are receiving breast milk need supplementation with iron, vitamin A, and vitamin D. Infants who are receiving formula should have iron-fortified formulas (Yuen, 1998).

Current growth-rate recommendations for premature infants are parallel to those established for typically developing fetuses/infants of the same gestational age. In the first days after a premature birth, the infant's health is balanced with the need to control the onset of acute neonatal illnesses and the introduction of feeding. This balance is difficult because of the risks of infection for the premature infant and the need to obtain maximum growth rates (American Academy of Pediatrics, 1998). A critical point in the premature infant's feeding development is the successful transition to solid foods. "The successful transition to solid feeding has been postulated as a critical period for feeding development" (Burklow, McGrath, Valerius, & Rudolph, 2002, p. 378).

Feeding Issues in Premature Infants   One of the main feeding issues for premature infants is their inability to coordinate oral-motor behaviors, which limits their ability to suck and feed orally. During development, a fetus begins sucking in utero between 15 and 18 weeks of gestation. By 34 weeks, sucking is usually "stable and well-patterned" (Poore, Zimmerman, Barlow, Wang, & Gu, 2008, p. 920). The transition from gavage feedings (in which a tube is inserted down the throat into the stomach and gravity carries the feeding to the stomach) to oral feed-ing is essential for premature infants, because it shows the reliability of the motor system and allows the infant to be released from the hospital. If the preterm infant cannot feed orally, he may be sent home on gavage feedings, but this is not a pre-ferred practice because it further impedes development of coordinated oral-motor behavior. One sign of readiness for oral feedings is nonnutritive sucking.

A premature infant who has early difficulties with feeding is likely to have later feeding problems. In fact, half of the population of feeding disorder clinics is made up of children who were born prematurely (Poore et al., 2008). The major-ity of premature infants continue to have feeding problems after release from the hospital and may be unable to manage the transition to a solid food diet.

Strategies and Specialized Interventions

According to Greer (2001), a prevalent concern in working with premature infants is what to feed them and when to begin feedings. Feeding issues present a unique challenge to mothers who may struggle to competently feed their premature infants (Pridham, Saxe, & Limbo, 2004; Singer et al., 2003; Thoyre, 2000, 2001). The ability to provide basic care for an infant is an important part of parenting. When an infant is born premature and the parent, especially the mother, is unable to feel competent feeding the infant, there could be consequences related to the infant's health, in-cluding problems with typical growth (DeWitt et al., 1997; Pridham, Brown, Clark, Sondel, & Green, 2002); infant's reactions to stress (Hane, Fox, Polak-Toste, Ghera, & Guner, 2006); and the quality of the mother–infant relationship (Lucarelli, Ambru-zzi, Cimino, D'Olimio, & Finistrella, 2003; Lumeng, Patil, & Blass, 2007).

Types of Feeding Interventions   Several methods can be used to feed pre-mature infants, including gavage, breastfeeding, and bottle feeding. In some in-stances, all three methods may be used in a sequence. In any case, these feeding techniques are still being studied along with preterm infants' abilities and delays that may enhance or detract from feeding.

Gavage Feeding   Gavage feeding is usually recommended when an infant does not have coordinated sucking and swallowing or when the energy used for sucking requires more energy than the calories the infant will consume. A problem-atic cycle can occur if a child's weight loss causes stress that, in turn, causes further weight loss.

Premature infants can sometimes root and grasp a nipple as early as 28 weeks gestation, with some ability for nutritive sucking by 32 weeks gestation. However even by the ages of 32 to 36 weeks gestation, premature infants may have an im-mature sucking pattern that prevents feeding abilities that are typical of full-term newborns (Bragelien, Rokke, & Markestad, 2007). "Most VLBW infants cannot be fed at the breast at birth, and feeding with expressed breast milk through a gastric tube is recommended, sucking skills mature at ~ 34 weeks, when nipple-feeding is introduced" (Berger, Weintraub, Dollberg, Kopolovitz, & Mandel, 2009, p. 1149).

An orogastric tube (inserted through the mouth) is the usual method for ga-vage feedings because infants are usually nose breathers, and a nasogastric tube (NG-tube; inserted through the nostril) can sometimes obstruct breathing. In ad-dition, the repeated insertion of an NG-tube can be irritating. However, orogastric tube feeding can cause other problems. It is sometimes an orally aversive experience for infants, and this can interfere with later feedings if the infant becomes orally defensive. For this reason, when oral feedings are started following use of orogastric tube feedings, an occupational therapist usually works with premature infants to help avoid feeding problems.

Data supports the development of sucking as an "inborn conditioned reflex dependent primarily upon physiological maturation, and [a response that] is capable of being strengthened or changed in accordance with learning experiences" (Bernbaum, Pereira, Watkins, & Packham, 1983, p. 44). Again, nonnutritive sucking is a sign of readiness for oral feedings. In the Bernbaum et al. study (1983), infants who were provided with nonnutritive sucking (a pacifier) during gavage feedings gained more weight even when taking in about the same number of calories as infants who were not provided with nonnutritive sucking. The researchers determined that premature infants provided with a pacifier during gavage feedings may develop more mature sucking reflexes, including better organization and efficient sucking, which facilitates the transition to oral feedings. They posited that the weight gain may be influencing "energy expenditure, or nutrient absorptions, or both" (p. 45).

Breast Milk and Breastfeeding   In 1912, Grulee stated,

> In feeding the premature infants, only one food is to be considered, i.e., breast milk. Any attempt to feed these infants artificially is practically certain to meet with failure. This is so true that success with food other than breast milk may be regarded as the result of good luck rather than good judgment. (p. 233)

The breast milk of mothers of preterm infants is thought to be higher in protein than milk of mothers with full-term infants (Gross, 1983). However, when this information was disseminated in the 1980s, preterm infants still did not have a growth rate similar to intrauterine growth rates. Commercial fortifiers for human milk were developed in the 1990s. Fortifiers are specialized, multinutrient mixtures that are added to breast milk for premature infants in order to provide nutrients for the premature infant (Clark et al., 2003); these supplements come in liquid and powdered formulas. Separate preparations (used in addition to breast milk, but not added to the breast milk) are also available to provide extra nutrients for infants who are receiving primarily breast milk. However, even today, there is no understanding of the precise nutritional needs of infants who are born premature.

The American Academy of Pediatrics supports the use of breast milk for premature infants with one caveat: the premature infant's nutritional status needs to be carefully monitored (2005). Some of the benefits cited by Schanler, Shulman, and Lau (1999) were "host defense, digestion and absorption of nutrients, neurodevelopment, gastrointestinal (GI) function, as well as psychological effect on the mother" (p. 1150). Goals for weight gains in premature infants are based on intrauterine growth rates, and supplements are essential to support the use of breast milk in order to reach those goals. When an infant receives unfortified breast milk, the risks are reduced growth rates and nutritional issues after leaving the hospital (Schanler et al., 1999).

Even though breast milk is beneficial for the preterm infant, breastfeeding a premature infant is not always easy. A premature infant's suck is not as strong that of a full-term infant, and premature infants may not have the coordinated rhythm of breath–suck–swallow. One concern with breastfeeding is the amount of energy expended during the meal. However, measures of resting energy expenditure have found little difference between rates after feeding from the breast versus a bottle of breast milk (Berger, Weintraub, Dollberg, Kopolovitz, & Mandel, 2009).

Not only do premature infants receive all of the same benefits of breastfeeding that term infants receive. Premature infants receive several additional benefits, including anti-infective properties and reduced rates of infections such as necrotizing enterocolitis and bacterial meningitis (Schanler et al., 1999). These benefits are especially important for preterm infants who are more likely to have immature immune systems compared with infants born at term and for whom infections are the major cause of illness and death (Silva, Jones, & Spencer, 2004; Wheeler, 2009). Other benefits include those recognized for full-term infants as described in Chapter 1.

Breastfeeding a premature infant can be difficult. However, these difficulties can be overcome if hospitals provide a family-centered atmosphere for parents. A study by Swift and Scholten (2009) encouraged family-centered care for parents of premature infants and cited several "trigger points" where dynamics between staff and parents can encourage more positive parent–child interactions to enhance infant feeding. The qualitative study results revealed that the parent–child relationship often took a back seat to the child's weight gain. Parents of premature infants are anxious to get their infants home and become frustrated if nursing staff provide inconsistent information (Swift & Scholten, 2009). Many times the mother's health is an issue. Furthermore, the mother's health issues may be related to why the infant was born premature and may affect breastfeeding. However, successful breastfeeding is possible with appropriate supports and help with breastfeeding challenges (Wheeler, 2009). Breastfeeding support must be continued after the mother is released from the hospital.

Bottle Feeding   Bottle feeding a premature infant is very different from bottle feeding a term infant. Unlike an infant born at term, a premature infant may be very sleepy at feeding times, may not be strong enough to drink enough milk to sustain growth, and may have a hard time swallowing and breathing at the same time. NICU nurses help teach parents how to bottle feed premature infants. Premature infants need to be fed within a certain time period or the calories gained from feeding are used up during the feeding. Premature infants also have specific nutrient needs that require different formulations of artificial milk. Several companies offer formulas for premature infants that contain more calories and nutrients than formulas for term infants. With many infant formulas on supermarket shelves, parents may be confused about the best type of formula for their premature infant. Most neonatologists or pediatricians make decisions about the formula an infant should be on. Another bottle feeding option is to get breast milk from a milk bank.

Strategies and Specialized Interventions

To provide safe and efficient oral feedings for infants, the coordination of sucking, swallowing, and breathing needs to be developed (Bullock et al., 1990; Gryboski, 1969). Nutritive sucking is when an infant draws out fluid from the alternation of both suction and expression or only expression (Lau, Sheena, Shulman, & Schanler,

1997). Suction is achieved with negative intraoral pressure when the tongue and jaw are lowered and the naso-pharynx is closed to pull milk out (Dubignon & Campbell, 1969; Lau et al., 1997). Milk is ejected or expressed when the nipple is compressed between the tongue and hard palate (Dubignon & Campbell, 1969; Lau et al., 1997; Waterland, Berkowitz, Stunkard, & Stallings, 1998). Most oral feeding strategies are directed at improving oral feedings by way of the sucking skills (Fucile, Gisel, & Lau, 2005). The next section examines strategies and specialized interventions aimed at improving the premature infant's oral feedings, which is not a simple issue.

Massage   Infant massage has been around in Asian cultures for almost 3,000 years, but it is a relatively new addition in the United States, having arrived in the 1990s. Infant massage offers great benefits to premature and low birth-weight infants because it lowers stress levels (Field, 2001; Field, Hernandez-Reif, & Freedman, 2004). Once the infant is stable and no longer in medical jeopardy, massage may be a recommended treatment. Infants who receive massage gain weight more quickly and are discharged from the hospital sooner than those who do not receive massage (Field, 2001; Field et al., 2004). Infant massage was introduced for premature infants after researchers discovered that nonnutritive sucking, or stimulation of the intraoral cavity, increased weight gain. Researchers hypothesized that by stimulating pressure receptors all over the body, the infant would gain even more weight (Burroughs, Asonye, Anderson-Shanklin, & Vidyasagar, 1978). Infants who received stroking with pressure gained more weight compared to those infants who had light stroking (Fucile & Gisel, 2010; Scafidi et al., 1990). This evidence has increased the amount of tactile–kinesthetic stimulation from almost none to daily massage for premature infants in NICU units.

Occupational Therapy Supports   Pediatric occupational therapists (OTs) are health care professionals who often work with premature babies, young babies, and children with physical problems caused by prematurity, serious illness, and birth defects in order to help them overcome these issues and grow and develop properly. Their goal is to help decrease the impact of disability on children, enhance their quality of life, and enable functional independence. An occupational therapist works with premature babies in several ways. First, an OT can help premature infants learn to breastfeed or drink from a bottle by working on oral stimulation. An OT can also help caregivers position the infant correctly for feeding and assist the parent in encouraging good sensory development in the infant.

Finger Feeding   Other strategies include various feeding methods. An infant can be fed using a finger with a soft, flexible feeding tube attached to it with tape. At the other end of the tube, a container has formula or breast milk for the infant to eat. The infant can suck on the finger, which approximates breastfeeding. Some experts think that the infant is more likely to breastfeed (and to breastfeed more effectively) when finger feeding is used instead of bottle feeding because of the skin-to-skin contact during the feeding and the immediate reinforcement of sucking. The tube can be taped to the breast when the infant is working on transitioning to the breast and also can provide supplemental nutrition to meet the premature infant's unique needs as the infant learns to breastfeed.

Tube Feeding   Tube feedings are a direct way to provide the necessary nutrition for the premature infant. In general, tube feedings are viewed as an interim feeding method until the infant can develop a coordinated suck. Tube feedings are intrusive and can be maladaptive sensory experience for the infant. The following section discusses tube feedings for premature infants.

Bolus Feeding Versus Continuous Feeding   With regard to early GI priming with human breast milk, the bolus tube-feeding method, may supply the best benefit for the preterm infant because premature infants are often unable to synchronize the suck–swallow–breath that is necessary for breastfeeding and bottle feeding. A bolus feeding provides the entire amount of the feeding in a short period of time rather than a delivered it over a long period of time. Recent studies have examined the tube feeding method used with premature infants and found the two most common methods are continuous infusion and bolus feedings (intermittent feedings about every 3 hours; Schanler, Shulman, Lau, Smith, & Heitkemper, 1999). Continuous infusions are given for an unlimited period of time, while bolus feedings usually last about 15 to 30 minutes and deliver the entire meal at one time. The bolus method presents more typical feeding intervals and fasting intervals, which may promote intestinal development and nutrient partitioning or the manipulation of the macronutrient content of the diet (Schanler et al., 1999). Typically, meals are eaten during one sitting, and there is a fast between that meal and the next one. Time between meals helps with the uptake of nutrients and may allow premature infants time for development of the intestines.

Oral Stimulation   The survival of preterm infants has increased immensely over the past 20 years (Guyer et al., 1999; Jadcherla & Shaker, 2001; Kramer et al., 2000). Failure to take oral feedings is one of the most common problems in preterm infants (Fucile, Gisel, & Lau, 2005; Jadcherla & Shaker, 2001; Lau & Hurst, 1999), and oral stimulation has been researched as a way to address this issue. Oral stimulation or oral sensorimotor input is stroking of the perioral and intraoral structures. The structures include the lips, jaw, cheeks, tongue, palate, and gums. Sucking on a nonnutritive pacifier also provides oral stimulation. This stimulation has been shown to improve oral feeding skills in preterm infants.

There are various oral-motor stimulation intervention techniques usually performed by professionals to assist in the oral feeding process. A common technique consists of sensorimotor input and includes cheek and/or chin support along with oral, auditory, kinesthetic, vestibular, and/or visual stimulation (Fucile, Gisel, & Lau, 2002; Gaebler & Hanzlik, 1996; Hill, Kurkowski, & Garcia, 2000; White-Traut et al., 2002). Supporting the infant's chin and/or cheeks during a feeding has been shown to increase the volume the infant takes (Einarsson-Backes, Deitz, Price, Glass, & Hays, 1993). Furthermore, infants have been found to achieve full feedings earlier, to gain weight more quickly, and to be released from the hospital earlier when the oral structures were stroked before or after oral feedings (Gaebler & Hanzlik, 1996; Fucile, Gisel, & Lau, 2002). White-Traut et al. (2002) found that auditory–tactile–visual–vestibular stimulation shortened the infant's hospital stay by assisting in the transition from tube feeding to full oral feeding. Fucile and Gisel (2010) stated that oral and tactile kinesthetic stimulation provides better growth outcomes. Oral-motor stimulation should be performed by a trained professional to avoid sensory and feeding issues that might occur from incorrect procedures.

Perioral Stimulation   This type of stimulation occurs just outside of the mouth and is associated with sensations that might occur during feedings. A qualified professional can tap the infant's cheeks with an index finger, stroke the cheek moving the index finger from the base of the nose toward the ear, and stroke back to the corner of the infant's lips. This should be done on both sides. Another area to stimulate is the lips. A professional can place the index and middle fingers in the middle of the upper then lower lip, gently but quickly stretch the lip outward, and stroke around the lips in a circular manner from one corner to the other.

Intraoral Stimulation   Intraoral stimulation involves stimulation of the tissues inside the mouth. For example, a professional can rub the upper gum with a pacifier to provide gentle, firm pressure. Then the pacifier is moved from the center of the gums to the back and from the back to the center. This series of movements is performed on each side of the infant's mouth for the upper and lower gums. To stimulate the tongue, a pacifier can be used to apply gentle downward pressure on the tongue while moving the pacifier forward. However, if the infant has a protruding tongue, the therapist will only apply downward pressure. To stimulate the premature infant's sucking, a pacifier should be placed in the center of the hard palate and moved forward to bring about a sucking response. Then the infant should be allowed to suck on the pacifier for a short time.

Intraoral stimulation has been shown to be beneficial for oral feeding, but more research is needed because there is inconsistent evidence to document whether oral sensorimotor stimulation is related to weight gain in premature infants (Fucile & Gisel, 2010). An underdeveloped cardiorespiratory system, central nervous system, and/or oral musculature may lead preterm infants to experience oral feeding difficulties. Research studying oral stimulation programs has found positive benefits relating to feeding behaviors in preterm infants (Tenhaaf, 2008). An infant born before 30 weeks remains in the hospital for about 11–12 weeks on average. Often, medical procedures—such as placement of a nasogastric or orogastric tube, placement of endotracheal tube, and suctioning—provide the infant's only oral-motor stimulation experiences during this hospitalization. These experiences are often aversive, and they fail to prepare the infant for later feeding. This puts the premature infant at greater risk of a feeding disorder. More research is needed to better understand the role of early oral feeding (Fucile, Gisel, & Lau, 2002).

To summarize, most efforts to enhance the acceptance of oral feedings are aimed at the infant's sucking skills. Children who have medical complications that are related to their prematurity and that require respiratory support should have "ongoing oral-motor feeding intervention" to optimally prepare them for oral feeding (Burklow, McGrath, Valerius, & Rudolph, 2002, p. 373). Daley and Kennedy (2000) asserted that for the best oral feeding outcomes in premature infants, care providers should consider the infant's gestational age and development, attempt to minimize the period of time during which the infant is not receiving oral feedings, and make sure the infant is receiving oral stimulation and oral support.

FAILURE TO THRIVE

Olsen, Skovgaard, Weile, Petersen, and Jorgensen (2010) wrote the following about failure to thrive (FTT):

It is recognized that a common characteristic in pediatric weight faltering is relative undernutrition, and clinical studies have found FTT closely linked to feeding problems and parent–child relationship difficulties; population studies have found associations between weight faltering and oral-motor difficulties, early feeding problems, compromised appetites and eating behavior problems, and difficult parent–child interaction and maternal psychopathology. (2010, p. 370)

The idea that it is not the food that makes a child healthy, but the process of feeding, was recognized by the pediatric world more than 100 years ago, when Henry Chapin carried out a trial on babies and young children in institutions for the destitute (Rudolf, 2008). "Chapin revealed that babies placed in institutions in 10 different cities in the United States had virtually a 100% death rate despite food and medical care, dying from what the doctors called 'failure to thrive' or 'marasmus'—wasting away" (Montagu, 1986, p. 97). To deal with this problem, Chapin created a new system for caring for infants by finding homes for them rather than having them remain in institutions (Antunovic, 2009). This was a marked change from previous processes, so studies were performed to determine the causes of marasmus. It appeared that infants were commonly affected by it even in the "'best homes, hospitals, and institutions and among babies receiving the best and most careful attention'" (Montagu, 1986, p. 99). Finally, Chapin found that those infants in the poorest home seemed to be "thriving" because mothers in these homes held, cuddled, patted, and nurtured their infants (Autunovic, 2009, p. 6). Mortality rates dropped precipitously once hospitals implemented programs where nurses were to "pick up the infants, carry them around, and 'mother' them" at least three times a day (Montagu, 1986, p. 99). Chapin's study provided one of the first understandings that infants can have adequate food and still die if they are not nourished emotionally.

In the 1970s, there was an emphasis on the critical nature of the home environment to promote optimum development. This emphasis led to the belief that failure to thrive could be an important indicator of child abuse and neglect, and as a result, according to Rudolf (2008), "poor weight gain in infant/child is still commonly equated with poor parenting and parents are blamed and responsible for weight gain" (Rudolf, 2008, p. 232). Furthermore, Rudolf pointed out that eating issues observed in children with FTT are not "unique," but are more severe than those not diagnosed with FTT (p. 230).

Pediatricians divided FTT into organic (OFTT) and nonorganic (NOFTT) varieties. For the condition to be classified as OFTT, a child has to have a diagnosis or clinical symptoms (e.g., prematurity, cleft lip and palate, cystic fibrosis, or heart disease) that increase the likelihood of being underweight due to feeding issues. Some such diagnoses show energy expenditure in the children that compromise caloric intake. For example, some children with cerebral palsy require more energy than they can consume to produce that energy.

FTT is not just a diagnosis for infants who are underweight, it can be applied to newborns who appear to be healthy. This is because an oral-motor dysfunction can lead to feeding problems ranging from a poor or disorganized suck to behavior issues involving resistance to feeding due to gastroesophogeal reflux disease. In toddlers, FTT can be related to texture issues (Ramsay, Gisel, McCusker, Bellavance, & Platt, 2002). There is also evidence that, like other developmental issues, feeding issues can emerge over time in infants and toddlers who did not previously exhibit these issues (Locklin, 2005).

Developmental Considerations and FTT   A study by Core (2003) found that "nutritional problems occurring earlier in life may have subtle effects later in an area of the brain that controls much of our behavior, thought, and emotion" (p. 17). The first years are critical for later mental development, and early problems can have permanent negative effects. Researchers found that many children with FTT, particularly boys, have difficulties with reading, spelling, and arithmetic as they age, and that the children who developed typically were more efficient at processing information. Children with FTT were found to have slower word recognition and were seen questioning their own decisions during testing, indicating an element of uncertainty in information processing (Core, 2003). The frontal lobe is involved with behavior, social judgment, reasoning, planning, speech, movement, emotions, and problem-solving: important functions that are referred to by psychologists as "executive functions." Research has found reduced responses to environmental stimulation in children who have FTT, which may show a relationship between the brain's frontal lobe functioning and FTT (Core, 2003).

Symptoms of Failure to Thrive

OFTT refers to a condition in which—due to a diagnosed condition or disability such as cerebral palsy—a child does not gain sufficient weight or maintain growth as appropriate for his or her age. There are a number of differential diagnoses in children who may have FTT. These include "normal child of short stature, idiosyncratic growth pattern, breastfeeding failure, formula feed errors, nonorganic failure to thrive, severe developmental delay, chronic infection (urinary tract, lung), gastrointestinal disorders, metabolic disease, and congenital heart disease" (Marcovitch, 1994, p. 35).

NOFTT refers to infants whose growth is "faltering," but for whom no identified organic condition has been diagnosed (Batchelor, 2008). Issues that may precede a diagnosis of NOFTT, as cited by Panetta, Magazzu, Sferlazzas, Lombardo, Magazzu, and Lucanto (2008) include "vomiting, diarrhea, poor appetite, food restriction and/or feeding rituals, recurrent abdominal pain, vivacity, constipation, irregular bowel movements, and abdominal distension" (p. 1281). Furthermore,

> Symptoms of failure to thrive may include: Lack of appropriate weight gain, irritability, easily fatigued, excessive sleepiness, lack of age-appropriate social response (i.e., smile), avoids eye contact, lack of molding to the mother's body, does not make vocal sounds, delayed motor development. (Lucile Packard Children's Hospital at Stanford, 2011, p. 1)

Other researchers have stated that symptoms of NOFTT include "minor infections, vomiting, diarrhea, behavioral problems and altered eating behavior" (Maggioni & Lifshitz, 1995, p. 792), along with "fist-clenching, apathy toward their caregivers, decreased motor activity, infantile anorexia" (p. 800).

NOFTT has a negative connotation when referring to the condition of a child who has parents who are neglectful or abusive and when the NOFTT has no specific causes (Lucile Packard Children's Hospital at Stanford, 2011; Rudolf, 2008). A caregiver's success feeding an infant depends mainly on the intricate interaction between the caregiver and child. However, problems can arise due to temperamental characteristics or a lack of a goodness-of-fit between a parent and child (Wright, Parkinson, & Drewett, 2006). Most physicians, when no physical reason or diagnosis can account for the infant's faltering growth, look for a cause external to the infant. Sometimes NOFTT is viewed as a syndrome that consists of slow weight gain or growth, delayed development, behavior that may not be typical of the infant, and/or interaction difficulties within the caretaker–infant relationship (Maggioni & Lifshitz, 1995). In over half of children in one NOFTT study, the infants' history, weight gain patterns, and food diaries provided evidence that the infants were undernourished. In fact, by a little over 1 year of age, children who are diagnosed with FTT have a delayed progression from purées to solid foods, poorer than expected appetites, and a diet that is restricted to a small number of foods (Wright, 2000).

Prevalence of Failure to Thrive

Only about 1% to 10% of infants are diagnosed with failure to thrive, and the most common cause of the diagnosis is undernutrition (Daniel, Kleis, & Cemeroglu, 2008; O'Brien, Heycock, Hanna, Jones, & Cox, 2004; Wright, Callum, Birks, & Jarvis, 1998). According to Dunne, Sneddon, Iwaniec, and Stewart (2007), FTT may account for 50% of the growth-faltering pediatric population. This is a fairly common problem (Daniel et al., 2008; Panetta, Magazzu, Sferlazzas, Lombardo, Magazzu, & Lucanto, 2008).

Causes for Organic Failure to Thrive

An infant or young child whose growth is faltering is diagnosed with OFTT if the cause of the faltering growth is a medical or physical condition such as genetic syndrome, endocrine disorder, neurological dysfunction, complications of premature birth, or other medical illness that hampers feeding and typical bonding interactions between parents and infants (Dunne et al., 2007; Lucile Packard Children's Hospital at Stanford, 2011; Sheila, 2006). Deficient intake is one cause of OFTT. This can be related to breastfeeding failures, errors in artificial feeding, impaired intellectual or motor development, or anatomical anomalies such as cleft palate or congenital heart disease (Marcovitch, 1994).

Rabinowitz, Katturupalli, and Rogers (2010) cited the following prenatal and postnatal causes of OFTT. Prenatal causes included prematurity with complications, maternal malnutrition, toxic exposure in utero, maternal alcohol use, maternal smoking, maternal use of medications, infections, intrauterine growth retardation, and chromosomal abnormalities. Postnatal causes included inadequate caloric intake, lack of appetite (such as that caused by chronic illness), inability to suck or swallow, vomiting, therapy used to treat a primary illness (e.g., chemotherapy), developmental delay, GI pain or impaired peristalsis, poor absorption and/or use of nutrients in the GI tract, increased metabolic demand, HIV infection, malignancy, cardiopulmonary diseases and inflammatory conditions, renal failure, and hyperthyroidism (p. 8). Gastro-esophageal reflux also has been found to be a common specific cause of OFTT.

Causes for Nonorganic Failure to Thrive

In order for a child to be diagnosed with NOFTT, all other diagnoses are excluded, and the child shows poor growth without a medical condition.

> Suggested causes for nonorganic failure to thrive have included emotional deprivation, inadequate nutrition, and a complex interaction whereby the difficulties of rail-

ing a 'sickly child' may contribute to parental psychological distress and thus to a disrupted mother–child relationship (Marcovitch, 1994, p. 37).

Maternal anxiety, depression, or disorganization may lead to the incapability to satisfy a difficult child's nutritional needs (Marcovitch, 1994). In general, "families of infants with FTT are highly stressed with poverty, violence, substance abuse, criminality, and dysfunctional relationships" (Benoit, 2005, p. 344). NOFTT can start prenatally as malnourishment during pregnancy, which could be due to poverty or an eating disorder (Rabinowitz, Katturupalli, & Rogers, 2010), causing the fetus to be smaller than normal or small for gestational age. The most commonly cited reason for NOFTT is inadequate nutrition for age. Postnatal causes suggest that environmental conditions are responsible, rather than biological, genetic, or organic disease causes (Sheila, 2006).

These environmental conditions include, but are not limited to, psychological, social, and/or economic problems within a family. Parents, most notably the mother, may not be able to care for the infant for reasons such as a lack of knowledge of caretaking, emotional issues related to upbringing, or addiction to alcohol or drugs (Lucile Packard Children's Hospital at Stanford, 2011; Sheila, 2006). NOFTT can also be related to "distorted social stimulation" that leads to poor weight gain, developmental delay, and inappropriate behaviors (Maggioni & Lifshitz, 1995). The onset of feeding problems and NOFTT before the age of 2 months have been associated with early child-related vulnerability and poor regulatory ability in combination with sociodemographic risk factors. Feeding, eating problems, and NOFTT after the age of 2 months may be linked to problematic mother–child relationships (Olsen et al., 2010). Much still needs to be investigated because children who are diagnosed with NOFTT may have a metabolic issue that is related to inefficient processing of nutrients compared to typically developing children. This in turn could lead to defects in the central nervous system, such as attention deficit disorder and other problems that affect attention and learning (Core, 2003).

Risk factors related to the parent–child relationship and the infant's ability to regulate feeding and eating should be explored (Olsen et al., 2010). Skuse, Gill, Reilly, Wolke, and Lynch (1995) found that an NOFTT diagnosis may precede poor parenting in some parent–child dyads in a small number of cases. Therefore, it is important to investigate behaviors at meals and psychosocial interactions in relation to the child's intake. "Poor parenting and family dysfunction can negatively affect a child's energy intake" (Olsen, Skovaard, Weile, Petersen, & Jorgensen, 2010, p. 380). Families with dysfunctional behaviors are also associated with infants who may have a NOFTT diagnosis. Some problems may include maternal depression, maternal substance abuse, family conflict, and low levels of emotional support for the mother (Olsen et al., 2010).

Sometimes, the reasons for failure-to-thrive are related to the infant's behaviors. NOFTT can develop in infants who do not express hunger to caregivers, infants with poor suck or coordinated oral-motor abilities, or infants who refuse to eat (Olsen et al., 2010). Younger children diagnosed with NOFTT are more likely to have an organic reason that is associated with the disordered eating. The following account demonstrates the link between an organic cause and feeding difficulties.

Amaya (who has full trisomy 18) was born full-term by cesarean section. Because she would not eat at birth, an NG-tube was inserted. About a week after she was born, she began to take a little bit from the bottle. Nursing was attempted, but she did not have a strong enough suck, so the parents went back to the bottle. Amaya started off drinking less than an ounce of formula every 3 hours. The remainder of the feeding was put through the NG-tube. Once she began eating an ounce at every feeding (when she was about 2 weeks old), the NG-tube was removed.

Strategies and Specialized Interventions for Failure to Thrive

Physicians often push families to increase caloric intake for children who are not gaining weight. Often these suggestions are made with little or no understanding of reasons why the child has poor eating skills. However, according to Marcovitch (1994), if the child is admitted to the hospital, a multifaceted approach is used

> to observe the infant's feeding behavior and mother–child interaction; to see whether the infant's weight gain returns to normal when he or she is removed from the family; to decide whether laboratory investigation is indicated after all; to gather evidence for use in child protection proceedings. (p. 38)

FTT is often a multifaceted problem requiring the skills of a feeding team. It is imperative that a team approach be used for this diagnosis because of the complicated nature of FTT. Strategies for both OFTT and NOFTT are discussed in the following section. However, because the two conditions are treated differently, each condition is also discussed separately.

Due to the complicated nature of the diagnosis, a feeding team is a must for treatment of both OFTT and NOFTT. A feeding team for a child with FTT should include a pediatrician, a nutritionist, a social worker, a physical or occupational therapist, a pediatric feeding therapist, and a qualified mental health provider. (See Chapter 5 for a more complete discussion of feeding teams.) A pediatric feeding therapist is usually a speech-language pathologist (SLP) who has additional training in the physiology of the oropharyngeal phase of swallowing. Although most children with FTT can be treated as outpatients, many sequential visits are necessary (Rabinowitz et al., 2004). During these visits, weight gain and daily calorie intake are documented. Once problems are identified, courses of therapy (e.g., behavioral feeding programs) can be assigned.

Screening   The appropriate diagnosis of OFTT or NOFTT needs to be made so that appropriate treatment can be provided. Prior to a diagnosis of NOFTT, a child should have a thorough neurological and developmental assessment to rule out issues that might be tied to OFTT. Several studies (e.g., Reilly, Skuse, Mathisen, & Wolke, 1995; Reilly, Skuse, Wolke, & Stevenson, 1999) have found an association between children diagnosed with NOFTT and significant oral-motor dysfunction (OMD).

It is important to have a developmental feeding therapist do an oral-motor evaluation in terms of feeding. An OMD can be subtle, but have significant impact on a child's development and neurological functioning. Some children do well with formula or breast milk, but experience feeding problems when solids are introduced. Such issues can be related to an OMD that only comes to light with the need for a mature feeding pattern that includes solid foods.

Treatment at Feeding Clinics/Feeding Centers   For severe feeding issues that cannot be resolved with the previously described strategies, there are inpatient, out-patient, and day clinics. These programs are interdisciplinary and provide treatment for patients with impaired oral intake. Goals for the child may involve one or more of the following: decreasing oral defensiveness; selecting appropriate feeding bottles, nipples, and utensils; developing or identifying compensatory strategies to increase the child's food intake; and increasing the amount and variety of foods accepted.

The first step is to determine whether nutrition is the central issue. Supplements are often added to the child's diet. Also, negative feeding behaviors are addressed, and parent education is provided. In some programs, underlying feeding problems are addressed separately from the parents; then the parents are brought in, and the child is transitioned to eating with the parents. Some changes might include the child being fed an accepted food, which then is modified in some way—taste, texture, or quantity—for each trial. Each session ends on a positive note so all associations with food are positive. Consequence-based procedures are also conducted with the child. Consider the following example, which describes a typical sequence of events.

Anthony was diagnosed with FTT when he was 8 months old and weighed only 12 pounds. He had to have an NG-tube and then a G-tube. However, when he was transitioned to formula he was not eating enough. Next, his parents found an intensive feeding program were they trained on how to deal with his feeding behaviors, such as refusals (turning his head, throwing food, vomiting, etc.). They also learned how to use motivation (e.g., a high-energy toy) to create a fun eating atmosphere. The eating program was intensive, being performed 5 times a day, but it helped to break his pattern of refusing to eat. He had an occupational therapist who worked on sensory issues with his mouth and textures for an hour each day. The first successful event was when he started drinking one ounce. So far he has never taken more than 5 ounces, but his feedings are much better now. The current goal is for Anthony to consistently take about 4 ounces at each meal.

Treatment of Organic Failure to Thrive

As indicated previously, OFTT is caused by a medical issue. Therefore, a good understanding of the etiology of the condition and its effects on feeding and nutrition is crucial to the development of a treatment plan. Once the organic reason for OFTT is diagnosed, specific therapy should be immediately started.

Oral-Motor Care   A feeding therapist is likely to be part of the feeding team. A feeding therapist is especially helpful for developing an understanding of the child's oral-motor abilities and limitations. This specialist helps to identify the child's feeding strengths and challenges as related to oral-motor capabilities. For example, a child may be able to take thicker liquids, but not pureed solids. It is critical to the child's weight gain to have a comprehensive understanding of the child's feeding deficits (Rabinowitz et al., 2010). Planning for feedings should commence with the team to discuss the possible outcomes.

Nutrition/Diet Supplements   Some breastfed infants may be supplemented with formula. Young infants may not be making the appropriate weight gains after birth. Therefore, pediatricians often suggest formula for supplementation, and/or they may suggest more frequent feedings. For toddlers, foods that are higher in fats (e.g., sour cream, heavy cream, ice cream, butter, cheese, and oils) are often added to the child's diet. Young children with cerebral palsy often eat without consuming enough calories to meet their needs, so calorie-dense foods are identified. (See Chapter 8 for more information on supplements.) Sometimes when there is no weight gain, a trial of NG-tube feeding is the next plan of action to see if the child can absorb enough energy in order to grow (Rabinowitz et al., 2004).

Even when a medical issue is resolved, the feeding difficulties (e.g., negative interactions) it caused may continue. Batchelor (1999) discussed a negative feeding cycle in which difficulties with feeding lead to weight loss, which leads to stress in those who care for the child, which leads back to difficulties in feeding. (This cycle is illustrated in Figure 9.1.)

Treatment of Nonorganic Failure to Thrive

Treatment for NOFTT is complex and often addresses the nature of the child's environmental and psychosocial deprivation (Venkateshwar & Raman, 2000). Treatment may range from dietary advice to intensive home-based work with parents. The nature of treatment depends on the outcome of observations and understandings about the central issues related to the child's faltering growth. Although nutrition should be the basis for any intervention, it is not the sole answer in NOFTT.

Treatment of NOFTT is dependent on factors such as the child's age, overall health, medical history, extent of symptoms, and tolerance for medical interventions, along with the expectations for the course of the condition and the causes of the condition. For psychological causes, treatments should include improving the interactions between family members and the home environment (Batchelor, 2008). In NOFTT, it is important to understand the parents' views of what is going on with their child, but observations (especially in the home) are necessary for improving outcomes. Therefore, strategies include observation and follow-up discussions with caregivers to facilitate better a feeding environment. If these strategies are not helping, more intensive therapies can be employed.

Feeding Teams for NOFTT Treatment planning for NOFTT usually requires the involvement of a feeding team. For the NOFTT feeding team, a psychiatrist, psychologist, or family therapist should be included because there is likely to be a psychosocial issue. NOFTT is a complex, multifaceted issue and with an appropriately specialized feeding team, these issues can be addressed.

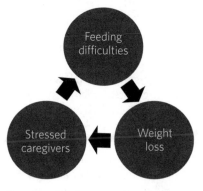

Figure 9.1 Cycle illustrating difficulties in feeding

Parent Education   Some cases of NOFTT are related to parents' lack of knowledge and inexperience. Young parents, parents with less education, and inexperienced parents do not always understand the nutritional and developmental needs of infants and young children. Parents must be educated regarding not only their child's nutritional needs, but also their social, emotional, cognitive, and physical needs. One study found that parents were feeding their children only 60%–94% of what the children needed nutritionally because the parents were concerned about obesity and other health related issues (Pugliese, Weyman-Daum, Moses, & Lifshitz, 1987). In light of such deficiencies in understanding, professionals working with the family need to consider the parents' ability to respond appropriately to the child's needs as well as the child's developmental level. Some parents may misread an infant's cues and try to play with an infant who is actually expressing hunger. During a meal, adults may misread signs that children are full or want more, creating a negative association with meals that may interfere with the infant's feeding.

Parents may also need education on how to properly mix formulas, breastfeeding techniques, interactions during feedings between the infant and caregiver(s), and caloric intake. Sometimes parents may add too much water to formula, thus providing inadequate nutrients for the growing infant. Also, breastfeeding problems should be investigated. If the mother is breastfeeding, an observation should be performed to make sure proper technique is used so that the infant is getting enough to eat. If the technique is incorrect, education and consultation with a breastfeeding educator might help ameliorate the problem. Observations during feedings should also provide adequate information to help the parents with their interactions with their infant. A team member can improve mealtimes by educating the parents on appropriate behaviors and desirable changes.

Parent Psychosocial Support and Therapy   Mothers who have mental illnesses, such as depression or anxiety, that are related to psychological trauma or parent–child issues are more likely to have problems responding appropriately to their infants or young children. The mother's mental health is associated with eating problems in very young infants as well as young children with more severe issues leading to NOFTT (Benoit, 2005). A parent may need psychological counseling to deal with issues that affect her ability to properly care for the child. For example, a parent who shows disgust at the typical feeding habits of a 2-year-old would need to learn to accept these behaviors in order to avoid problems with the parent–child relationship which may affect feeding. Enhancing the parent–child relationship can improve outcomes leading the mother to better nurture her child and to be less disgusted by typical behaviors.

Teams should also facilitate access to formal and informal support resources within the community, such as child care and parent health resources in order to help parent to become more self-sufficient (Belsky, 1984). Parents need support and guidance in problem-solving and decision-making for themselves and their children, and this is especially true for parents who are having problems. This kind of support improves the quality of parenting.

In working with parents in providing psychosocial support, professionals need to observe parent–child interactions and define issues that are of concern. These issues may be related to the infant, the parent's past history, or current relationships. For example, parents may need help resolving familial conflicts. Skills and supports for the parents will assist them in taking care of conflicts and attending to the parenting role. Also, parents may need help understanding their feelings, reactions, and defense strategies. Such an understanding helps parents develop healthier patterns of interaction. An infant mental health specialist is a professional who can help promote positive parent–child interactions and healthy development in the infant and young child while encouraging parental competencies.

Behavioral Feeding Programs   Due to the complicated nature of NOFTT, a behavioral feeding program is often necessary. Maladaptive feeding behaviors are frequently a part of the infant or young child's repertoire, even though these behaviors have negative consequences on development and health. When NOFTT is related to the parent–child relationship, the associations between the child's actions and the parent's actions have formed the disordered feeding that lead to NOFTT. These associations must be extinguished while new ones are being created.

Principles of learning such as those discussed in Chapter 2 (following the heading "Behaviorist Theory") are used to treat NOFTT. For example, positive behaviors may be rewarded, and negative reinforcement may be used to increase more positive eating behaviors. For example, a child may receive a desired reward after showing a behavior that is related to positive eating, such as touching a fork to the lips. Over time, this behavior becomes associated with positive, rather than negative, events. Approximations also may be rewarded. A child who avoids sitting at the table and eating may be rewarded for small steps toward that goal. The child may be rewarded first for looking toward the table, then for getting closer to the table, then for sitting at the table, then for eating a bite at the table, and finally, for eating a meal at the table.

Rewards are also given when children demonstrate a desired behavior like taking a bite of food. Gradually, the difficulty of the task that is rewarded is increased. For example, rewards may be provided for sitting in a highchair or accepting a feeding utensil. Later, the reward may be given only after the child dips the feeding utensil into the food. Negative behaviors—such as vomiting, head turning, and refusing to take food—are ignored. Often when a behavior that was formerly rewarded with attention (even negative attention) is ignored, it will initially increase before it decreases. The child will increase the behavior in an effort to gain the same response because it is reassuring and comfortable, but once the child realizes that the behavior no longer gets attention, the behavior will decrease.

NOFTT is difficult to resolve. Sometimes there are short-term nutritional gains in weight, but improvement in social-emotional well-being and developmental benefits continue to lag (Benoit, 2005). NOFTT is a multidimensional issue with serious impacts on a young child's development, health, and social-emotional functioning (Benoit, 2005). It is not easily or simply resolved.

SUMMARY

This chapter discussed two issues related to feeding and to future development: prematurity and FTT. For premature infants, nutrient content and weight gain are primary concerns. Massage and oral stimulation may help the infant with weight gain, and specialists such as occupational therapists are usually available in the NICU.

On the other hand, FTT—especially NOFTT—may be more complicated and difficult to treat. One quote from Wright, Parkinson, and Drewett (2006) stands out: "The challenge for clinicians in the future is to establish and formally evaluate preventive and treatment approaches that reduce, rather than increase, maternal anxiety, while maintaining or increasing their child's dietary intake" (p. 1269). FTT is a complicated issue that defies simple solutions such as simply having the child eat more. Professionals must recognize the interpersonal issues that may be related to an infant's lack of weight gain and subsequent growth faltering. As discussed in Chapter 2, family dynamics and parent–child attachment may be an issue. FTT is a complex issue with many questions still needing answers.

TABLE TALK

Jim and Judy were elated at the birth of their second daughter, Madison, a vigorous 8-pound, 8-ounce infant. Judy had successfully breastfed her first daughter for 2 years, so it did not occur to her that Madison might have difficulty breastfeeding. However, within a week, things were not going as expected. Madison was not latching or sucking well, and when she did take in a significant amount of breast milk, it came right back up.

At 2 weeks of age, Maddie weighed only 7.4 pounds. She had lost almost 10% of her birth weight. At a weekly monitoring appointment, the pediatrician, Dr. Williams, expressed concern over Maddie's poor weight gain and her vomiting soon after each feeding. She suggested that Maddie be positioned at a 30-degree angle in her crib for sleep. Judy reassured Dr. Williams that she would continue to nurse frequently around the clock. Within a few weeks, it became apparent that nothing had improved. Maddie stayed hydrated because Judy nursed her almost hourly. She had plenty of wet diapers saturated with urine, but few bowel movements. Maddie had a poor latch onto Judy's breasts, but Judy's abundant milk supply, which she could express into Maddie's mouth, allowed Maddie to gain at least 1 or 2 ounces prior to each pediatric visit.

Jim and Judy were becoming more and more concerned about their daughter's lack of sufficient weight gain, but felt they were doing everything they could. They considered stopping breastfeeding, but they knew that breastfeeding is one of the best sources for feeding an infant and wanted to make sure Maddie got the nutrients she needed.

Discussion Questions

- What do you think about Jim and Judy's situation?
- What suggestions do you have for increasing Maddie's weight?

FEEDING NUGGETS

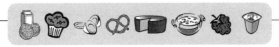

Books

Primary Care of the Premature Infant by Dara Brodsky and Mary Ann Ouellette (2008)

Neonatal Nutrition and Metabolism by Patti J. Thureen and William W. Hay (2006)

Feeding and Nutrition in the Preterm Infant by Elizabeth Gowan Jones, Caroline King (2005)

Children who Fail to Thrive: A Practice Guide by Dorota Iwaniec (2004)

Failure to Thrive and Pediatric Undernutrition: A Transdisciplinary Approach by Daniel
   B. Kessler and Peter Dawson (1999)

Web Sites

For information about breastfeeding premature infants:
www.preemie-l.org/bfaq.html
www.llli.org/nb/nbpremature.html

For information about massage for premature infants:
http://video.about.com/preemies/Preemie-Infant-Massage.htm

For information about failure to thrive:
http://kidshealth.org/parent/growth/growth/failure_thrive.html
http://www.umm.edu/ency/article/000991.htm

10

Young Children With Sensory-Based Feeding Issues

What You'll Learn in This Chapter

This chapter provides

- An overview of sensory integration issues and issues related to feeding
- An overview of autism and issues related to feeding
- Examples of strategies and specialized interventions to address these issues

■ ■ ■ FOOD FOR THOUGHT ■ ■ ■

"Jed's parent and teacher were very concerned with his eating behaviors. At 14 months, he would soon be advancing to the 15–24-month classroom, where all the children are self-fed and served only table foods. A specialist from Archway (an early intervention program) visited the center and explained that Jed has sensory processing issues with textures of foods. She suggested that Jed have one-on-one interaction during meals. Jed also has negative behaviors with foods and throws them on the floor. The specialist explained that

when she works with him in the home, he puts foods that he does not want off to the side."
Wendy, Child Care Provider

"Nate, who is 6 years old, has severe autism, many dental problems, and a very restricted diet. He refuses food, has tantrums at meals, and eliminates items from his diet when the brand, shape, color, size, texture, or taste of a preferred item is unfamiliar or altered in any dimension. Currently, he eats 27 out of 91 foods listed on a Food Inventory. Most days his diet consists of soda, flavored water, Little Debbie Nutty bars, cookies, granola bars, crackers, and chips."
Holly, Board Certified Behavior Analyst

"Billy, who is 48 months old, has autism and peanut allergies. He is also unable to hold a fork, so he uses his hands. He doesn't have access to special cutting utensils. He also flaps his hand while he eats, so we challenge him to focus and try to help him with his fine motor skills."
Whitney, Early Childhood Student and Child Care Provider

Each of the previous examples illustrates the uniqueness of sensory systems. People experience taste, texture, color, size, and smells in very different ways. Three people might describe the flavor of a particular food differently. The first person might find it intense, the second person might think it perfect, and the third person might describe it as bland. Our senses also help us understand our environment (Dunn, 2001). When a person walks downstairs, but can't see her feet, she is more likely to stumble than if she can see her feet. Sensation, then, affects our behavior. If a smell does not meet our expectations, that food may not be appetizing. For example, if your tomato soup smelled of potatoes and celery or smelled of meat, it might be unappetizing. This chapter describes strategies and outcomes related to feeding problems with underlying sensory processing problems including sensory integration dysfunction and autism spectrum disorders.

SENSORY INTEGRATION

Each of us has environmental sensitivities, but for the most part they do not interfere with daily living. Some people are sensitive to room temperature, but they dress appropriately so that their sensitivity does not interfere with daily tasks. Others have certain food preferences and are sometimes referred to as "picky eaters," but selective eating does not interfere with their ability to lead normal lives. However, when an individual's sensory information does not integrate in a productive way, there can be problems leading to sensory integration dysfunction. The term *sensory integration* was defined by Ayres over 30 years ago as "the neurological process that organizes sensation from one's own body and from the environment and makes it possible to use the body effectively within the environment" (1979, p. 11). The five main senses are touch (tactile), sound (auditory), sight (visual), taste (gustatory), and smell (olfactory). Two other sources of sensory stimulation are: vestibular (movement and balance) and proprioception (joint and muscle sense).

SENSORY INTEGRATION DYSFUNCTION

There is a growing knowledge base regarding sensory processing problems and the possible effects on daily routines and activities (Kranowitz, 2005; Lynch &

Simpson, 2004). Sensory processing problems occur when an individual is unable to process incoming environmental stimuli in a productive way (Dunn & Westman 1997; 2001). For example, one child may find clothing feels really itchy; tags may need to be removed from clothing before this child can wear it. Another child may get lost or panic easily with small changes in the arrangement of a room. Sensory processing issues can also be manifested as feeding problems. For example, a child may refuse to eat foods that feel too lumpy, such as oatmeal or yogurt with added fruit. Also, a child may claim that a food smells really bad or overstate information about the temperature of foods. These reactions may seem extreme, but usually are true to the experiences of the child.

Dunn and Westman (1997) proposed a conceptual model describing how sensory processing issues may affect development in young children. The model describes the interaction between the child's neurological threshold and the child's behavioral response to the environment. The central nervous system is responsible for how information from the environment is interpreted. In Dunn's model, a neurological threshold is the amount of stimulation needed for a child's nervous system to respond to the environment. Everyone has different thresholds, and some people have lower thresholds, requiring very little variation in environmental stimuli for that individual to notice and respond (Dunn, 2007). Other people have higher thresholds, requiring a great deal of stimulation to notice changes in the environment. For example, one child may need a great deal of texture or very intense flavors in her foods to evoke responses from the nervous system, while another child would be overstimulated by those same foods and experience a nervous system response to very slight changes. A child's neurological threshold guides behavior and sensory integration during daily routines and activities (Dunn, 2001; Dunn & Westman, 1997).

An individual's neurological threshold may or may not be paired with a behavioral response which is the "manner in which the young child responds in relation to the thresholds" (Dunn, 1997b, p. 24). The responses are on a continuum. "At one end of the continuum, persons have a passive strategy" (Dunn, 2007, p. 85). In other words, they do not change their setting, but rather remain in the situation even though it may make them uncomfortable. On the other end of the continuum, "persons utilize an active strategy" (Dunn, 2007, p. 85); the person leaves an uncomfortable setting or changes it in some way to fit better with their neurological threshold. For example, if a child with a passive behavioral strategy was being fed a food with too much texture, he or she would eat it, but become very irritable and fussy. On the other hand, a child with an active strategy would refuse to eat and try to leave the situation. In this comparison, the sensory responses of the two children are similar, but the behavioral responses are different. Children have unique responses to the environment and to their sensory perceptions of that environment.

A child's responses only become a problem when they interfere with his or her ability to engage in typical daily activities, such as eating. Sensory modulation— the ability to regulate information in order to generate an appropriate response— is an important part of appropriate interactions in any environment. Infants and toddlers with poor sensory modulation are likely to have maladaptive feeding behaviors or behaviors that negatively affect feeding behaviors. For example, a child might cry every time he or she comes to the dining table and fuss during a meal or play with food instead of eating it. The next discussion will review the different components of sensory modulation.

Components of Sensory Modulation

In relation to children's sensory processing, Dunn (1997a) proposed four different components of sensory modulation related to problems with sensory processing: 1) poor registration, 2) sensitivity to stimuli, 3) sensory seeking, and 4) sensory avoiding. The following section describes how each component of sensory modulation can affect feeding (see also Table 10.1). Each person has more than one pattern of sensory processing, and each sensory system may be affected differently. For example, a single individual may be sensory-seeking for touch but sensory-avoiding for olfactory stimulation.

Poor Registration   Infants and toddlers with poor registration have "high thresholds and passive responding strategies" (Dunn, 2001, p. 611). These children need a great deal of stimulation to attract them. They tend to be disinterested in their environment and activities, including mealtimes. Foods may not be attractive or tasty to these children. At mealtimes, toddlers with poor registration may do everything but eat. For example, a toddler may place her fingers in the food, examine the texture of the fabric on the highchair, throw food on the floor, or rub food into the highchair tray.

Strategies for Children With Poor Registration   Children with low registration need more stimulation. Try the following techniques to engage these children:

- Provide textured paint for fingerpainting. Children with low registration need more to stimulate them, so add sand or other textures to finger paint to increase the sensory experience.

- Allow children with low registration to play with their food. Children with low registration need a lot of stimulation, so if they can engage with their food in more than one way, they are sometimes more willing to eat it.

- Provide massage using lotion. Massaging lotion onto the skin of children with low registration provides stimulation. Stimulating their feet or hands or other areas helps these children 'wind up' their sensory system and become more receptive to outside information.

- Add strong smells. In the same way that adding texture to paints adds stimulation, adding strong smells to the environment will increase the level of stimulation provided by the environment. Boil cinnamon and orange peels or burn a candle to add scents to the air.

- Add scent, glitter, or sand to play dough. Again, this increases levels of sensory information and is more likely to stimulate the child.

- Add flavors to foods. For example, add vanilla or cinnamon to foods such as pancakes and yogurt to increase the sensory stimulation of the food.

Sensitivity to Stimuli   In contrast, young children who demonstrate sensitivity to stimuli have low thresholds with passive responding (Dunn, 2001) and tend to be "distractible or hyperactive" (Dunn, 1997b, p. 31). Children with sensitivity to stimuli may not be able to settle down to eat, may have trouble remaining at the table, or may fuss to get out of their highchairs. They can also be very cautious or negative about trying new foods, such as those with novel colors, flavors,

Table 10.1.   Feeding-related sensory processing issues

Sensory modulation component	Characteristics	Feeding strategies
Poor registration High neurological threshold Minimal behavioral response	Requires stimulation in order to eat or drink Withdrawn/difficult to engage/self-absorbed Uninterested in environment and/or dull appearances Has difficulty noticing what is happening in the environment Content to lie on a blanket in a noisy, busy classroom Later development of motor skills compared with sensation-seeking peers	Offer foods with texture (e.g., crunchy foods) Offer foods with intense flavors, textures, and/or smells Add temperature to foods and beverages (e.g., very cold water, warm apple sauce)
Low neurological threshold Weak behavioral response	Needs less input to get a response Difficulty focusing on a task and learning from their experiences Hyperactive/distractible Fidgets with "itchy" clothing, refuses to try new foods, or complains about the "itchy" carpeting Covers ears or becomes upset in response to loud noises	Allow the child to eat at a quiet table or in a quiet room Decrease distractions during mealtime (e.g., by turning off lights, turning off music)
Sensory seeking High neurological threshold Active behavioral response	Requires more input—such as movement, touch, sound, and visual stimulation—to respond A desire to touch, taste, smell, see, and hear everything around them—explorers of the world. Fidgets Plays with food/handles everything Chews on nonfood items Very active, continuously engaging, and excitable Frequently move until they drop	Provide physical activity before mealtime Add texture to food (e.g., raisins to oatmeal) Provide brighter lights, more noise, and more scents at meals Offer adapted positioning, such as therapeutic ball or sit pad in chair Suggest that the child bring preferred object to mealtimes (e.g., favorite book, fidget toy)
Sensory Avoiding Low neurological threshold Active behavioral response	Very sensitive to changes in routine and may become upset by deviations from a schedule Expends a great deal of energy to avoid stimulation Appreciate routine and consistency Easily overwhelmed by smells and flavors or other sensory input from the environment Develops rituals for daily activities especially to avoid situations that might be overwhelming Actively avoids stimulation that is overwhelming	Use a picture schedule to indicate what is coming next or what to expect during the day Provide transition object during mealtime Sit child at the end of the table or alone Create calm environment at meals Minimize odors related to food preparation

or textures. Sensitivity to stimuli may be first observed in a child when moving from breast or formula to solid foods. The child may gag and spit during this transition and will take longer to accept new foods compared with children who are not sensitive.

Strategies for Children With Sensitivity to Stimuli   Children with sensitivity to stimuli are easily overwhelmed, but do little to help themselves. Try these techniques:

- Provide a feeding environment that is quiet, has low lighting, and is free of distractions. The less stimulation the better. Loud eating places, like restaurants, may inhibit eating.
- Give ample warning when change is coming. Children who are sensitive to stimuli will not actively avoid stimuli, but it is best to let them know what is coming so they are somewhat prepared. Even though they still may find the stimuli aversive, they are likely to have a less of a negative reaction if they are forewarned.

Sensory Avoiding   Children who are sensory avoiding have low neurological thresholds, but active response strategies (Dunn, 2001, p. 612). For example, a child who is sensory avoiding may try to leave the dinner table or other feeding-related activities by withdrawing or throwing a temper tantrum because there is too much stimulation from the overhead lights, smells, textures, and so forth. Additionally, children who are sensory avoiding often create rituals for typical daily activities to help meet their sensory needs. They will actively avoid situations that are overly stimulating.

Strategies for Children Who Are Sensory Avoiding   Children with this sensory integration dysfunction need support to remain engaged in activities because their behavioral response is to escape. Try the following techniques:

- Provide a picture schedule and/or a transitional object for mealtimes and snacks. This technique helps children with sensory avoidance to prepare for what is coming.
- Provide plans for when the child may be faced with new sensory challenges. Because these children avoid stimulating situations, being proactive helps the child deal with the environment more effectively.
- Introduce new foods and drinks slowly, adding one at a time so the child has time to accommodate to new flavors and textures. This technique helps children with these difficulties deal with the overstimulation of new flavors. The more slowly these children are faced with more stimulation, the better they will handle new sensory inputs.

Sensory Seeking   Children who are sensory seeking "have high thresholds, but have active responding strategies" (Dunn, 2001, p. 611). Because these children have high neurological thresholds, they engage in behaviors to increase their sensory experiences. These children fidget, play with their food, touch everything, and chew on nonfood objects such as clothing to increase sensations, but they may be so busy with these behaviors that they do not eat. They actively try to meet their sensory needs.

Strategies for Children who are Sensory Seeking   These children enjoy stimulating activities. Therefore, stimulating them before eating and while they are eating is helpful. Try these techniques:

- Engage children in physical activity before eating, like carrying heavy items, i.e., jugs of water. Because children with this issue are looking for more stimulation, just sitting at the table to eat can be underwhelming and understimulating. So if the child is worn out before sitting down to eat, he is more likely to sit still instead of trying to seek out more stimulation.

- Keep a fidget toy nearby. If a sensory-seeking child is having trouble focusing on the meal or snack, having something to play with will help him to focus on the meal.

- Add texture to preferred foods. For example, add berries to yogurt and pancakes. More stimulation is better, and these children are constantly looking for more input.

- Burn scented candles. This will add to the sensory environment.

- Play music. Music provides input to another sensory system and increases the level of overall stimulation.

FEEDING AND SENSORY PROCESSING PROBLEMS

Every young child has specific feeding-related likes and dislikes. One toddler prefers spicy foods. Another child prefers bland foods and finds spicy foods overwhelming. If such variations are extreme, they may be due to sensory processing issues. If a child has a sensory processing problem, developmental feeding difficulties may persist and produce challenges for the child and caregivers. For example, one infant may need highly flavorful foods like grapefruit to elicit a willingness to eat. In contrast, a sensitive toddler may eat only bland foods.

Signs of feeding difficulties or "red flags" may be observed initially when an infant or toddler does not meet developmental feeding milestones, such as weaning from breast to bottle or from bottle to cup. (See Table 10.2 for more examples.) Providing parents and other caregivers with information about feeding-related sensory processing issues can help both caregiver and child.

Table 10.2.   Red flags indicating feeding-related sensory processing problems

- Avoids putting objects near or in the mouth (especially when developmentally appropriate)
- History of feeding problems (usually starting at birth)
- Accepts a limited variety of foods
- Dislikes having faced washed (much more so than most children)
- Overly sensitive sense of taste or smell
- Reactions to spicy foods are either too extreme or lacking
- Avoids certain textured foods
- Excessive gagging, coughing, retching, or vomiting that interferes with eating or nutrition
- Loss of weight or not gaining weight for 2–3 months
- Does not progress to solid foods within developmentally appropriate timelines
- Inadequate intake of foods and liquids
- Power struggles during meals, making mealtimes unpleasant and stress-filled
- Behavior problems at mealtimes that defy most solutions (e.g., spits out food; throws plate)
- Persistent food refusal
- Taking an extended amount of time to eat (30–45 minutes)
- Does not transition from puréed foods to solid foods
- Holding and/or storing food in cheeks or under tongue interfering with food intake

Adapted from "Feeding Developmental Milestones," by Chatterboxes Pediatric Speech-Language Pathology, 2008. Retrieved from www.teamchatterboxes.com/milestones_feeding.html.

Assessments of Sensory Issues

Several assessments of sensory irregularity are available. The Sensory Profile is based on interviews with parents of children with disabilities and was developed by Dunn and Westman (1997). The Sensory Profile has 125 items in eight areas: 1) auditory, 2) visual, 3) taste/smell, 4) movement, 5) touch, 6) activity level, 7) body position, and 8) emotional/social. For each item, parents rate the frequency of times the child displays a behavior on a Likert scale ranging from 1 (*always engaging in the behavior*) to 5 (*never exhibiting the behavior*).

A shorter version of this profile, the Short Sensory Profile (SSP) was developed by McIntosh, Miller, Shyu, and Dunn (1999). The SSP has only 38 items and is completed by the caregiver. It is a screening tool designed to determine whether a child between the ages of 3 years and 10 years is developing typically or may have sensory modulation disruptions. There are seven factors on the profile: 1) tactile sensitivity, 2) taste/smell sensitivity, 3) visual/auditory sensitivity, 4) movement sensitivity, 5) underresponsive/seeks sensation, 6) auditory filtering, and 7) low energy/weak. The profile has good reliability for differentiating among sensory processing difficulties. The responses to items are on a Likert scale ranging from 1 (*never responds in this manner*) to 5 (*always responds in this manner*). This profile helps clinicians and other professionals to better understand a child's sensory issues. Because the instrument has only 38 items, it is more efficient than the longer version.

The Infant/Toddler Sensory Profile (Dunn, 2002) is a questionnaire designed for parents to assess children's responses to everyday sensory events in order to look at patterns in young children who may be at risk for sensory processing problems. This profile has 36 items for infants up to age 6 months, and it has 48 items for children ages 7–36 months. It has scores for the quadrants similar to those found in Dunn's model of sensory processing. The caregiver completes the profile, rating the frequency of behaviors on a Likert scale ranging from 1 (*nearly never*) to 5 (*almost always*; Dunn & Daniels, 2002). Scores correspond to Dunn's model of sensory processing (i.e., sensation avoiding, sensation seeking, sensory sensitivity, and low registration), along with information about each sensory system (tactile, auditory, etc.). Information from the profile provides information for professionals who work with the child.

Strategies For Children With Sensory Integration Problems

In order to select strategies for treating or assisting children with sensory integration problems, professionals must know which dysfunction the child has because the approach is different depending on the individual's neurological threshold and behavioral responses. One of the simplest ways to begin addressing a sensory integration dysfunction is to vary food items. For example, if the child is a sensory seeker, caregivers can provide foods that have more texture and are therefore more stimulating (e.g., oatmeal with raisins, pancakes with toppings). For a child who is sensation avoiding, caregivers can provide bland foods, such as plain pancakes or plain yogurt. These simple adjustments can alleviate some of the causes of mealtime stress.

Another solution to try is oral massage. Occupational therapists (OTs) should be included on feeding teams to assist children who have sensory integration dysfunction to improve their feeding issues. OTs can recommend techniques for facial and oral massage to prepare the child for eating. For a child who is sensory defensive, massage can begin with the face and work toward the mouth. Washcloths or swatches with other various textures, such as cotton or satin, also can be used.

A NUK oral massager for the gums can help children who may be extra sensitive to oral stimulation or who need extra stimulation to prepare for eating. Children who need more oral stimulation can bite on "chewies," items that allow the child to chew on something often meeting a sensory need. The child may be given a toothbrush to chew on for stimulation. Oral stimulation can be provided with a range of foods that have different textures (e.g., pretzels, yogurt, Jell-O, crackers, carrots, and ice cream). It can also be useful to vary the temperature of liquids by serving warm liquids and ice water.

A child with aversions to eating due to sensory issues should be allowed to play with food because this sometimes increases the likelihood that the child will eat it. Children who have difficulties with textures should be gradually introduced to thicker, coarser textures; slowly changing the texture gives the child time to adjust and increases the likelihood that the food will be accepted.

For more stimulation, provide ketchup to dip foods into. Sometimes the dipping and licking is stimulating to the child. Use peanut butter for a more challenging food to lick. Sometimes dipping food entices the child to eat not only the dip, but also the food that is being dipped. Distraction is another way to help with sensory integration problems that affect feeding. Reading a book while eating or playing soft music may help some children. However, other children may be overwhelmed by this "noise."

CHILDREN WITH AUTISM SPECTRUM DISORDER

One disorder in which sensory integration issues are common is autism (e.g., Nate's story at the beginning of this chapter). Autism "is a complex developmental disability that causes problems with social interaction and communication. Symptoms usually start before the age of 18 months and can cause delays or problems in many different skills that develop from infancy to adulthood" (National Institutes of Health, 2010). Autism symptoms include problems in three areas of development: communication, social interactions, and routine or stereotypic behaviors (see Table 10.3). Children with autism have communication problems that include issues with eye contact, smiling, pointing, and spoken communication. Children with autism have social problems usually dealing with emotions, such as sharing their own emotions and understanding the emotions of others. Children with autism also may have difficulties holding a conversation, making it difficult to establish and maintain friendships. Children with autism often have issues with rigid routines and repetitive behaviors. Routines are invariably followed; if such rigidity is not allowed, the child with autism will exhibit extreme responses (National Institutes of Health, 2010). Children with autism may repeat words or actions over and over, and they tend to play in repetitive ways, using toys in the same ways or engaging in the same scenario.

The number of young children diagnosed on the autism spectrum has increased sharply in recent years. Kogan et al. (2009) estimated that the prevalence of autism is 1 in 91 births; The National Center on Birth Defects and Developmental Disabilities estimated the prevalence to be 1 in 110 births (n.d.). Because autism is a spectrum disorder, there is a range in severity among children who are diagnosed. One young child may have mild symptoms while another has severe symptoms.

Table 10.3.   Traits exhibited by young children with autism

Behavior	Example
Trouble expressing needs	Uses only gestures, such as pointing or leading
Resistant to change	Throws tantrums if changes are made in furniture, foods, clothing, and so forth
Echolalia	Repeats words or phrases instead of using unique or original utterances
Exhibits inappropriate affect	Laughing/crying/distressed without apparent cause
Preference for being alone	Plays without seeking the company of others
Trouble interacting with same-age peers and adults	May try to interact but often unsuccessfully
Resistance to being cuddled	Wiggles out of embraces
Little or no eye contact	When speaking to others looks in another direction
Engages in ritualistic play for long periods of time	Spinning objects; lining up objects
Abnormal attachment to objects	Seems to prefer a specific toy over people
Overly or under-sensitive to pain	May react as though something that should not be painful is; may not react to something that should cause pain
Unresponsive to environment	Behaves as though he or she cannot hear, even though hearing is typical

Autism and Feeding Issues

Grandin (1995) stated, "Many children with autism are finicky and will eat only certain foods. Their eating problems usually have a sensory basis. They are unable to tolerate the texture, smell, taste or sound of the food in their mouth" (p. 75). Ermer and Dunn (1998) conducted a study that compared 679 typical children with 38 children diagnosed with autism (using sensory profiles) and with 61 children diagnosed with attention-deficit/hyperactivity disorder (ADHD). They found that children diagnosed with autism had higher levels of oral sensitivity, fine motor or perceptual problems, and inattention and/or distractibility when compared with both of the other groups. They also had lower levels of sensory seeking when compared with the other groups. Because they lack sensory seeking, the children with autism were less likely to exhibit typical responses, such as enjoying strange noises, and less likely to exhibit typical behaviors, such as seeking movement. In fact, a majority of children diagnosed with autism are either hypersensitive or hyposensitive to light, sound, temperature, and other external stimulation (Reynolds & Dombeck, 2006). Some children with autism have both hypersensitivities and hyposensitivities. As a result, children with autism diagnoses often cover their ears, avoid or react negatively to bright lights, or crash hard into sofas and crave strong bear hugs (Rudy, 2011).

Feeding Difficulties

Kanner (1943) was the first to define and identify autism in children, and he listed feeding problems as one of the characteristics describing the syndrome. Although atypical feeding patterns are not a diagnostic symptom for autism, 60%–90% of children with autism demonstrate difficulties around mealtimes (Ahearn, 2003; Flanagan, 2008; Ledford & Gast, 2006; Piazza et al., 2002). In fact, researchers have found that children with autism spectrum disorders (ASD) eat fewer foods from every food group (Schreck, Williams, & Smith, 2004). Ledford and Gast (2006) reviewed 16 studies published between 1994 and 2004 and found that children with ASD were selective in their food choices by type or texture and also by brand

and presentation. Eating disorders are complex and often require multiple trials of multiple possible solutions, which leaves children with ASD at risk for health and growth problems (Cornish 1998; 2002). The following are some of the feeding issues common among children with autism.

Physiological Feeding Issues   Two main feeding issues for children with autism are gastrointestinal (GI) issues such as constipation, diarrhea, gastroesophageal reflux disease and food allergies (Arvedson, 2008). Schwarz (2003) noted the incidence of undernutrition tied to physiological issues affecting intake and absorption of nutrients in children with ASD. Additionally, young children with autism may experience food allergies that can further impede intake, GI functioning, and age-appropriate weight gain (Adams & Conn, 1997; Volkmar, Wiesner, & Westphal, 2006).

Behavioral Feeding Issues   The literature on autism-related feeding issues has focused on three categories of feeding difficulties: 1) selective behaviors based on texture and type of food, such as eating only low-texture foods, 2) refusing to eat; and 3) disruptive behaviors at mealtimes (Bandini, Anderson, Curtin, & Cermak, 2010; Flanagan, 2008; Johnson, Handen, Mayer-Costa, & Sacco, 2008; Kedesdy & Budd, 1998; Macht, 1990; Matson, Fodstad, & Dempsey, 2009; Morris & Klein, 2000; Schwarz, 2003; Schreck et al., 2004). Although typically developing young children often demonstrate comparable behaviors, children with autism typically exhibit food refusal for a longer period of time, which increases the potential for interference with daily activities and nutritional status (Dovey, Farrow, Martin, Isherwood, & Halford, 2009; Laud, Girolami, Boscoe, & Gulotta, 2009; Volkert & Vaz, 2010). For example, a child may eat only preferred foods that are prepared a specific way (e.g., temperature), foods that are a specific brand, or foods that are presented on a preferred plate (Matson, Fodsad, & Dempsey, 2009). Many young children with autism are sensitive to textured foods such as oatmeal, yogurt with fruit, and pasta (Bandini et al., 2010; Matson & Fodstad, 2009; Thompson, Bruns, & Rains, 2010).

Some young children with autism choose foods with powerful flavors such as spicy, sour, bitter, or salty, while other children with autism insist on very bland flavors (Twachtman-Reilly, Amaral, & Zebrowski, 2008). Children are said to be hyporesponsive (or "underresponsive") if they prefer strong flavors that activate the underresponsive oral receptors. A hyporesponsive child may, for example, prefer sour or bitter foods, eating grapefruit without showing any sign that it is sour. On the opposite end of the spectrum are children who are hyperresponsive (or "overresponsive"); these children prefer bland foods with little flavor, like crackers or oatmeal (Dunn, 2007; Twachtman-Reilly, Amaral, & Zebrowski, 2008). In addition, some children with autism may have a preference for puréed foods. Other children may consume only crunchy foods, and other children may entirely avoid specific food groups. (See Dunn, 2007; Roche, Martorana, Eicher, & Daukas 2007; Thompson et al, 2010.)

STRATEGIES AND SPECIALIZED INTERVENTIONS

The following specialized strategies and interventions include environmental modifications, changes to food preparation and food presentation, changes in diet, and specialized behavioral interventions. Strategy and intervention choice depends on the issues that the specific child exhibits. Not all of these options will be appropriate for an individual.

Environmental Modifications

Making changes to the environment is one of the first and most basic ways to begin helping a child with eating issues. Space around the meal area—including walkways, the table and chairs, lighting, and noise level—can affect mealtimes (Flanagan, 2008; Kedesdy & Budd, 1998; Lowman, Kientz, & Weissman, 1999). For example, if a child finds the brightly lit dining room to be overwhelming, he or she may leave the room or refuse to eat, or a child with autism may eat only when a specific television show is playing at a particular volume. To better understand the impact of the environment on a child's behavior, interviews and observations may be necessary. Some formal assessment instruments include items that address the feeding environment (e.g., Children's Eating Behavior Inventory, (CEBI), Archer, Rosenbaum, & Streiner, 1991). Assessment results should be used to ensure a match between the child's preferences and his or her environment.

An appropriate environment for a child should have sufficient space, appropriate furniture, and a place for a plate, a cup, utensils, and other necessary materials. The space should contain the child if he is prone to running and climbing, but the space should not feel restrictive to the child. An OT can help to develop a seating system that provides support for the child but also encourages interaction with others and self-feeding during the meal.

Another aspect of environment is lighting. Lighting should be moderate and not overly bright or dim (unless the child prefers very bright or dim lighting). Dimmers are helpful so that the lighting level can be adjusted appropriately for the child. Noise, especially an overly noisy environment, may interfere with eating. A young child with autism may be distracted by the hum of a computer, musical toys, or conversation. Environmental modifications can facilitate successful mealtimes. It is important to be aware that the environmental issues that affect a child with autism may be very subtle.

Meal Preparation

A modification to meal preparation is a naturalistic way to increase acceptance of foods and beverages. Simple modifications include changes to the temperature, texture, portion size, and other components of a meal (Flanagan, 2008). For example, a child may prefer all foods puréed and refuse to eat when a food item is thick or has lumps. This can create difficulties in a child care classroom, prekindergarten classroom, or restaurant setting because in these settings, meals are prepared according to typical development. Parents can work with caregivers and program staff to address some of these issues, but child care centers are often unable to address specific needs. Therefore, children with autism need to learn to accept food items, especially when eating in a community setting. It is important for EC/ECSE administrators and educators to know each child's preferences, including foods the child likes, those the child dislikes, and textures that are preferred or refused.

Other issues with food should also be recognized so that mealtime difficulties can be avoided. This information should include foods the child absolutely refuses, allergies, and other pertinent information. Because children with autism often have sensory issues, providing caregivers with information before they plan meals benefits the child as well as the caregivers. For the most part, meals can be served to children with autism in a similar manner as that used to serve other children who serve as a model of people who eat other foods. However, modifications should be made according to each individual child's preferences and needs.

Many young children with autism are sensitive to textured foods such as oatmeal, yogurt with fruit, and pasta (Bandini et al., 2010; Flanagan, 2008). Texture can be adjusted in several ways. The term *texture manipulation* refers to changing the texture of food items by chopping or puréeing (Ledford & Gast, 2006). A blender can be used to blend familiar and novel foods to the child's desired consistency. Often this can be a starting point to moving the child to more developmentally appropriate textures. Accepting a new food if it is finely chopped often means the child may accept a coarsely chopped version in the future. The child may also be more likely to accept novel foods if they are first presented in a smoother version then presented in a coarser version.

Another environmental adjustment is the modification of portion size. This technique can be especially useful with children who put large amounts of food in their mouths, causing gagging and choking. Offering more, but smaller portions, can address this issue (Arvedson, 2008). Offering smaller portions also can help children to eat more because they will be less likely to feel overwhelmed. It is best to work with a speech-language pathologist or nutritionist and to be mindful that settings such as a child care center must follow state regulations and guidelines regarding portion size. Changes in portion sizes should be noted in food diaries or other recordings on a consistent basis because if portion size is reduced, there needs to be an increased number of food presentations (i.e., a higher number of smaller portions). To ensure that this occurs, the child's feeding team should develop a plan with a schedule and specified portions for each mealtime.

Many children with autism display ritualistic behaviors such as lining up toy cars in a particular order or removing items from a box and then replacing them over and over. Ritualistic behaviors can be exhibited during mealtimes, as when a child insists on using the same cup, plate, or utensil at every meal (Dunn, 2007; Murphy & Caretto, 1999). Additionally, a child may favor specific foods and, in some cases, eat only particular brands of these foods. It is common for toddlers and preschoolers to favor particular dishes or specific foods, but these preferences are often developmental in nature, do not last for an extended period of time, and are not demanded with the tenacity exhibited by many children with autism. For example, a young toddler might only eat bread, cheese, and bananas for a couple of weeks or a month. In contrast, a child with autism might eat the same foods for an extended period with little variation (Dovey et al., 2009; Schreck et al., 2004).

In light of these behaviors, children with autism must be offered a range of foods and an array of eating utensils across all settings, including child care and professional settings. During a meal, caregivers, parents, and peers, can model appropriate behaviors, encouraging children with food issues to explore and/or attempt to use a new item or eat a new food (Flanagan, 2008; Johnson, Handen et al., 2008; Martins, Young, & Robson, 2008). Consistently offering new and different foods, cups, plates, and utensils may help children with autism to expand their preferences. Changes should be made gradually. For example, if a child will drink only out of one specific cup, another cup might be set on the table one day, pushed closer to the preferred cup on the next day, pushed right next to the preferred cup on the following day, and finally be offered in place of the other cup. Gradual introductions of new items alongside the preferred items are best. This sequence sometimes takes weeks rather than days.

Functional Analysis

A functional analysis is a method used to collect information to understand the reason or function behind inappropriate behavior (Fischer & Silverman, 2007; Olive, 2004; Piazza et al., 2003). This method can be very useful when trying to understand and alter feeding problems. First, information is accumulated about the antecedents (what occurs prior to the behavior) and the consequences (what occurs after the behavior) of a child's eating behaviors. Additionally, a variety of environmental and physiological conditions (e.g., alertness, hunger, illness) are explored and data are collected. Parents, caregivers, and others who are close to the child help provide descriptions of the child's behavior during mealtimes at home, at child care, and in the community (Najdowski et al., 2008). Behavior analysts are individuals with training in functional analysis. These professionals (or other qualified professionals) should collect and examine data to identify the function of the behavior and to help develop strategies to increase appropriate feeding behaviors (Piazza et al., 2003).

Specialized Diets and Supplements

Casein and gluten-free diets are often employed by some parents for their young children with autism (Adams & Conn, 1997; Levy & Hyman, 2003). However, regarding the efficacy of these regimens, published results are contradictory at best (Cornish, 2002; Elder et al., 2006). Volkmar, Weisner, and Westphal (2006) noted that "controlled scientific studies with groups of cases are not yet widely available" about casein and gluten-free diets (p. 364).

Nevertheless, with a casein-free diet, foods that contain casein, a milk protein, are removed. With a gluten-free diet, wheat products are removed. These modifications require parents and caregivers to be vigilant in order to keep children from consuming these items, which can be difficult because these ingredients may not be readily apparent in some foods and because these modifications drastically limit the child's diet (Silberberg, 2009). As with other changes, these dietary restrictions should be used only with professional supervision, such as in collaboration with a nutritionist (Elder, 2008).

Supplements can be added to a child's diet as an additional means of meeting nutritional needs. Supplements should be selected based on the child's unique feeding needs. Pediasure and Ensure pudding provide additional calories, and multivitamins can be added to a child's limited diet to ensure adequate vitamins and nutrients. A pediatrician or nutritionist can provide advice about supplementing a child's daily intake in order to make up for a missing vitamin or nutrient if there is a specific deficiency, such as iron deficiency. One deficiency that is beginning to get attention with regard to children who have autism is omega-3 fatty acid deficiency. Research is examining the introduction of omega-3 supplementation (e.g., Amminger et al., 2007; Meiri, Bichovsky, & Belmaker, 2009).

Behavioral Interventions

Behavioral interventions to address feeding issues in children with autism are varied and range from simple to complex. Some of the techniques that can be utilized to address a variety of feeding challenges include extinction procedures, systematic desensitization, fading, and differential reinforcement. Several authors note that all interventions must be implemented consistently across all caregivers who participate in mealtimes with the child (Arvedson, 1997; Flanagan, 2008; Piazza & Addison, 2007). Behavioral interventions sometimes seem easy to perform, but training is required to ensure that interventions are implemented uniformly and that they follow established procedures and protocols.

Escape extinction (nonremoval, physical guidance, and representation) is based on negative reinforcement. When escape extinction is used to address feeding issues, a nonpreferred food will be removed after a refusal behavior. Therefore, the child is not allowed to escape from eating. Children may want to leave because of the food, but because it is removed, they do not try to escape. The nonremoval technique would be holding a bite of food in front of the child until he takes a bite. Once he takes a bite, the food is removed from in front of him. He is praised or provided with tangible positive reinforcement. Physical guidance is used when an adult physically helps guide the eating utensil into the child's mouth, possibly physically opening the child's mouth. Once the bite is accepted, the child is given positive reinforcement.

Another technique used to get children with autism to eat is differential reinforcement. This is a positive reinforcement method in which the desired behavior is coupled with removal of reinforcement for undesired behavior. Usually, children gain attention for not eating. With differential reinforcement, the child would be ignored when not eating and gain attention only when eating. This method has been proven useful in at least one study by Gutentag and Hammer (2000). The authors were able to get a 3-year-old with mental retardation and a gastronomy tube to eat. Several research studies (Coe et al., 1997; Didden, Seys, & Schouwink, 1999; Hoch, Babbitt, Coe, Krell, & Hackbert, 1994) have shown that combining differential reinforcement with escape extinction can be successful in improving feeding behaviors in young children with medical problems who are dependent on tube feedings and in young children with varying cognitive abilities.

The Premack principle is the premise that the child will perform the nonpreferred activity (eating certain foods) so that he or she can engage in the preferred activity (playing with a favorite toy). This is also called "Grandma's Law." Many parents use this without realizing they are doing so by saying, "After you finish your peas, you can have some cake." It is similar to the escape extinction method except that it adds another component. In addition to the removal of something negative, the child is given something positive.

In behavioral momentum, the order of the activities is reversed so that "You can have cake" comes before "you eat your peas" so the preferred activity precedes the less preferred activity. This technique is shown to be effective only in combination with other methods for feeding problems (Dawson et al., 2003). Dawson found it to be effective only when combined with escape extinction to treat food refusal.

Systematic desensitization is often used when a child will not accept textured foods. During this procedure, the food item that the child will not accept is systematically presented until the child is first willing to touch it, then taste it, and then finally, eat it. Each step is reinforced as the child makes gains in accepting the texture of certain foods. Kahng, Boscoe, and Byrne (2003) discussed a token economy, which can be used to increase acceptance of rejected foods. The tokens are given to the child when the child exhibits desired behaviors and can be traded for items such as stickers or toys. The number of tokens can vary for purchase of tangible items. For example, five tokens may buy a sticker, but ten are necessary to purchase a small car.

It is critical to note that any time a change is made in the way challenging behaviors are handled, the child may demonstrate an extinction burst, or an increase in the undesirable behavior. This means that the child is aware (usually unconsciously) of the changes and may increase the undesirable behavior in an attempt to elicit the response that has been provided in the past. In other words, when a behavior does not prompt the familiar response, a child may increase the behaviors. Parents, caregivers, and professionals should be aware of this phenomenon and not be discouraged. The extinction burst indicates that the intervention is effective. In the past, the child has learned that the established behavioral response (e.g., food refusal) is effective. Once the child understands that the old behavior does not work, he or she will begin using the new ones that have been offered by the feeding team (see Fischer & Silverman, 2007; Lowman & Murphy, 1999).

SUMMARY

The strategies and interventions discussed here should be implemented by trained professionals across settings, including the child's home and child care site. It is important to collect data that tracks feeding changes (e.g., in the amount of each type of food accepted) as part of a child's feeding plan. A food diary, observation, and formal instruments can be used to collect data, and the child's progress can be substantiated by comparing assessment results from one point in time with those from another period of time (e.g., every two weeks, three months).

▪ ▪ ▪ TABLE TALK ▪ ▪ ▪

When Reese was 22-months old, he was diagnosed with autism by a developmental pediatrician. His parents had sensed for awhile that something was wrong. Reese's parents have had trouble getting him to eat foods other than puréed baby food. Reese had been eating puréed baby food for about 10 months when his parents tried to move him up with solid pieces of food and had little success. He would eat the puréed foods, but kick and cry while spitting out the chunks of the solid foods. Reese's parent continued to feed him the puréed foods because they worried that otherwise he would not get enough to eat. They are now concerned about his inability to transition to solid foods, especially when they go out.

After Reese's diagnosis, early intervention specialists gave his parents suggestions, but nothing worked. Soon Reese was 3 years old and still eating puréed baby foods and refusing to feed himself. His parents have to prepare separate meals for him because the food has to be puréed. They are able to purée the foods they eat, so they have stopped purchasing baby food. However, when they go out to eat, they have to bring Reese his own foods. Also, he insists on eating in front of the television with a specified show playing. If he does not have puréed foods and his preferred show on the TV, he throws tantrums and will not eat. His behaviors have gotten increasingly worse.

Reese's feeding habits are putting stress on his family. Mealtimes have become dreaded experiences. Reese's feeding problems are controlling the whole family.

Discussion Question

■ Based on the information discussed in the chapter, what suggestions do you have for Reese's parents?

■ What are they doing correctly?

■ What should they change?

■ Which professionals should they seek out for help?

FEEDING NUGGETS

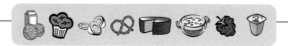

Books

Building Bridges Through Sensory Integration by Ellen Yack, Shirley Sutton, and Paula Aquilla (2003)

Sensory Integration: A Guide for Preschool Teacher by Christy Isbell and Rebecca Isbell

The Out-of-Sync Child: Recognizing and Coping with Sensory Processing Disorder by Carol Kranowitz and Lucy Miller (2006)

Raising a Sensory Smart Child: The Definitive Handbook for Helping Your Child with Sensory Processing Issues by Lindsey Biel and Nancy Peske (2009)

Ten Things Every Child with Autism Wishes You Knew by Ellen Notbohm (2005)

Web Sites

Autism Link
http://autismlink.com
135 Cumberland Rd., Suite 105
Pittsburg, PA 15237
(412) 364-1886
info@autismlin.com

Autism Society
www.autism-society.org
4340 East-West Hwy, Suite 350
Bethesda, Maryland 20814
1.800.328.8476

11

Young Children with Oral-Motor Difficulties

What You'll Learn in This Chapter

This chapter provides

- An overview of oral-motor difficulties including dysphagia, aspiration, and gastroesophageal reflux
- A description of pica
- Examples of strategies and specialized interventions to address these issues

■ ■ ■ **FOOD FOR THOUGHT** ■ ■ ■

"Before Kareef, who is 10 months old, attended the child care facility, he was fed all puréed food. One day at the child care center he was fed mashed green beans. As he tried to swallow the food, he gagged on the food, and it came back up. Currently, he only eats baby food and cannot eat any food with texture."

Yolanda, Child Care Provider

"At 18 months, Harrison couldn't keep a bottle down. He would choke or vomit after feeding, and he weighed only 10 pounds. He was also not eating solid food. The doctor decided to install a G-tube. He tolerated the G-tube feedings well and gained 5 pounds in a month. He was fed every 3 hours and had a continuous drip at night."

Noelle, Undergraduate Early Childhood Student

"Sam was born at 34 weeks gestation, weighing 5 pounds, 12 ounces. He was in the NICU for 2 weeks. He has had feeding problems since birth. He had bad reflux as an infant. His formula was changed five times during infancy. He vomited five to eight times per day until he was 14 months old, and he remained on formula until he was 18 months old. Sam gagged on foods of various textures and refused many foods (had a very limited diet) until he was 3 years old. Now Sam is 42 months old. He still occasionally gags and/ or vomits when food becomes 'stuck' on the middle of his tongue."

Angela, Parent and Certified Behavior Analyst

"During the holiday season of 2009, when Scott was 3 years old, it came to the attention of Scott's parents that he would eat nonfood items when he consumed three light bulbs from the Christmas tree. After this occurrence, child care teachers began to watch him more closely and found he would eat items such as chalk, paper, crayons, cardboard, paint, and rocks from the playground. During a weekend with grandpa, Sam ate pieces of two DVD boxes."

Laura, Child Care Provider

The children's experiences that open this chapter illustrate several types of feeding issues in young children. Oral-motor disorders, such as dysphagia, aspiration, gastroesophageal reflux (GER) and pica, interfere with the eating and drinking process. Manikam and Perman (2000) discussed "difficulty consuming adequate nutrition by mouth...and those who eat the wrong thing" (p. 34). The condition in which an individual eats nonedible items such as dirt, paint chips, clay, and chalk is called pica. Manikam and Perman also noted, "treatment...requires careful analysis of proper seating and positioning, appropriate textures for easy chewing and swallowing" (2000, p. 42). The strategies and interventions used to address these issues often require training for their implementation and must be closely monitored in order to ensure positive child responses and progress in feeding skills and intake.

WHAT THE LITERATURE SAYS

Oral-motor difficulties affect one or more components of feeding. Swallowing and digestive disorders are often manifested concomitantly because the systems involved must operate together to achieve effective and efficient feeding, including movement of the tongue, chewing patterns, swallowing mechanism, and esophageal function. Singly or in combination, oral-motor difficulties can range in severity (from mild to extremely discomforting or painful) as well as chronicity (from rarely to once per day or multiple times per day). As described by Manikam and Perman (2000), young children may experience "difficulty consuming adequate nutrition by mouth...and...eat the wrong thing" (p. 34). In typically developing children, these issues usually stem from limited intake and inappropriate mealtime behaviors, such as a young toddler who will not stop play activities to consume a full meal. This type of behavior will ease as the child gains an understanding and practice with age-appropriate mealtime expectations (see Chapters 1 and 3).

The focus of this chapter is infants, toddlers, and preschoolers with oral-motor difficulties resulting primarily from problems with the swallowing mechanism or process. The difficulties may be compounded by the environmental and/or social context surrounding mealtime, such as hurried mealtimes and a mismatch between the child's cues during feeding interactions and the parent or caregiver responses to those cues. In addition, the ability to swallow requires a foundation of sensorimotor skills. If one or more of these skills is compromised, the intake of foods and fluids can become an upsetting or uncomfortable experience (Gisel, Birnbaum, & Schwartz, 1998; Morris & Klein, 2000; Schwarz, 2003).

A team approach is necessary in order to address oral-motor difficulties by identifying causation and developing, implementing, and evaluating interventions. Reducing discomfort and the successful resolution of the problem are the ultimate goals. Team members may include a speech-language pathologist (SLP), occupational therapist (OT), otolaryngologist (ear, nose, and throat doctor), behavior analyst, early childhood teacher, child care providers, dietitian, and parent(s). Each team member's expertise contributes to the development and consistent implementation of an effective plan (e.g., Boesch et al., 2006; Haddad & Prestigiacomo, 1995; Lefton-Greif, 1994; Palmer, Drennan, & Baba, 2000; Roche, Martorana, Eicher, & Daukas, 2007).

The following sections provide an overview of the causes and characteristics of dysphagia, aspiration, and GER. Pica is also described. Table 11.1 offers a side-by-side comparison of indicators of dysphagia, aspiration, and GER.

Table 11.1.   Indicators of oral-motor difficulties

Indicator	Dysphagia	Aspiration[a]	Gastroesophageal reflux disease[b]
Respiratory distress (e.g., increased breathing rate, change in skin color)	Yes	Sometimes	Sometimes
Arching head or back during feeding	Yes	No	No
Difficulty coordinating lips, tongue, and jaw	Yes	Sometimes	No
Excessive drooling	Yes	No	Yes
Frequent coughing and gagging	Yes	Yes	Yes
Choking on food, fluid or saliva	Yes	Yes	Yes
"Wet" burps	Sometimes	No	Sometimes
Frequent hiccups	Sometimes	No	Sometimes
Difficulties with fluids in mouth	Yes	Sometimes	Sometimes
Spitting up more than twice a day	Sometimes	No	Yes
Fussy before, during and/or after feeding	Yes	Yes	Yes
Pocketing food in cheeks	Yes	Yes	No
Prolonged feeding time (>30 minutes)	Yes	Sometimes	Sometimes
Poor appetite	Yes	Sometimes	Sometimes
Poor or no weight gain for a minimum of three months	Sometimes	Sometimes	Sometimes
Refusal of foods and/or fluids	Yes	Yes	Yes
Sore or irritated throat	Sometimes	No	Yes
Pain in and around chest or abdomen (heartburn)	Sometimes	Sometimes	Sometimes
Regurgitation through nose and/or mouth	Yes	No	Yes
Failure to thrive	Yes	No	Sometimes
Nasal congestion	No	Sometimes	Yes
Fever or excessive perspiration	No	Sometimes	No
Ear infections	No	No	Sometimes
Difficulty sleeping	No	Sometimes	Yes

[a]Includes symptoms of silent aspiration. [b]Includes symptoms of GER.

ORAL-MOTOR DIFFICULTIES

The literature indicates that the majority of oral-motor difficulties are caused by damage to one or more areas of the brain responsible for oral muscle control. Oral-motor skills are critical to the child's progression from sucking on a bottle or breast to drinking from a cup and from munching to chewing various textures (Murphy & Caretto, 1999). Buswell, Leslie, Embleton, and Drinnan (2009) discussed issues that may arise for premature infants. This group, especially infants born before 32 weeks gestation, often experiences intraventricular hemorrhage (IVH; bleeding inside the fluid-filled areas of the brain). When a brain bleed is severe, brain functioning can be adversely affected for the long term. For example, the child may exhibit atypically high tone (hypertonicity) in the limbs as well as the mouth and jaw. Tongue thrust when trying to clear a spoon may also be observed. The converse is hypotonicity which is "floppy" muscle tone. A child with hypotonicity may not be able to fully close the mouth during a feeding, causing fluids and foods to escape during nursing, bottle feeding, and solid-food feeding. Sometimes hypotonicity may also result in increased saliva production.

These atypical responses are not limited to premature infants. They can also be present in young children with cerebral palsy or genetic syndromes such as trisomy 21 (Down syndrome), trisomy 18 (Edward syndrome), and Alpert syndrome (Cooper-Brown et al., 2008; Jones, 2006; Kumin & Bahr, 1999; Pereira, Sacher, Ryan, & Hayward, 2009).

As mentioned earlier in the chapter, symptoms of oral-motor difficulties vary. In addition, symptoms may occur individually or in combination. However, oral-motor difficulties generally involve problems coordinating the necessary parts of the mouth, tongue, and jaw to accept fluids and solids. Breastfeeding can also be affected when the muscles of the lips, tongue, jaw, and cheeks do not fully coordinate their movements. These problems can be further complicated by difficulties with deglutition or swallowing (Bernard-Bonnin, 2006; Darrow & Harley, 1998; Derkay & Schechter, 1998; Link, Rudolph, & Willging, 1999; Miller, 2009). With growth and maturation, some young children may cease to have these difficulties, while other children will continue to experience them. For example, Buswell et al. (2009) examined 15 preterm infants (born between 24–36 weeks gestation). Three infants (20%) were found to have oral-motor difficulties at 10 months corrected age. (Corrected age is determined by subtracting the number of weeks of prematurity from the child's chronological age. A 12-month-old child who was born 8 weeks early has a corrected age of 10 months.)

Dysphagia

Difficulties with swallowing are termed *dysphagia* and "can result from structural anomalies of the mouth and pharynx or from central nervous system defects or injury" (Manikam & Perman, 2000). There are three interrelated types of dysphagia: 1) oral dysphagia (the difficulty in the mouth to coordinate chewing and swallowing the food bolus), 2) oropharyngeal dysphagia (difficulties as the food bolus leaves the mouth and enters the pharynx, and 3) pharyngeal dysphagia (problems with timing and/or coordination to move the food bolus through the pharynx). Throughout this book, all types of swallowing disorders will be described using the term *dysphagia*. (For an in-depth discussion of dysphagia, refer to Arvedson & Brodsky, 2002, and Prasse & Kikano, 2009).

Premature infants may demonstrate dysphagia due to immature oral-motor development as well as short or prolonged enteral feeding (i.e., tube feeding; Bell & Alper, 2007; Fraker & Walbert, 2003; Prasse & Kikano, 2009). Other young children experience swallowing issues associated with specific medical diagnoses or conditions that affect the anatomy of the mouth or jaw (e.g., cleft palate) or that weaken or damage the muscles and nerves necessary for swallowing (Derkay & Schechter, 1998; Newman et al. 2001; Prasse & Kikano, 2009; Pereira et al., 2009; Rosenthal et al. 1995; Swigert, 1998).

A young child with dysphagia may feel pain when swallowing fluids, foods, or saliva. In severe cases, eating becomes a negative experience, making it difficult to consume sufficient calories for nourishment. It is imperative to collect information from parents and caregivers to learn if the dysphagia is in response to specific fluids and food items or related to the time and/or location of feeding and other variables. The most critical step is identifying the combination of causal factors so that appropriate interventions can be used (Field, Garland, & Williams, 2003). A thorough feeding assessment is necessary to pinpoint swallowing difficulties so that appropriate strategies and interventions can be developed and implemented.

Sheppard (1995) discussed clinical evaluation of dysphagia, which he said should include a detailed medical history, examination of the mouth and jaw, observation of respiratory function, and measurement of oral secretions. Prasse and Kikano (2009) stated the requirement of "a careful physical examination to assess the nutritional status, growth, and development or to identify structural abnormalities is important" (p. 249). In addition, diagnostic tests such as a *videofluoroscopic swallow study* (VFSS) or a flexible endoscopic examination of swallowing (FEES) can examine pharyngeal transit time, which is defined as the time necessary for the movement of the bolus over the base of the tongue into the esophagus (Bell & Alper, 2007; Duca, Dantas, Rodrigues, & Sawamura, 2008; Link et al., 1999; Lowery, 2001; Marquis & Pressman, 1995; see Chapter 6 for a full description of VFSS and FEES). An extended transit time is often an indicator of dysphagia—for example when the bolus does not immediately proceed past the tongue but sits in a pocket in the back of the mouth. The author further recommends observation during feeding (e.g., child's posture, presented food textures, utensils, environmental distractions). Newman et al. (2001) cautioned that some young children may demonstrate swallowing difficulties only toward the end of a bottle or solid food feeding. For this reason, observation and diagnostic testing must continue throughout the entire feeding episode.

Many authors, including Arvedson, Rogers, Buck, Smart, and Msall (1994), Benson and Lefton-Greif (1994), and Rogers and Arvedson (2005) have recommended the evaluation of all phases of swallowing (oral, pharyngeal, and esophageal) to determine the presence and severity of dysphagia and aspiration. The VFSS modified barium swallow study (MBS) is able to examine all phases. Arvedson et al. (1994) found that approximately one quarter of the young children in their study aspirated fluid before or during swallows. The majority of these occurrences (90%) were classified as silent aspiration. Silent aspiration is especially dangerous because the child does not actively cough to dispel the item (Ramsey, Smithard, & Kalra, 2005).

Aspiration

Aspiration occurs when solids or fluids that should go into the stomach travel instead into the respiratory system. Stated another way, aspiration is when ingested items go into the lungs rather than the stomach. Aspiration is caused by improper coordination of one or more parts of a child's swallowing mechanism (Schwarz, 2003; Schwarz, McCarthy, & Ton, 2006). Most young children are able to cough in order to expel an item that has "gone down the wrong way" or "down the wrong pipe," but a child who aspirates may not be successful at clearing these items. It is important to emphasize that young children with dysphagia do not aspirate, but the majority of children who aspirate also have dysphagia (Boesch et al., 2006).

Repeated aspiration can have a negative effect on the lungs, and some substances can be more harmful than others. For example, fat molecules (e.g., in milk) are difficult to clear, but water can be more easily expelled. Sometimes bacteria in the mouth (due to poor oral hygiene and/or medication) reach the lungs during aspiration. Inflammation of the airway to the lungs and of the lungs themselves that is caused by mouth secretions, food, or fluids is a lung infection known as aspiration pneumonia (Arvedson & Brodsky, 2002; Boesch et al., 2006; Field et al., 2003). Repeated bouts of aspiration pneumonia can affect overall lung function. Frequency of aspiration and the amount of material aspirated both vary depending on the underlying cause of the aspiration. Regardless of amount or frequency, all types of aspiration endanger overall lung function.

Arvedson, Rogers, Buck, Smart, and Msall (1994) discuss the risk for silent aspiration resulting from dysphagia. In contrast with aspiration that is characterized by attempting to clear the airway of a foreign object, fluid, or food item, silent aspiration (as briefly described in an earlier section) does not produce any demonstrable signs of distress and often results in the aspirated item or material reaching the lungs. This type of aspiration can lead to a host of respiratory complications, including recurring pneumonia and chronic lung disease (Ramsey et al., 2005). A swallowing study (often a modified barium study; see Chapter 6) can identify children who experience silent aspiration. Children with neurological conditions such as cerebral palsy or seizures should be closely monitored for silent aspiration. Sometimes, oral feeding must be greatly reduced or stopped due to incidences of silent aspiration. In this case, tube feeding is indicated and provides a safer method of feeding.

Gastroesophageal Reflux

Hyman (1994) described gastroesophageal reflux (GER) as the movement of stomach contents back into the esophagus. GER causes irritation to the esophagus as well as to the child's mouth or nose. Gastroesophageal reflux disease (GERD) is the clinical manifestations of GER. Approximately half of infants under 3 months of age experience at least one episode of regurgitation per day. At 6 months, many infants no longer experience GER episodes because they have developed improved neuromuscular control, which helps them sit up. Only 5% to 10% of 12-month-old infants experience GER; this reduction is tied to maturation of the digestive system and reduced intake after rapid growth during the first year (Arvedson & Brodsky, 2002; Bernard-Bonnin, 2006; Orenstein, Izadnia, & Khan, 1999).

Infants with GER often display excessive crying, irritability, and refusal of breast milk, formula, or solid foods. Dovey, Farrow, Martin, Isherwood, and Halford (2009) focused on GER and food refusal. Specifically, the authors discussed the possible interplay of behavioral and medical components of food refusal. For instance, if the child finds the sensation of GER frightening, he or she may refuse some or all foods. Swallowing may also be painful due to irritation from repeated GER episodes. Infants may also exhibit arching of the back, frequent spitting up, hiccupping, coughing, and even respiratory problems. Toddlers and preschoolers with GER generally display similar symptoms (Pulsifer-Anderson, 2009; Tsou & Bishop, 1998; Tuchman, 1994) and can often describe them to parents and caregivers.

A study by Mathisen, Worrall, Masel, Wall, and Shepherd (1999) examined 20 infants, (ages 5–7 months) with GER. The infants were found to be more difficult to feed and displayed more food refusals compared with infants without GER. The authors also described the infants' mothers experiencing negative feelings and less enjoyment in their feeding interactions with their infants. It is interesting that the infants also displayed oral-motor difficulties such as immature lip, tongue, and jaw control as well as symptoms of dysphagia. A number of factors can contribute to GER in young children, especially those with developmental delays, including decreased muscle tone in the mouth and digestive track, and the presence of a motility disorder (in which movement through the digestive track is not rhythmic, causing delays in the breakdown of food and negatively affecting nutrition; Schwarz, 2003).

For all oral-motor difficulties described in this chapter, an assessment must be conducted to ascertain causation and to develop a treatment plan. Reilly, Wisbeach, and Carr (2000) recommended an observation of a feeding session along with one or more diagnostic tests such as an upper GI barium study, gastroesophageal scintigraphy, or a 24-hour pH probe (see Chapter 6). Authors in the field also emphasize thorough assessment in the identification of GER (Sandritter, 2003; Pulsifer-Anderson, 2009; Schwarz, Corredor, Fisher-Medina, Cohen, & Rabinowitz, 2001). There is also the possibility that GER may be caused by a sensitivity or allergy, such as lactose intolerance (allergy to milk and milk-based products). These causes can be easily remedied once the specific allergen is identified and eliminated from the child's diet. If a formula-fed infant is found to have food sensitivities or allergies, many alternative hypoallergenic formulas are commercially available (e.g., Alimentum, Elecare, Nutramigen).

Silent GER, which is similar to silent aspiration, may also occur. With silent GER, the child may not vomit or appear uncomfortable after a feeding (Orenstein, Izadnia, & Khan, 1999). There are also instances in which children swallow the refluxed material. Symptoms of this condition include the child arching the neck and back during or after a feeding, food refusal, frequent hiccups, frequent ear infections, and difficulty sleeping.

As noted earlier in this chapter, Table 11.1 provides a side-by-side list of indicators for dysphagia, aspiration, and GER.

Pica

According to Parry-Jones and Parry-Jones (1992), the first published statement on the ingestion of nonfood items (pica) is attributed to a French physician in the late 1400s. Mansbacher (2009) defines pica as "swallowing non-food objects" such as dirt, clay, sand, paper, paint chips, chalk, glue, and soap (p. 32). This behavior must be exhibited for more than 1 month in order for a diagnosis of pica to be made. Pica has been attributed to nutritional deficiencies, mental illness, and an inability to distinguish between edible and nonedible items. A typically developing toddler may ingest nonfood items, but ends that behavior upon understanding the difference between edible and nonedible items or when the behavior does not attract adult attention. For a young child with a developmental delay, such understanding may develop much later. In fact, some children with significant disabilities may never progress to that point. Lacey (1990), who focused on adults, pointed out the adverse effect of pica on eating appropriate quantity and quality of nutritive foods and fluids. For example, ingesting a large amount of dirt or clay can satiate hunger for several hours without providing any nutritive value. The author also noted, "physiological, psychological, and sociological explanations each provide some understanding of pica, [but] no single explanation is likely to provide sufficient rationale for all the behaviors associated with pica practices" (p. 34).

It is important to note that pica can cause a range of medical problems, including blockages in the digestive tract, tears in the intestines, and constipation (Rose, Porcerelli, & Neale, 2000). The primary method to reduce pica is to deny the child access to nonedible items (e.g., keep the items out of reach) and to provide close supervision when the child comes into contact with the items (e.g., monitor when child plays in the yard). Chatoor (2009), Chatoor and Khushlani (2006) also described an exclusion criteria for pica: nonnutritive eating is sometimes part of culturally or religiously sanctioned practices wherein inedible items may be offered as part of a religious ceremony.

STRATEGIES AND SPECIALIZED INTERVENTIONS

Sheppard (1995) and other authors (e.g., Arvedson & Brodsky, 2002; Sandritter, 2003; Siktberg & Bantz, 1999; Woods, 1995) recommend a range of strategies to address oral-motor difficulties, including altering the presentation of foods and fluids, using adapted utensils, and implementing behavioral strategies and changes in positioning. Medications may also be required for young children with compromised swallowing. As described earlier in the chapter, the child's feeding team works collaboratively to develop and implement appropriate strategies and specialized interventions to reduce dysphagia, aspiration, and GER. The transdisciplinary team model (see Chapter 5 for a description) is especially conducive for addressing the breadth and depth of interventions because the professionals share their individual expertise to provide coordinated treatments. A team approach is also called for to design a plan to reduce and, ultimately, eliminate pica.

Oral-Motor Exercises

Kumin et al. (1999), Kumin, Von Hagel, and Bahr (2001) describe oral-motor exercises to improve overall muscle tone and assist eating and swallowing. The exercises, collectively known as the Beckman Oral Motor Protocol, include lip and cheek stretches, gum massage, and pressure to the gums and tongue. The protocol can be adjusted to the specific oral-motor strengths and needs of an individual child based on the results of a feeding assessment (see Chapter 6). For example, exercises can be tailored to assist a child with Down syndrome who has low muscle tone throughout his body as well as for a toddler with high muscle tone in his face, arms, and torso due to cerebral palsy (Manno, Fox, Eicher, & Kerwin 2005). An infant or young toddler may only tolerate one or two exercises a session due to a lower threshold for oral stimulation.

Exercises to help young children blow bubbles and drink from a straw are also effective when presented consistently over time and with adult supervision (see Rosenfeld-Johnson, 1999 for a full description of these exercises). Fast tapping, light touch, and gentle vibration can increase tone around the mouth, while slow tapping, deep pressure, and intense vibration tends to decrease tone (Morris & Klein, 2000). As with other feeding interventions, recommended oral-motor exercises must correspond to a child's specific needs and the recommendations of his feeding team. For example, Mathisen et al. (1999) reported that infants with GER often display "resistance to feeding and oral hypersensitivity which reduces the infants' desire to use the mouth for exploratory play or the intake of food" (p. 168). The oral-motor recommendations for a young child with the behaviors described previously will often be markedly different from a program aimed at a toddler with swallowing difficulties.

Oral-motor exercises are sometimes used to strengthen the muscles of the face, tongue, lips, and palate for feeding as well as to improve coordination and range of motion (active and passive stretching exercises result in greater mobility in affected areas including arms, legs, and neck; Prasse & Kikano, 2009). The exercises described here and previously should be completed in front of a mirror so the child can see her mouth, tongue, and jaw movements. Labeling the movements can help the child remember to use them in multiple settings such as child care, home, and in the community. Always consult with the feeding team for the optimal set of exercises for an infant, toddler, or preschooler. The regimen will vary by age and oral-motor needs (Bell & Alper, 2007; Gisel, Birnbaum, & Schwartz, 1998; Lefton-Greif, 1994; Murphy & Caretto, 1999).

There are a variety of commercially available items to address oral-motor difficulties. Toothettes and NUK toothbrushes can provide oral stimulation to the inside of the cheeks and the gums. It is best if the child can do this independently with adult supervision. For an infant or younger toddler, it is important to offer the Toothette and NUK toothbrush several times so the child becomes familiar with it and is not fearful when it is initially placed in her mouth. This is an especially critical consideration for infants with GER. Small tastes of formula and food items can be placed on these items and on pacifiers. Pacifiers can also be used to encourage coordination of sucking and swallowing. As a similar strategy, if a young child mouths his or her fingers, small tastes of food can be applied to the fingers.

Input from the child's feeding team is necessary to determine developmental readiness and appropriate texture/consistency and to consider allergies before presenting items to the child. Once cleared by the feeding team, a variety of food items can be placed on the lips or tip of the tongue to promote tongue movement and related skills. Lollipops, apple sauce, frosting, and whipped cream are examples. Some children may require assistance at the jaw line (Manno et al., 2005). Tastes of juices can also be offered. It is important to point out that tastes of foods and food smells can increase the flow of saliva. Therefore, young children with dysphagia should be closely monitored during oral-motor activities.

After successful tastes, the child can be offered food items or fluids from a spoon (see description of spoons in the following section). This provides a larger bolus for the child to work with and encourages additional oral-motor skills to clear the spoon, move the item around the mouth, and swallow. Providing preferred items facilitates in the establishment of successful oral-motor movements. Offering these items encourages their consistent acceptance which, in turn, can lead to improved mealtimes (Sheppard, 1995). Bernard-Bonnin (2006) cautioned to wipe a child's mouth and face only after completion of oral-motor exercises (not during the exercises) because the stimulation involved in cleaning the oral area may be overwhelming for some young children. Examples of oral-motor exercises are provided in Table 11.2.

Table 11.2. Examples of oral-motor exercises

Massage and stretches to the cheeks and mouth
Move fingers or soft cloth over lips, touch top of upper and lower lip, push straight out and push against cheeks
Imitate yawning, smiling, and similar mouth movements
Use a Toothette or NUK toothbrush around the gums and on the tongue or other areas of the mouth
Offer chewy tube, Chewelry, Knobby Chew, or similar item
Place bite size pieces of cereal on a table and ask the child to pick up a piece with his tongue without using
  his hands or lips
Blow bubbles through a bubble wand or straw or use another type of blow toy such as a whistle
Drink fluids through a straw (thicken as needed)
Place tastes of food items (e.g., puréed fruit or frosting) on lips and assist child to clear
Suck or chew on licorice strips or similar food item

Environmental Considerations

Visual stimuli, noise level, and environmental temperature are variables that can affect the feeding abilities of young children with oral-motor difficulties (Fraker & Walbert, 2003; Morris & Klein, 2000; Wolf & Glass, 1992). The feeding environment should have minimal distractions so that the child can focus on the approach and intake of food and liquid. In addition, a child with high muscle tone may startle to loud or unexpected noises, which can interrupt swallowing. If the child is too cold or too warm, oral-motor coordination may be affected. An additional consideration related to the environment is dressing the child appropriately for the setting (e.g., sweater in a cold room). It is also important to be sure a child wears loose-fitting clothing around the neck, torso, and abdomen because tight clothing can put pressure on the lower portion of the esophagus and increase GER.

A change in feeding schedule may be called for in order to address feeding difficulties related to dysphagia, GER, and aspiration. Smaller, more frequent feedings reduce some young children's GER episodes (Bernard-Bonnin, 2006). The family's preferences and child's feeding needs must be taken into account when adjusting a feeding schedule. For example, a parent with several young children may prefer one evening mealtime rather than several snack times. Authors also recommend reducing the amount of food items and fluids offered approximately 1 to 2 hours before a nap or bedtime (e.g., Arvedson & Brodsky, 2002; Palmer, Drennan & Baba, 2000; Tsou & Bishop, 1998). This schedule change is meant to reduce dysphagia symptoms and GER and potentially to allow for more restful sleep.

If changes to the feeding schedule are recommended, all child care providers and program professionals should be included in order to develop the most optimal mealtime schedule. For example, if a child receives breakfast and a snack at prekindergarten, the staff at the afternoon child care may need to provide lunch at a later time. The previous suggestions concerning lighting, acoustics, and temperature are also relevant when examining the multiple settings in which a young child participates in snack and mealtime activities. The feeding team can also recommend additional modifications to feeding times in order to address oral-motor difficulties and maintain the child's overall nutritional status (Camp & Kalscheur, 1994; Klein & Delaney, 1994).

Changes to Foods and Fluids

Formula, Bottles and Nipples   If an infant experiences one or more of the conditions described in previous sections of this chapter, the child's feeding team may recommend a change of formula. For example, a formula with higher fat content such as Enfamil Lipil may help a child swallow more effectively. A formula that addresses protein sensitivity and related digestive issues, such as Alimentum, can reduce GER and, potentially, aspiration. Conversely, Borowitz and Borowitz (1997) indicated that the type of formula does not affect GER. There may be a reduction when a new formula is introduced, but the GER often returns after this initial reduction. The authors recommended adding infant cereal to thicken feeds; doing so can facilitate swallowing and reduce GER. It may be necessary to try several types of infant cereal in order to establish which one is most effective and most preferred by the infant (Arvedson & Brodsky, 2002; Klein & Delaney, 1994).

Wolf and Glass (1992) discuss bottle nipples in terms of shape (e.g., round or flat), the size of the hole, and their effect on flow-rate and coordination with a young child's suck–swallow–breathe pattern. The size and shape of the bottle must also be considered. For example, an older infant with dysphagia may favor and be more successful with a 4 ounce bottle rather than an 8 or 9 ounce bottle. An angled bottle also helps limit the swallowing of air and maintain the child's head in a more upright position. Commercial examples of angled bottles are the Evenflo Purely Comfi and Playtex Comfortflow.

Foods   Swallowing problems, GER, and aspiration can be at least partially addressed through changes to food texture or the reduction or elimination of specific foods. The benefits of providing more highly textured foods include increasing saliva production, improving muscle tone in and around the mouth, decreasing oral sensitivity, and strengthening overall chewing and swallowing (Miller & Willging, 2003; White, Mhango-Mkandawire, & Rosenthal, 1995). Oral-motor swallowing difficulties and aspiration are best treated by a specialized diet (Sheppard, 1995). For a child who is eating solid foods, fruits, vegetables, and grains cause less damage to the lungs if aspirated compared with orange juice. Fruits with juice or syrup are more easily chewed and swallowed than fresh fruits, but the child should still be monitored for aspiration while eating these items. Textured cheeses such as cottage cheese can be offered. Meats that are soft and moist or have gravy or sauce are preferred (e.g., meatballs) to stringy pieces of meat such as chicken breast. Foods that are "runny" (e.g., apple sauce) or change form (e.g., ice cream) should be avoided.

When reducing or eliminating foods or fluids from the diet of a young child with GER, it is important to identify the specific items that cause discomfort. Food sensitivity or allergies can be treated by eliminating the source. A formula-fed infant will require a new dietary source without the element(s) that trigger or intensify GER but one that still meets age-appropriate nutritional needs. Commercially available options include Alimentum, Elecare, Nutramigen, and Pregestimil. Breastfed infants may experience GER due to foods their mother eats such as vegetables, citrus fruits, spicy dishes and sauces, fatty foods, and dairy products (Smith, Ziegler, & Gladson, 2009). The mother's intake of caffeinated items such as coffee and chocolate can be another cause of GER in a nursing infant. Toddlers and preschoolers with dysphagia and GER should be monitored for these items.

An infant can also suck on a pacifier to reduce GER. Saliva is alkaline (a base), and increased saliva production helps neutralize some of the acid associated with GER. It is also necessary to read the child's cues such as turning his head or pushing the spoon away to indicate that the child is finished eating or that the child is experiencing pain or discomfort. Oral-motor coordination may also become increasingly difficult as the feeding continues and the infant becomes tired or distracted (Morris & Klein, 2000). As previously stated, a greater number of small meals and snacks (instead of fewer, larger feeding sessions) should be offered to reduce GER and dysphagia symptoms. Frequently burping infants (after they ingest of 1 or 2 ounces) can help alleviate GER and aspiration.

Fluids   The optimal method to address oral-motor difficulties is the addition of thickeners to fluids (Boesch et al., 2006; Hyman, 1994; Pulsifer-Anderson, 2009). Commercial thickeners are available in powder form. The amount of powder added is dependent on the severity of the child's swallowing difficulties. Thin fluid can be thickened to a nectar, honey, or pudding consistency. Fluids that are mixed to a nectar consistency can be poured; the thickness is similar to that of a cream soup. Fluid with a nectar consistency can be offered from a cup. Honey consistency is thicker and not as easy to pour, but it can be presented in a cup. Pudding consistency requires a spoon.

Garcia, Chambers, Matta, and Clark (2005) examined commercially available thickeners including Thick-It and Thicken Up alongside the National Dysphagia Diet guidelines (described in National Dysphagia Task Force, 2002). The guidelines specify texture (Level I purées, Level II ground foods, Level III ground foods, and Level IV chopped foods) and fluid consistency levels. The guidelines specify the use of pudding consistency before moving to a less viscous level. The authors found that 10 and 30 minutes after preparation, gum-based thickeners (e.g., Simply Thick) maintained their viscosity or thickness better than starch-based products (e.g., Thick-It and Thicken Up). The starch-based products continued to absorb fluid and changed viscosity (becoming thicker over time).

Water, apple juice, and milk pre-thickened to nectar consistency can be found at some retailers (e.g., Walgreens) or can be special-ordered through a pharmacy. In addition, household foods—such as infant cereal, unflavored gelatin, instant breakfast powder, and mashed potato flakes—can be added to fluids to increase their viscosity. Puréed baby foods, such as fruits, vegetables, and meats, are also an option. Given the array of thickeners, the child's feeding team will provide recommendations to meet the child's nutritional needs and to reduce GER and aspiration and/or to address dysphagia concerns.

Supplements   Some young children with oral-motor difficulties may require supplements (Camp & Kalscheur, 1994, Gisel et al., 1998; Schwarz et al., 2001). Supplements can be added to foods and fluids to alter their consistency and to provide necessary nutrients, including dietary sugars and oils. Commonly used supplements include Polycose (manufactured by Ross) and Moducal, Casec, and MCT Oil (all manufactured by Mead Johnson; White et al., 1995). Additional information about supplements is available in Chapters 8 and 12.

Changes to Feeding Utensils

The literature indicates the need to examine the spoons, cups, plates, and bowls that are presented to a child for feeding purposes (Gisel et al., 1998; Miller, 2009; Siktberg & Bantz, 1999). Changes to one or all of these items can be used to address oral-motor difficulties.

Spoons A Maroon spoon is often recommended for children with oral-motor difficulties. The spoon is made of hard, smooth plastic with a shallow bowl. This shape helps children more easily transfer foods into the mouth. A Maroon Spoon also stays the same temperature regardless of the food item's temperature. This is especially helpful for young children who are sensitive to food's temperature (Siktberg & Bantz, 1999). The use of spoons with a soft bowl is also recommended. The soft texture helps the child with oral-motor difficulties to clear the spoon. It can also facilitate bolus formation and the swallowing process.

Cups Toddler and preschool aged children use a variety of cups to consume fluids. Flow-rate is a critical variable. Flexi cut cups, for example, offer a cut out for the child's nose and do not require neck extension. These cups are available in multiple sizes (1, 2, and 7 ounces) to match child's skills and intake needs. An additional example is the Munchkin Mighty Grip Flip Straw Cup. This cup is easy to grip and can hold up to 10 ounces of fluid (see Chapter 8). The straw assists a young child with dysphagia or GER to coordinate sucking and swallowing and to minimize coughing, gagging and refluxing.

A more specialized example is the PROVALE Regulating Drinking Cup. This item offers a controlled flow of either 5 cc or 10 cc of liquid each time it is brought to the mouth. (Approximately 30 cc equals 1 ounce). No thickener is required and the cup's construction is such that the child's head remains in a neutral position during drinking. A Honey Bear (or Mr. Juice Bear) cup with straw is another alternative. In sum, a child should not use a cup that requires leaning his head back.

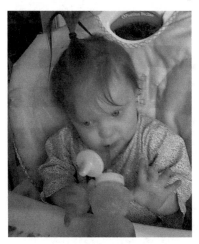

Molly (February)

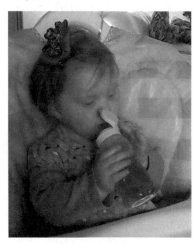

Molly (March)

Positioning

Regardless of the presence of a specific oral-motor difficulty, optimal positioning is necessary for any feeding activity (Gisel et al., 1998; Hyman, 1994). The first consideration is the child's range of motion in his arms, legs, and neck. Limited range of motion affects a body's alignment which is the ability to keep the head, neck, and trunk (torso) at midline (both sides of the body "meet" in the middle). It is also important to check for primitive reflexes which can impede alignment and also ingestion of foods and liquids. Typically, primitive reflexes such as the rooting reflex and the asymmetrical tonic neck reflex (ATNR; face is turned to one side, the arm and leg on the side to which the face is turned extend and the arm and leg on the opposite side bend), diminish and disappear as an infant gains control over her body. For some young children, these reflexes remain due to a neurological condition. For example, persistence of the ATNR impedes bringing hands to mouth and to midline which can limit an older infant's ability to self-feed.

Sheppard (1995) discusses the need for postural control to facilitate intake. Woods (1994) specified that the child must have his chin in a tucked position (slightly downward and toward the neck); must have stability through the trunk; must have the pelvis and hips aligned with his trunk; and must have his feet flat and secured. Woods's recommendations focused on treatment of dysphagia. However, they are also relevant to the feeding of infants, toddlers, and preschoolers with GER or to reduce the risk of aspiration (Boesch et al., 2006). In addition, Redstone, and West (2004) focus on improving jaw control and trunk alignment to address oral-motor difficulties present in some young children with cerebral palsy (see Chapter 12).

Siktberg and Bantz (1999) state that

> the optimal body position is an upright 90-degree sitting position with hips, knees, and ankles flexed at a 90-degree angle and feet flat on a surface. The child's head should be midline of the body with the chin slightly flexed with arms and hands near midline of the body. (p. 226)

It is sometimes necessary for the child to have a headrest added to a highchair or, if decided by the feeding team, a specialized feeding seat to facilitate midline orientation. There may also be a need for a strap to secure the shoulders and a foot rest or foot plate. Dysphagia can be exacerbated by the child's body being out of alignment.

It is helpful to keep young children, especially infants, in an upright or semi-upright (slightly inclined) position after feeding. Experts recommend keeping some young children upright for most waking hours, aiding in the swallowing process and in passage of the bolus along the digestive track and possibly reducing or preventing reflux (Sandritter, 2003; Woods, 1995). There are also indications that propping children while they sleep aids in preventing GER. However, Borowitz and Borowitz (1997) noted that "avoidance of undesirable positions" may be preferable to placement in a more optimal position that causes a young child discomfort (p. 22). For example, if an infant with GER is placed in an infant seat after a feeding and then cries for 10 minutes, swallowing a great deal of air, the likelihood of a GER episode is increased.

When an infant or young toddler is held for a feeding, chin tuck can be assisted by holding the child in a manner that encourages flexion (bending). Furthermore, supporting the child's trunk and hips, along with facilitating chin tuck, can help reduce swallowing difficulties (Woods, 1994). Towels and small Tumbleform rolls can be used to position an infant with GER. In addition, an acid reflux (AR) pillow is commercially available. The pillow provides support for the child to maintain chin tuck and a midline orientation during and after feeds.

To feed a toddler or preschooler in a highchair or similar seating, a parent or caregiver should feed from a seated position in front of the child. Standing can cause hyperextension of the child's head and neck which adversely affects swallowing. An adult may also sit at a slight angle to the child with one arm around the child to provide support to the jaw, cheeks, and lips as appropriate. Members of the child's feeding team must be consistent regarding positioning interventions to effectively address oral-motor difficulties.

Behavioral Strategies

Behavioral strategies have been described by many authors for treatment of dysphagia (e.g., Manno et al., 2005; Sheppard, 1995). Kerwin (1999) and Piazza, Patel, Gulotta, Sevin, and Layer (2003) emphasized using positive reinforcement for appropriate feeding behaviors and ignoring or guiding inappropriate behaviors. Manno et al. (2005) discussed the use of task analysis and altering what occurs before the specific feeding behaviors (antecedent condition). Specifically, the desired feeding behavior is first broken down "into small, discrete steps, [then] manipulating the antecedent condition by presenting food or fluid in a way that allows the child to complete the behavior expected successfully and clear consequences for completing or not completing the task" (p. 153). Consequences (responses to behavior which can be positive, such as praise or preferred food item, or negative, such as ignoring or removing a favorite toy) are also planned with input from parents, caregivers, and other members of the child's feeding team. For young children with dysphagia, aspiration, or GER, behavioral strategies can also address mealtime anxiety. For example, because of repeated coughing and choking, a young child may withdraw from mealtimes; the child may require shaping procedures and positive reinforcement before tasting foods, approaching the mealtime table, and so forth.

Behavioral treatment for pica often includes the presentation of an unpleasant taste (e.g., hot sauce), smell (e.g., bleach) or sensation (e.g., light pinch) before or after eating a nonfood item. In this way, the child learns to associate the disagreeable sensation with the nonfood item. Over time, this association will reduce and then eliminate ingestion of the nonfood item and increase intake of appropriate, edible items (Mansbacher, 2009). In behavioral terms, this is an example of the use of negative reinforcement or gaining removal of an unpleasant stimulus when a desired behavior occurs. Another technique was reported by Kern, Starosta, and Adelman (2006) who studied two children with pica. An inedible item was paired with a preferred food item; then the children were given verbal cues to exchange the edible item for the nonfood item (e.g., "if you want a chip, hand me the paper," p. 144). Positive reinforcement was also provided. Both children displayed a decrease in pica episodes with an increase in eating preferred food items across settings. Often, several behavioral strategies implemented by all members of the child's feeding team are necessary for long-term change in behavior.

Bell and Stein (1992) identified the use of aversives and punishment to reduce pica. For example, Fisher et al. (1994) utilized a combination of positive reinforcement (preferred edible items or toys) and punishment (e.g., water mist, holding child's hands, and time out) to address the pica behaviors of three preschoolers with pervasive developmental delays. In addition, children were taught to discriminate edible items by their arrangement on a plate or placemat. It must be pointed out that, presently, punishment is not recommended or used to reduce inappropriate behaviors.

Table 11.3. Strategies and specialized interventions to address oral-motor difficulties

Environmental considerations
    Adjust light and sound to minimize distractions
    Observe child for optimal temperature for feeding
    Adjust feeding schedule to provide an increased number of smaller meals and snacks
    Provide final meal of the day at least 1–2 hours before bedtime
Changes to formula, bottles, and nipples
    Use specialized formula as necessary
    Add rice cereal or other infant cereal to thicken breast milk or formula
    Adjust size and/or shape and texture of nipple
    Adjust size and/or shape of the bottle
Changes to foods
    Modify food texture
    Reduce or eliminate foods that cause or contribute to dysphagia, GER, and aspiration
    Offer a pacifier to infants to increase saliva production and reduce acid
Changes to fluids
    Use commercial thickeners to increase thin fluids to nectar, honey, or pudding consistency
    Add household foods (e.g., infant cereal, potato flakes) to increase viscosity
    Offer supplements as directed
Changes to feeding utensils
    Offer spoons that assist with bolus formation and the swallowing process
    Use cups that do not require the child to lean the head back
    Use cups that offer controllable flow rate and include a straw if needed
Positioning
    Encourage chin tuck
    Promote midline orientation and postural control
    Address primitive reflexes if present
    Position the child in an upright or semi-upright position before, during, and after feeding
    Secure feet as needed
    Specialized seating or equipment as indicated such as Baby Acid Reflux pillow, bolster or wedge
Behavioral strategies
    Positive reinforcement
    Negative reinforcement
    Task analysis
    Shaping
    Systematic desensitization
    Limited use of aversives
Medications
    Antacids
    Proton pump inhibitors
    Histamine-2-receptor antagonists
    Check for medication interactions and side effects

Medications

There are several types of medications to address GER. Antacids such as TUMS can be tried first (if the child can chew and swallow the tablet). Another type of medication is prokinetics, which work to increase gastrointestinal motility or the movement of food bolus and fluids down the digestive tract. This type of medication helps reduce heartburn and vomiting. Prilosec and Prevacid are prokinetics and are available over the counter (OTC). Proton pump inhibitors such as Zantac or Tagamet are medications that reduce the production of gastric acid. A similar class of medications is the histamine-2-receptor antagonists, which also decrease acid production. Reglan is used to improve digestion and requires a prescription. These medications may be used in combination. Medication requires ongoing supervision from a pediatrician for drug interactions, especially if the child receives additional daily medications (e.g., antibiotics, antiseizure medications). In addition, some of these medications were not originally intended for administration to young children (Schwarz et al., 2001; Strople & Kaul, 2003). All of these medications should be given approximately a half an hour before a feeding or meal.

Sandritter (2003) advocated the use of GER medication only after a thorough physical examination, a 24-hour pH probe, and trials of less invasive methods such as changes to foods and positioning strategies. Sandritter cautioned that only few types of medications are intended for infants and to be aware of possible side effects such as stomach pain and constipation.

Oral-motor difficulties may be manifested in several ways, but all of these difficulties converge in feeding issues that greatly affect food intake. Young children with dysphagia require an array of strategies and specialized interventions to make mealtimes enjoyable for themselves, their caregivers, and feeding team members. See Table 11.3 for an overview of the strategies and specialized interventions described in this chapter. Aspiration must also be addressed with appropriate methods of assessment (see Chapter 6) and intervention. The potentially harmful health outcomes of these conditions, as well as pica, necessitate a systematic approach to treating and reducing their symptoms and manifestations.

■ ■ ■ TABLE TALK ■ ■ ■

Jamie is 27 months old. As an infant, he had difficulty with GER. With assistance from his pediatrician and SLP, he was able to accept 2–3 ounces of breast milk without experiencing discomfort. Jamie's mother and father (Gabbie and Matthew), worked closely with him to ensure that his feedings were enjoyable and met his needs. He was burped several times during a feeding and kept upright for at least 30 minutes following a feeding.

When Jamie began solid foods, he enjoyed fruits with thicker consistency, such as bananas and apricots, and finger foods, such as cheese cubes and bite-size crackers. He took several ounces of juice from a Sippy cup with some coughing. Jamie's mother noted that Jamie was willing to taste foods such as apple sauce and puréed vegetables, but after several spoonfuls he would turn his head away and grimace.

When Gabbie asked the SLP about Jamie's behavior, the SLP asked if Jamie had ever aspirated fluids or liquids, but Gabbie couldn't recall this happening. The SLP told Gabbie that some children aspirate without coughing or gagging. After learning this information, Gabbie and Matthew presented Jamie only his preferred food items. They were hesitant to offer additional age-appropriate foods. Mealtimes were quickly becoming a source of anxiety for the entire family.

At Jamie's 36 month well-visit, he was at the 25th percentile for weight. On previous visits, his weight was between the 50th and 75th percentiles. The pediatrician told Jamie's parents that they must give Jamie more table foods and introduce an open-mouth drinking cup. The doctor was concerned that without these changes in his feeding, Jamie would move to an even lower weight percentile.

Discussion Questions

■ Do you agree with the pediatrician's recommendations?

■ What types of foods and fluids would you recommend offering to Jamie?

■ How would you approach the issues described?

FEEDING NUGGETS

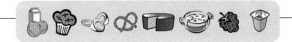

Books

Oral-Motor Assessment and Treatment: Ages and Stages by Diane Chapman Bahr (2000)
http://www.pearsonhighered.com/educator/product/Oral-Motor-Assessment-and-Treatment-Ages-and-Stages/9780205297863.page

Mouth Madness: Oral-Motor Activities for Children by Catherine Orr (1999)
clinicalcustomersupport@pearson.com
http://www.pearsonassessments.com/HAIWEB/Cultures/en-us/Productdetail.htm?Pid=076-1648-50X&Mode=summary

Reflux 101: A Parent's Guide to Gastroesophageal Reflux by Jan Gambino (2008)
refluxmom@gmail.com
http://refluxmom.com/?page_id=19

Web Sites

For more information about the Beckman Oral Motor Protocol:
http://www.beckmanoralmotor.com/index.html

Pediatric/Adolescent Gastroesophageal Reflux Association (PAGER)
gergroup@aol.com
http://www.reflux.org

Dysphagia Plus Progressive Therapy Solutions
Cust_Svr@dysphagiaplus.com
http://www.dysphagiaplus.com/

12

Young Children With Neurological Disorders

What You'll Learn in This Chapter

This chapter provides

- A description of cerebral palsy (the most common neurological disorder in young children)
- An overview of intraventricular hemorrhage and shaken baby syndrome (additional conditions resulting in neurological disorders)
- An examination of cerebral visual impairment
- Strategies and interventions to address mild to severe feeding problems associated with neurological disorders

■ ■ ■ FOOD FOR THOUGHT ■ ■ ■

"Aazim, who is 48 months old, has cerebral palsy and physical limitations. I have fed him several times in school. His meal contains milk with small pieces of soft bread. I mix them together and feed him with a spoon. His lips cannot close very well because of his physical disability, but he can swallow the food very well."

Shafia, Early Childhood Special Education Graduate Student

"Vinny, who is 14 years old, has full trisomy 13, balanced translocation of chromosomes 5 and 13, and is extremely visually limited. He has no lower field of vision and is blind in his right eye. He has never seen clearly. We tried several feeding utensils. Scoop plates and scoop bowls work best for him. He uses either an Avent Sippy cup or drinks through a straw. With regard to spoons, he has to have a large grip and a lightweight handle with not too big a reservoir for the food."

Nina, Parent

The preceding examples provide a context for feeding issues affecting young children with neurological disorders. There are many manifestations of neurological disorders, and primary among them are motor difficulties affecting the arms and legs as well as the neck and facial area. Singly, or in combination, these motor difficulties can interfere with intake of fluids and foods as well as with swallowing. Respiration can also be negatively affected, which can further impede feeding. Some young children also experience compromised vision and/or hearing as a result of neurological insult. Limited vision can also reduce self-feeding.

Cerebral palsy is the most commonly diagnosed neurological disorder requiring the services of a feeding team (Roger, 2004). Stevenson et al. (2006) discussed growth and overall health in children with moderate to severe levels of cerebral palsy. The majority of children with this condition require a wheelchair or other assistive device for mobility (e.g., walker, orthotics, braces), are underweight, and are at risk for a variety of medical complications, especially respiratory conditions such as pneumonia. The literature also indicates that children with cerebral palsy should participate in naturally occurring and age-appropriate home and community activities (Liptak & Accardo, 2004; Morrow, Quine, & Craig, 2007). Because cerebral palsy varies widely in severity (one child may have one limb mildly affected; another child may be severely affected, including severe vision impairment), it is important to focus on individually appropriate goals and interventions for overall development (Cooley and the Committee on Children with Disabilities, 2004). All of these recommendations affect the treatment of feeding difficulties in young children with cerebral palsy.

WHAT THE LITERATURE SAYS

Cerebral palsy is a set of neurological disorders affecting body movement and muscle coordination. The condition is diagnosed in infancy or early childhood and remains static during the child's lifetime (severity does not improve or worsen). Cerebral palsy is caused by injury to parts of the brain that control muscle movement. Most children with cerebral palsy are born with it but the condition may not be detected until months or even several years later. A small number of cases are caused by brain damage during labor and delivery or the first few months or years of life (e.g., anoxia; loss or restricted oxygen); some cases are caused when premature infants experience an intraventricular hemorrhage (IVH; brain bleed) after birth; and some cases are caused by brain infections such as bacterial meningitis or viral encephalitis and head injury (Burklow, McGrath, Allred & Rudolph,

2002; Jones, Morgan, Shelton, & Thorogood, 2007; Krigger, 2006; Venkateswaran & Shevell, 2008).

The most common signs of cerebral palsy are prolonged presence of primitive reflexes. For example, the asymmetrical tonic reflex (ATNR) is demonstrated by infants up to 6 months of age. When the infant's face turns to one side, the arm and leg on that side extend and the arm and leg on the opposite side bend. Older infants, toddlers, and preschoolers with neurological disorders, especially cerebral palsy, may continue to exhibit an ATNR. This reflex can affect a child's ability to bring her hands to midline as well as to her mouth. Over an extended period of time, ATNR may cause scoliosis (curvature of the spine) and hip dislocation. Other primitive reflexes that can affect feeding are the startle reflex and the gag reflex.

Young children with neurological disorders display muscle tone abnormalities. Children with spastic cerebral palsy have stiff, tight, or high muscle tone (hypertonicity). Approximately 10%–20% of children with cerebral palsy experience slow, writhing muscle movements or athetoid cerebral palsy. Some children have ataxic cerebral palsy, which affects balance and coordination. Finally, a small number of children are diagnosed with a mixed type of cerebral palsy that includes symptoms of two or all three of the other types (Krigger, 2006). Some children also display low muscle tone (hypotonicity) which affects head control, trunk stability, and overall body movement. Some children with cerebral palsy are mobile and need very little assistance to interact with their environment, while others are totally dependent on caregivers for all of their daily needs and activities (See Palisano et al., 1997, for information about use of the Gross Motor Function Classification Scale for children with cerebral palsy).

It is important to note a relationship between the muscles and movements affected by cerebral palsy and oral-motor development (Krigger, 2006). For a typically developing child, the transition from sitting to standing, for example, is accompanied by changes in the ability to move food around in the mouth. In addition, stability in the trunk and pelvic area is critical to maintaining an upright position for meals (Lowman, 2010). Noterdaeme, Mildenberger, Minow, and Amorosa (2002) examined similar issues in young children with autism and speech-language disorders and found a correlation with oral-motor difficulties in speech production and feeding skills. Other authors focused on children with speech-only disorders and language-only disorders with similar impact on current and future motor skills (Visscher, Houwen, Scherder, Moolenaar, & Hartman, 2007). In sum, the literature reveals associations among these developmental pathways and the need to provide interventions as early as possible to promote optimal development. The motor skills developed during an infant's first year are critical to future skills. Table 12.1 provides an overview of gross-motor, oral-motor, and speech development during the first year along with possible complications due to neurological disorders.

The following statement points to the need for examination and dissemination of feeding strategies and interventions for young children with cerebral palsy:

> There is increasing recognition of the range and significance of feeding disorders in childhood. In spite of this, there is a paucity of information concerning the development of feeding efficiency and the prevalence of feeding impairments in the general population and in children with cerebral palsy. (Rogers, 2004, p. S28)

Table 12.1. Examples of the interrelationship of gross-motor, oral-motor, and speech development during the first year and possible complications due to neurological disorders

	Gross motor	Oral-motor	Speech
Newborn (birth–3 months)			
Typical development	Total body movement	Suckling pattern	Reflexive sounds
	Limited range of motion	Needs pressure to cheeks, lips, and jaw	Differentiated cries (hungry, tired)
	Head turns to maintain airway	Accepts fluids and breathes at same time	Displays some facial expression
	Shoulder elevates to assist head control	Some coordination in breathing and sucking	Produces vowel sounds
Possible complication	Minimal head control	Unable to suckle	Undifferentiated cries
	Limited head turn	Limited coordination	Limited vowel sounds
Infant 4–6 months			
Typical development	Pushes up on elbows on belly	Moves objects to mouth	Produces open vowel sounds
	Supported sitting to independent sitting	Better coordination at breast or with bottle	Babbling emerges (various sounds)
	Moves hands/plays in side-lying position	Introduce spoon feeding	Some intonation of sounds
	Rolling (back to belly and belly to back)	Tongue moves laterally in mouth	Some sound imitation
Possible complication	No independent sitting	Limited coordination	Limited babbling
	Little voluntary movement	Limited mouthing of food or objects	Limited ability to form sounds
Infant 7–9 months			
Typical development	Commando-crawls and creeps	Lip closure around spoon	Continues babbling; some combinations
	Rotates trunk	Munching emerges	Vocalizes more
	Stands with wide base	Tongue and jaw move separately	Clearer articulation of sounds
Possible complication	Unable to crawl	Limited lip closure	Little babbling
	Cannot rotate trunk	Limited jaw movement	Limited articulation
Older infant (10–12 months)			
Typical development	Cruising	Drink from cup	Approximates words
	Stands independently for longer periods	Bites and chews soft foods	Produces consonant-vowel combinations
	Takes steps with or without assistance	Finger feeds	Produces jargon (babbling and words)
Possible complication	Unable to cruise	Ineffective bite	Limited vocalizations
	Cannot stand alone	Difficulty self-feeding	Does not use jargon

However, the use of feeding strategies and interventions must be tempered with accurate assessment information that describes the type and extent of feeding problems due to prenatal or postnatal neurological injury. In this regard, the literature does provide some guidance on methods to assess feeding problems in young children with neurological disorders.

The first step is to complete a physical examination that evaluates muscle tone and voluntary movement and that includes an imaging study such as magnetic resonance imaging (MRI). An MRI produces images of organs and structures inside the body (Aneja, 2004; Ashwal et al., 2004; Jones, Morgan, Shelton, & Thorogood, 2007). Results can be used for diagnosis of structurally based feeding conditions. Literature also describes the use of videofluoroscopy (video X-ray imaging study) to examine the swallowing mechanism (Aneja, 2004; Jones et al., 2007). A videofluoroscopic swallowing study (VFSS) provides detailed information about the movement of food and fluids from the mouth to the stomach. Rogers, Arvedson, Buck, Smart, and Msall (1994) found that VFSS results for almost all children with cerebral palsy in their sample (97%) indicated difficulties with textured food items including purées and solids and many episodes of silent aspiration of fluids. Similar results were described by Baikie et al. (2005) and Wright, Wright, and Carson (1996). Dysphagia (swallowing disorders; see Chapter 8) is also common as mechanisms in the pharynx and esophagus are affected when a young child has a neurological disorder (Alper & Manno, 1996).

Ashwal et al. (2004) supported assessment of oral-motor skills including jaw control and tongue movement. The Schedule for Oral-Motor Assessment (SOMA) examines these types of skills and is widely used (Reilly, Skuse, Mathisen, & Wolke, 1995). In addition, Kenny et al. (1989) developed the Multidisciplinary Feeding Profile (MFP). This instrument's strength lies in its focus on the feeding skills and behaviors of children who are dependent feeders. Items focus on facial features such as the structure of the lips, tongue placement, and features of the soft and hard palate. In addition, the MFP considers the presence of the gag reflex, voluntary oral-motor movements (e.g., jaw), and patterns in spoon feeding, biting, chewing, cup drinking, and swallowing including observing lip retraction and tongue thrust. The SOMA and MFP can also assist in identifying problems with mastication (biting, crushing, and grinding food), swallowing, and breathing (Redstone & West, 2004).

There is also concern about nutritional status and overall growth in children with cerebral palsy. Half the children in Schwarz et al. (2001) sample ($n = 79$) were diagnosed with cerebral palsy and required gastrostomy feedings and/or supplements to meet their nutritional needs. Trier and Thomas (1998) also suggested that enteral feeding (i.e., tube feeding) be considered when oral feeding becomes unsafe, when oral feeding becomes unenjoyable for child and parent or caregiver, and/or when oral feeding becomes overly time consuming (see Chapter 14). The authors also offer thickening of liquids and adjusting food consistency to reduce or eliminate gastroesophageal reflux (GER) and aspiration (Thomas & Akobeng, 2000). Finally, Strauss, Shavelle, Reynolds, Rosenbloom, and Day (2007) noted, "gastrostomy and oral feeding can be complementary rather than mutually exclusive" (p. 90). Improved survival was identified for children receiving both types of nutrition. This finding also points to the importance of maintaining oral feeding after the introduction of enteral methods. Gisel and Alphonce (1995) indicated that "oral feeding may then focus on the pleasurable, social aspects of the meal while gastrostomy feeding provides necessary calories for growth" (p. 272).

Some children with cerebral palsy require placement of gastrostomy tubes (G-tubes) to increase intake and reduce respiratory difficulties such as pneumonia (Fung et al., 2002; Gisel et al., 2003; Redstone & West, 2004; Samson-Fung, Butler, & O'Donnell, 2003). Sullivan et al. (2005) identified positive outcomes for children with neurological disorders with only minor complications 12 months post-surgery (e.g., irritation of the G-tube site, leakage, tube blockage). However, in a review of the literature, Sleigh and Brocklehurst (2004) found evidence of a variety of problems after G-tube surgery, including aspiration (food items and fluids into the lower airway or lungs) and infection at the G-tube site. The authors also noted that the reintroduction of food and liquids by mouth requires much team input and collaboration for its success. Sullivan et al. (2005) asserted that "published evidence supporting gastrostomy tube feeding as an effective nutritional intervention in children with CP is weak" (p. 84).

Weight gain can be facilitated with oral feeding interventions. This is critically important because many children with neurological disorders have difficulty attaining and maintaining age appropriate growth (Motion, Northstone, Edmond, Stucke, & Golding, 2002; Sullivan et al., 2000). Sullivan et al. (2000) found that the majority of children in their study (n = 271; range = 4–13 years of age) were underweight or struggled to gain weight. In addition, parents reported spending approximately 3 hours daily to feed their children with cerebral palsy. In addition, some children may take medication for other neurological issues such as seizures. Feeding may be affected if, for example, the medication causes drowsiness so that the child is not fully awake at mealtimes. Finally, children with cerebral palsy may exhibit excessive amounts of drooling which can interfere with eating and drinking (Van der Burg, Didden, Jongerius, & Rotteveel, 2007).

Intraventricular Hemorrhage

Cerebral palsy is sometimes a manifestation of intraventricular hemorrhage (IVH). Premature infants are at risk for this condition, which involves bleeding into the fluid-filled areas (ventricles) surrounding the brain. This condition occurs frequently in premature children because blood vessels in the brain are not fully developed and are extremely fragile (Burklow, McGrath, & Kaul, 2002). An ultrasound of a premature infant's heads is recommended to determine if an IVH has occurred because there may be few outward symptoms (e.g., breathing pauses, excessive sleep, weak suck; Futagi, 2006).

IVH varies from Grade 1 to 4. Higher grades are associated with a greater severity of bleeding. For example, a Grade 2 IVH involves a small amount of bleeding and does not usually cause long-term problems. A Grade 3 or 4 IVH, on the other hand, has the potential to affect overall brain function and produce chronic problems in feeding. Burklow et al. (2002) recommend a team approach to address the needs of infants and young children with IVH. Specifically, the authors recommended "well-coordinated, interdisciplinary care, given the multitude of nutritional, physiologic, developmental, and behavioral factors that need to be assessed and managed simultaneously" (p. 28).

Shaken Baby Syndrome

Gutierrez, Clements, and Averill (2004) described shaken baby syndrome as the violent shaking of a child, often under 2 years of age, by an adult caregiver resulting in brain injury (p. 24). Most often, the child will experience a Grade 3 or 4 IVH and related neurological complications such as cerebral palsy and blindness. Impaired feeding and swallowing disorders may also result regardless of the extent of injury. Fulton (2000) and Smith (2003) stated that some children may require total or supplemental tube feeding after the shaking episode(s). In addition, sometimes treatment is not sought until days or weeks after the injury when an adult notices untypical behavior such as vomiting, increased sleeping, and lethargy. This can further affect the child's intake and overall growth and nutrition.

Addressing feeding needs must be part of a larger context of permanency planning because large numbers of shaken baby cases occur at the hands of a parent or a parent's partner (Smith, 2003). Input from medical professionals, such as an ophthalmologist and neurologist, is also required. These specialists can determine the extent of injury to the child's vision and overall neurological functioning, respectively.

Cerebral Visual Impairment

Many children with a neurological disorder are also diagnosed with cerebral visual impairment (CVI; Dutton & Jacobson, 2001; Fazzi et al, 2007). In fact, approximately 40% of brain function is related to vision (Dutton & Jacobson, 2001). CVI is a neurological disorder rather than a vision or eye disorder. Put another way, in CVI the structures of the eyes are not directly affected, unlike those of a child with cataracts or retinopathy of prematurity (ROP).

CVI occurs when one or more parts of the brain involved with vision (e.g., the occipital lobe) are damaged. Causation is similar to cerebral palsy—loss of oxygen at birth and perinatal meningitis—and co-occurrence of cerebral palsy and CVI is common. In addition, in a study by Ghasia, Brunstrom, Gordon, and Tychsen (2008), a correlation was observed between a higher GMFCS score and CVI. The presenting visual difficulties are due to damage to the neural pathways which affect how information is processed (Dutton & Jacobson, 2001; Lanners, Piccioni, Fea & Goergen, 1999). Damage to these pathways can affect the child's ability to focus on objects, use the entire visual field, and perceive the depth and distance. The condition does not worsen, but the child must learn to draw meaning from an often visually confusing environment. In addition, the manifestation of CVI often varies, so changes in visual functioning and peripheral vision are common (Teplin, 1995).

Several possible manifestations of CVI can influence feeding. Good, Jan, Burden, Skoczenski, and Candy (2001) discussed how "poor feeding skills and recurrent problems with aspiration are common because of difficulties encountered with food that require chewing (partly a visually learned skill) and swallowing" (p. 58). The authors also caution that some children with neurological disorders are easily overstimulated, which has implications for all activities of daily living including mealtimes. It is important to provide children with cerebral palsy and CVI with high-contrast feeding utensils and verbal cues to encourage self-feeding (see Vinny's experience at beginning of this chapter). Finally, Fazzi et al. (2007) and Venkateswaran and Shevell (2008) emphasized the need to accurately assess feeding issues so that appropriate interventions can be developed and implemented with this population.

Feeding Team

Input from a variety of professionals is needed to develop and implement an effective feeding program. Due to the neurological basis of these conditions and associated anatomical issues, input from a number of specialized professionals is often required for planning, implementing, and evaluating interventions. In addition to a speech-language pathologist (SLP), occupational therapist (OT), physical therapist (PT), dietitian, parents, caregivers, and early intervention (EI) or preschool professionals, a range of medical disciplines may be part of the team for a brief or extended period of time. A SLP or OT is often the professional who coordinates the work of the team (Anderson, 1998; Blacklin, 1998; Swigert, 1998). While diverse in composition, the feeding team for a young child with cerebral palsy must work in a coordinated fashion in both the short term and the long term (Cooley and the Committee on Children with Disabilities, 2004).

A child's team may include a pulmonologist or pulmonary disease specialist. This individual diagnoses and treats pulmonary (lung) conditions and diseases. A related specialist is a respiratory therapist (RT) who evaluates and works with individuals with breathing or other cardiopulmonary disorders. An RT works under the direction of a physician. An orthopedist is a surgeon focusing on the skeleton (bones of the body); one may be involved if a child requires surgical intervention such as hip surgery. The input of a physiatrist may also be necessary. This physician diagnoses a variety of medical problems and recommends treatment, including therapy and specialized equipment. In addition, a team may include a radiologist, a physician with specialized training in interpreting medical images, such as results from a VFSS. A neurologist focuses on the diagnosing and treating nervous system disorders including those affecting the brain and muscles. In addition, a gastroenterologist specializes in the diagnosis and treatment of disorders of the gastrointestinal or digestive tract, including the esophagus, stomach, small intestine, large intestine, pancreas, liver, and gallbladder.

STRATEGIES AND INTERVENTIONS

The following strategies and specialized interventions focus on encouraging young children with neurological disorders to participate in feeding activities, whether or not oral feeding is the primary source of nutrition or a supplementary source. The feeding team must be aware of the medical issues and complications outlined previously to ensure that all feeding experiences are both safe and enjoyable. For example, Anderson (1998) stated that a child may need to be fed prior to the family's mealtime to address intake needs. When the family eats, the focus can shift to socialization and offering tastes of table foods.

Oral-Motor Exercises

Oral-motor treatments have been described for many years as a means to address feeding problems (Alexander, 1987; Beckman, 2003; Kumin, Von Hagel, & Bahr, 2001; Morris, 1989). The most common oral-motor conditions in young children with cerebral palsy are gag reflex, tonic bite reflex, jaw thrust, tongue thrust, bruxism (tooth grinding), high or low tone in cheeks, and excessive drooling (Anderson, 1998; Motion et al., 2002). A variety of exercises can be used, such as massage that includes stroking, tapping, and applying firm pressure, vibration (e.g. electric toothbrush), and the application of hot or cold items (e.g., a warm cloth or ice pack) to the cheeks and lips. These types of oral-motor exercises can improve the coordination of tongue movements and increase muscle strength. Also, "Oral-motor skills may be particularly important when a decision is made for oral supplementation with calorically denser foods" (Gisel, Applegate-Ferrante, Benson, & Bosma, 1996, p. 70). This circumstance addresses young children with neurological disorders who are primarily tube fed and permitted to receive some foods or liquids orally.

Young children with both types of tonal difficulties (hypotonicity and hypertonicity) require input to the cheeks and mouth to prepare for food items and fluids. The difference in the provision of oral-motor exercises for children with hypotonicity versus hypertonicity lies in matching the type of touch or stimulation to the child's skills and needs. For example, Harry (2008b) describes spoon feeding her daughter with cerebral palsy involving hypertonicity:

> First, to get Melanie to open her tightly pursed lips, then to relax the trap-like jaw just enough to get the tip of the spoon in, then to get her to relax her tongue so that the spoon could be placed on the top instead of below it, thus allowing the milk to go down her throat instead of over her lips and down her chin. (p. 31)

This vignette illustrates the need for oral-motor intervention for the lips, mouth, and jaw to reduce muscle tone. Active (child participates) or passive (feeder provides) stretching encompasses exercises such as pursing lips, blowing bubbles, drinking from a straw, and licking food from the lips. These exercises can improve oral-motor skills such as lip closure, tongue lateralization (movement of tongue from side to side in the mouth), and chewing, and they can facilitate weight gain and meeting nutritional needs—for example, by limiting food loss from the mouth (Gisel, 1994). A child's daily regimen of oral-motor exercises will be developed by the feeding team to account for age, skills, and neurological status.

Oral-motor exercises can help a child to accept food from a feeder (e.g., parent, child care provider) as well promote self-feeding (Gisel et al., 1996). Gisel et al. (1996) described a study that included young children with cerebral palsy. After oral-motor exercises, improvements were noted in lip closure with food items, chewing, spoon feeding, and swallowing. The researchers also provided opportunities for the children to see and smell foods and to touch feeding utensils before their use. This was done to address sensory aspects of feeding that can affect the effectiveness of oral-motor exercises. Also, Anderson (1998) pointed out that a child with cerebral palsy may be over- or under-responsive to touch around the mouth. Accordingly, providing firm pressure or light touch will depend on the child's reactions. For example, a child with low tone may need firm pressure as well as adult assistance to be an active participant in oral-motor exercises (Kumin et al., 2001). Temperature of foods and liquids can also affect intake. Overall, a child's desensitization to tactile input (touch) around the face can improve coordination of the oral musculature which directly affects feeding.

Some oral-motor exercises require more active manipulations by the feeder. If a child has difficulty opening her mouth, the feeder can provide the exercises as described previously, as well as place the thumb of her nondominant hand on the child's chin and pointer and middle fingers under chin to gently open the child's mouth (Redstone & West, 2004). Another way is to place the thumb on one side of the jaw and the same hand's index finger on the other side of the jaw and gently to open the mouth. For a child with difficulty chewing food items, it is helpful to place the palm under the child's chin to help keep the mouth closed and to provide rotating movements to the chin and jaw to facilitate chewing. Due to the more intrusive nature of these oral-motor exercises, the feeding team must be consulted on their use. Exercises should facilitate feeding, not produce additional issues such as resistance to touch around the mouth and cheeks. In addition, the feeder must sit in front of the child because sitting to the side or behind cause tonal responses (e.g., primitive reflexes) that impede eating and drinking.

For some children, drooling interferes with feeding. Excessive saliva may disrupt the breakdown of food in the mouth and hamper swallowing (Motion et al., 2002; Sullivan et al., 2000; van der Burg et al., 2007; van der Burg, Jongerius, van Limbeek, van Hulst, & Rotteveel, 2006). Oral-motor exercises can help by encouraging lip closure, for example (additional strategies to address drooling are included in the Specialized Supplements and Calorie Boosters section). Results of a VFSS can pinpoint the muscles involved in swallowing and indicate the need for additional responsiveness to the presentation of foods and liquids. An additional strategy to address input to the face is to refrain from wiping the child's mouth and face frequently because this input can increase muscle tone and, over time, lead to heightened sensitivity around the mouth, cheeks, and chin.

Positioning

A child must be comfortable in order to participate in feeding activities. If positioning is not appropriate, a young child, especially a nonverbal one who cannot tell a parent or caregiver of her discomfort, may not eat or drink or may experience more episodes of GER or aspiration. Regardless of the stage of feeding development, a child with a neurological disorder requires support to many parts of the body, including the head, neck, shoulders, and hips. Breastfeeding can be facilitated by a more upright position. A highchair for a toddler may need rolled towels or specialized items to encourage midline orientation, especially if the child still exhibits an ATNR. A preschooler may need a specialized feeding chair or a wheelchair designed to meet motor needs. To facilitate intake of food and liquids through the mouth, movement of the bolus, and swallowing, positioning must focus on stability of the head, neck, trunk, pelvis, and hips while normalizing muscle tone and abnormal posturing (Donato, Fox, Mormon, & Mormon, 2008). Symmetry through the trunk and pelvis is also needed for feeding success. GER and aspiration can thus be reduced or eliminated through positioning, and corresponding pulmonary status can be improved (Gisel, 1994; Gisel et al., 2003).

For an infant or younger toddler with a neurological disorder, positioning must aid head control. For example, the child can be positioned facing the feeder on the feeder's lap. A pillow or wedge can also be placed behind so the child is semireclined and receives more support for the head and neck (Woods, 1995). With approval of the child's feeding team, prone position (on the belly) may be recommended. This position is thought to reduce hypertonicity and maintain an open airway. For older toddlers, a highchair with or without a customized insert can be used. A child can also be fed in a stroller with back support. If a child continues to be fed in a feeder's lap, the feeder should cradle the child as she would an infant and assist the child to maintain chin tuck along with alignment through the shoulders, torso, and hips. For all positions, feeders will need guidance from the feeding team to provide the proper amount of support to key areas (e.g., alignment through torso, flexion to hips).

Gisel et al. (1996) described positioning of 35 children aged 4–13 years with cerebral palsy in the following way:

> Children were observed at lunch/snack time in their accustomed room with the person (assistant) who was the child's regular feeder. Children were either seated in their custom-fitted wheelchairs or, if ambulatory, in a chair that permitted flexion of hips and knees at 90° with feet flat on the floor and the back well supported by a backrest. Special attention was paid to head alignment in a straight axis with the trunk, and a 30° chin tuck position. Arms were placed in a flexed position on the child's lap tray or

on the feeding table in front of the child. Children who were able to feed themselves had custom-prescribed feeding utensils to permit optimal independent function, i.e. a cup positioned in a support stand so that drinking was possible from a straw without the use of the upper extremities or a built up handle on a spoon to facilitate grip and thereby self-feeding. (pp. 60-61)

This illustration highlights the importance of facilitating trunk stability and flexion at the hips and knees to maintain a sitting position. An adductor may be necessary to encourage and maintain bending at the hips. In addition, a pommel can be used to keep knees apart. A feeding chair or wheelchair with a tray provides a surface on which the child's arms can rest. It also assists with trunk stability and promotes weight-bearing on the child's elbows. The child's feet must also be secured. For some, all that is needed is a surface to rest on such as the floor or a foot plate on a wheelchair. A child with more involved tonal issues may need "shoes" with straps (i.e., an outline of a shoe on a foot plate). The child's feet are placed in the shoes and secured with straps in a crisscross fashion to prevent extensor tone that straightens the feet at a 90° angle to the hips.

A child's head and neck may need additional support to facilitate intake. An OT and a PT are members of the feeding team with expertise in this aspect of positioning. A headrest can be made specifically to match an individual child's tonal needs. If a child still displays an ATNR, the PT and OT can help fashion a headrest so this primitive reflex is reduced or prevented. Improved swallowing has been found to be an additional outcome of proper head and neck positioning in children with cerebral palsy (Larnert & Ekberg, 1995). Gisel et al. (1996) advised positioning the child to facilitate chin tuck. Bringing the chin toward the chest assists the bolus to move down the digestive track rather than into the child's airway (Redstone & West, 2004; Snyder, Breath, & DeMauro, 1999; Woods, 1995).

Alignment of the pelvis is essential. Proper positioning of the pelvis provides a stable base and improves control of the head and trunk, which also assists with respiration and self-feeding. A child's pelvis must be fully upright and flush to the back of the feeding chair. If the seat depth prevents this, one or more members of the feeding team can make necessary adjustments. A foam insert, padding for one or both sides of the seat or nonslip material such as Dycem may be added. While maintaining a stable position, the feeding chair may need to be reclined or "tilted in space" to address tonal issues, typically hypertonicity (Lowman, 2010; Redstone & West, 2004; Snyder et al., 1999). Seat depth will need to be adjusted as the child grows and, potentially, as the child improves stability in her torso, pelvis, and hips.

Appropriate positioning promotes self-feeding for young children with neurological disorders who gain that developmental level (Redstone & West, 2004). Improved control of arms and increased ability to manipulate utensils may be an added outcome of postural stability and alignment. In sum, positioning is a dynamic component of feeding young children with neurological disorders. Modifications and adjustments are needed as the child grows physically and as he or she develops skills to compensate for tonal difficulties. Refer to Table 12.2 for positioning considerations in preparing for a feeding activity or mealtime, during a feeding activity or mealtime, and after a feeding activity or mealtime. In addition, Box 12.1 in the appendix offers a list of positioning equipment that may be used alone or in combination to help ensure alignment and normalize tone to aid eating, drinking, and swallowing.

Table 12.2.   Positioning a toddler or preschooler with neurological issues for feeding

Feeding phase and technique	How each technique facilitates feeding
Preparation for meal	
Stretching exercises	Prepares body for change in position
Orthotics for hands and feet	Promotes flexion or extension as needed
Transfer to feeding seat	Signals mealtime
Secure lap belt	Secures hips
Head upright and at midline	Prepares for presentation of food items
Trunk stabilized with chest harness	Promotes trunk alignment
Pelvis in upright position	Increases hip flexion
Hips flexed at 90 degrees	Promotes stability
Knees flexed at 90 degrees	Promotes stability
Ankles in neutral position	Provides stability to lower extremities
Feet secured with straps or "shoes"	Provides stability to lower extremities
Provide tray (if needed)	Assists weight-bearing on elbows
During meal	
Maintain upright, reclined or "tilt in space" sitting position	Maintains alignment and stability throughout body
Maintain body in symmetrical position	Assists intake
Feeder sits in front of or on side of child	Prevents head turn and primitive reflexes
Feeder provides assistance at jaw and mouth as needed	Assists intake
Feeder provides mealtime items with assistance from child	Encourages participation and independence
Feeder provides verbal cues, instructions, and descriptions	Assists intake
Feeder observes and responds to child's facial expressions	Assists intake
Completion of meal	
Feeder cleans mouth, cheeks, and chin with assistance from child	Indicates mealtime has ended
Feeder cleans plate, cup, and utensils with assistance from child	Encourages participation and independence
Prepare for transfer from feeding seat	Signals end of mealtime

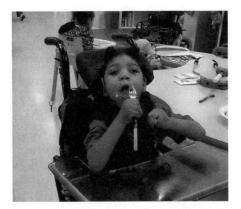 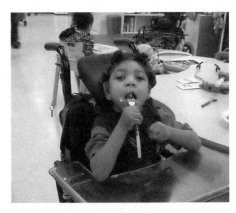

Child with cerebral palsy positioned in wheelchair feeding self using adapted fork

Specialized spoons, cups, and other adapted utensils are often needed. Refer to Chapters 11 and 13 for additional feeding items that address young children with tonicity issues affecting oral intake. It is also important to note that some commercially available cups can be used without adaptations. Assessment results and feeding team recommendations will guide decision-making.

Specialized Supplements and Calorie Boosters

The literature indicates that a majority of children with neurological disorders are underweight or malnourished (Fung et al., 2002; Gisel & Alphonce, 1995; Holland & Murray, 2004; Motion et al., 2002; Stevenson et al., 2006). Furthermore, Anderson (1998) outlined the progression from textured foods as smooth solids (strained and puréed foods), junior or mashed foods, finger foods, lumpy solids, coarsely chopped foods, and table foods. The author then points out that children with cerebral palsy may have difficulty attaining the developmental skills necessary to progress to more textured food items, which are more calorie-dense. Taken together, the information described points to the need to explore other alternatives to meet a child's nutritional and growth needs.

A young child's feeding team determines the need for specialized supplements and calorie boosters. Specifically, a dietitian can evaluate caloric needs. A medical professional such as a gastroenterologist or pulmonologist may also be asked to offer input. For example, some calorie dense foods may aggravate GER. Several household foods are readily available calorie boosters. Margarine or butter can be added to vegetables, rice, and pasta, and whole milk can be used to prepare hot cereals, shakes, and pudding. If tolerated, peanut butter adds a large number of calories to a child's daily diet as do age-appropriate portions of hard and soft cheeses. Custards and ice cream are additional options. Products such as Carnation Instant Breakfast powder can also be used to add calories to foods the child prefers (e.g., yogurt, custard, oatmeal).

Thickeners may need to be added to all or some of these items so they are a consistency the child is able to swallow with ease (see Chapter 8 for additional information after thickeners). Thickened fluids may cause excessive drooling, which can limit the intake of nutrients because drool mixes with the food, which then may be lost from the sides of the mouth. Drooling can be addressed with behavioral strategies, medication, or surgery, but results vary in their effectiveness (see Van der Burg et al., 2007). Again, the feeding team will assess the alternatives and work together with family members and other caregivers to ensure the most appropriate decision and corresponding interventions.

Supplements such as Ensure, Ensure Plus, Sustacal, and Pediasure do not require a prescription from a medical professional. PediaSmart is an organic alternative; it is similar in nutrition to Pediasure, but made without artificial colors or flavors. PediaSmart also does not contain lactose, corn, or gluten, which some young children cannot tolerate in their diet. Supplements such as Jevity and Osmolite require a doctor's prescription. The specific amount and schedule of a supplement (e.g., once a day, twice a day as a snack, at every meal) will be determined by a dietitian. Adjustments will be made to accommodate growth and any change in health or developmental status. For example, if a supplement causes GER, a different one can be tried for several days to a week while monitoring the child for this specific oral-motor difficulty.

Enteral Feeding

In reviewing the literature, Rogers (2004) stated that approximately 60% of children with cerebral palsy have feeding problems and half of those feeding issues are significant enough to necessitate short- or long-term enteral feeding. Fung et al. (2002) also cited poor weight gain and a high incidence of chest infections and pneumonia in some oral feeders. Smith, Camfield, and Camfield (1999) shared results showing fewer respiratory problems, dysphagia, and vomiting after gastrostomy (G-tube) placement in a sample of 40 children with severe cerebral palsy.

For a child receiving enteral feedings, oral supplementation is based on individual feeding abilities. Specifically, determining the amount and types of oral feedings for a child receiving enteral feeds is based on several factors. Rogers (2004) emphasized observation of oral feedings for instances of coughing, gagging, and related difficulties. Information also needs to be gathered from feeders about dysphagia and aspiration. Review of medical history regarding respiratory illnesses such as chronic asthma and hospitalization for pneumonia should also be completed. Rogers also stressed evaluation of the types of foods the child accepts, duration of feedings, and overall efficiency (intake compared to overall nutritional needs for growth and health). Even if results indicate that oral supplementation is not recommended, the decision must be tempered with an understanding of the importance many families place on oral feeding (Craig, Scambler, & Spitz, 2003; Petersen, Kedia, Davis, Newman, & Temple, 2006; Sleigh, 2005). Oral stimulation and/or tastes of foods may be permitted so the child can participate in family mealtimes. Parents refer to this as keeping a degree of "normalcy" in their lives. When medically approved, supplementary oral feedings is sometimes the compromise necessary to gain parent support for tube placement (Craig et al., 2003; Petersen et al., 2006). If supplemental oral feeding is not feasible, it is important to offer oral stimulation activities (see oral-motor exercises in the previous section for examples).

The feeding team must work together to weigh the benefits and risks of oral feedings. As previous cited, G-tube placement helps increase weight gain and overall nutritional status and reduce respiratory issues (Sleigh & Brocklehurst, 2004; Stevenson et al., 2006). Feeding times are also decreased. Some parents indicate that, with oral feedings, mealtimes take upwards of 1 to 2 hours (Sleigh, 2005; Sullivan et al., 2005). Parental anxiety often diminishes when enteral feeding is started because it is precisely measured and scheduled.

When tube feeding is initiated, parents and caregivers must learn the procedures to prepare the formula (homemade or store bought) and deliver tube feedings to the child by bolus or gravity feed. (Chapter 13 offers an extensive description of enteral feeding methods.) Monitoring the child to ensure that feeds are tolerated is critical. Because poor weight gain is a primary reason for placement of a G-tube, any digestive complication must be investigated. If a child is experiencing vomiting during or after tube feeding, for example, a Nissan fundoplication may be needed (Samson-Fang et al., 2003). This is a surgical procedure to tighten the opening from the esophagus to the stomach to prevent stomach contents from refluxing into the esophagus. A fundoplication is often completed at the same time as surgical (versus endoscopic) G-tube placement. However, the fundoplication can cause complications because it narrows the opening into the stomach. This narrowing can negatively affect oral feedings. In addition, although the child will not reflux or vomit, he or she retains the ability to retch (i.e., "dry heave"), which can be unpleasant and potentially harmful. Vomiting releases pressure. If the pressure builds sufficiently, it can damage the fundoplication. Again, the feeding team will determine the need for this procedure and evaluate its effectiveness. (See Chapter 13 for an in-depth discussion of tube feeding.)

Blacklin (1998) noted "children [with cerebral palsy] must learn to see the feeding routine as an orderly and predictable time to receive nourishment, as well as to receive the feelings of warmth and acceptance that help them feel loved and secure" (p. 221). Whether children are primarily fed orally or fed via an enteral tube, there are crucial considerations when feeding young children with neurological disorders. Mealtimes must focus on positive interactions between child and feeder, promote weight gain and well-being, and encourage independence to the degree possible.

▦ ▦ ▦ TABLE TALK ▦ ▦ ▦

Stefanie was diagnosed with cerebral palsy at 13 months of age. Her mother, Angela, and grandmother, Denise, were concerned about her delayed motor development and slow growth. On her first birthday, Stefanie weighed 14 pounds and was only able to hold her head up for 10–15 seconds at a time. She sometimes reached for toys and was observed attempting to roll from her back to her stomach. Most of her seemingly voluntary movements were, in fact, due to primitive reflexes.

Stefanie had feeding problems from the time she was a few weeks old. It was difficult for Angela to keep her daughter comfortable for bottle feedings. Stefanie would accept 2 or 3 ounces and then push the nipple out of her mouth and stiffen. It would take up to half an hour to resume a feeding. Most of the time was spent gently touching Stefanie's cheeks and lips and rubbing her arms and legs so they would relax. Stefanie began accepting puréed foods at 8 months of age but exhibited a strong tongue thrust. Angela and Denise, her caregiver during the day while Angela works, were never sure how much Stefanie accepted by mouth due to the tongue thrust and constant drooling.

Stefanie is almost two years old and is still struggling with feeding. She weighs only 21 pounds and frequently has colds and respiratory infections. Denise holds Stefanie to feed her. Angela usually uses either the corner chair that Stefanie's physical therapist provided or her adapted stroller. Stefanie still demonstrates some tongue thrust when eating mashed foods from a spoon. She is beginning to accept tastes of textured foods such as oatmeal and rice.

Stefanie is unable to feed herself finger foods due to the limited use of her arms. She also has trouble with liquids such as milk, juice, and water. Stefanie's speech-language pathologist, Jesse, suggested thickening liquids with Thick-it. He also suggested that Angela consider calorie boosters or some type of tube feeding to ensure Stefanie receives the calories she needs to grow and remain healthy. Angela spoke with Denise about Jesse's recommendations. They decided they are willing to try anything to keep their daughter/granddaughter eating by mouth rather than have a tube in her nose or stomach.

Discussion Questions

▧ Do you agree with Jesse's recommendations?

▧ What types of calorie boosters would you try with Stefanie?

▧ How would you approach Angela and Denise about tube feeding for Stefanie?

FEEDING NUGGETS

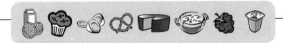

Books

Children with Cerebral Palsy: A Parent's Guide by Elaine Geralis (Editor), 1998
  info@woodbinehouse.com
  http://www.woodbinehouse.com

Cerebral Palsy: A Complete Guide for Caregiving by Freeman Miller and Steven J.
  Bachrach, 1995
  hfscustserv@press.jhu.edu
  http://jhupbooks.press.jhu.edu

Visual Impairment in Children Due to Damage to the Brain by Gordon Dutton and
  Martin Bax (Editors), 2010
  http://www.wiley.com

Web Site

United Cerebral Palsy
  http://www.ucp.org/

APPENDIX

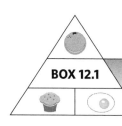

BOX 12.1   Frequently used positioning equipment

For infants:
   Infant seat (or carrier)
   Adapted infant seat
   Highchair/feeding chair
   Stroller
   Adapted stroller

For toddlers and preschoolers:
   Highchair/feeding chair
   Adaptive chair (e.g., Rifton, Tumbleform)
   Corner chair
   Floor sitter
   Prone or supine stander
   Sidelyer
   Stroller
   Adapted stroller
   Travel chair
   Wheelchair

Considerations for young children birth to age 5 years:
   Includes room for growth
   Use towels, cushions, and wedges to assist with hip and trunk stability and alignment
   Include chest harness, hip adductor, or pommel for knees as needed
   Provide a tray to assist arm stability and weight bearing with elbows
   Provide Velcro straps or "shoes" to secure feet

13

Young Children With Anatomical Anomalies

What You'll Learn in This Chapter

This chapter provides

- An overview of cleft lip and palate, the cleft feeding team, and parent perceptions
- An overview of jaw malformations, enlarged tongue, and feeding young children with tracheotomies
- Strategies and corresponding adaptations to promote successful feeding
- A description of surgical procedures to address anatomical feeding difficulties and associated after care

■ ■ ■ FOOD FOR THOUGHT ■ ■ ■

"Vinny, who is 14 years old, has full trisomy 13 and balanced translocation of chromosomes 5 and 13, has been eating orally since birth, even though he was born with a cleft palate.

When he was first born, feeding was a real challenge because, although he had a great sucking reflex, it was not a productive suck. He got very frustrated.

An occupational therapist tried several different bottle/nipple combos. The Mead cleft lip/palate nursers with silicone orthodontic nipples worked best for him. The Mead nurser is a kind of soft, flexible, squeezable bottle, so when Vinny sucked he got something for his troubles. At that time the Mead nurser was VERY hard to find!

By the time he had his palate repair at 9 months, he was up to about 5 ounces in 1 1/2 hours, and we thought that was super! Within 1 week following his palate repair, he could drink 6 ounces in 20 minutes. He was 12 pounds at 9 months when he had his palate repair. He weighed 15 pounds at 1 year, 25 pounds at 2 years, 35 pounds at 3 years, and 40 pounds at 4 years."

Nina, Parent

"Simon, who is 45 months old and has partial trisomy 9p, drank from bottles prior to his cleft surgeries. He was in the NICU for 1 week, and they placed a nasogastric tube through his nose/mouth immediately after he was born. We also insisted that we work with the feeding specialist to teach him how to bottle feed. There was no reason why he shouldn't— almost all babies with cleft lip and palate bottle feed unless they have additional issues like Pierre Robin sequence or low muscle tone. We wanted him to learn to eat orally as soon as possible and not develop an oral aversion issue. It was a bit of a struggle for him to bottle feed. We learned to place the nasogastric tube (NG-tube) prior to his leaving the hospital and a nurse came out a few times to check on him for us. We used the NG-tube for a total of 3 weeks to supplement his bottle feeds until both we and he had the skill to solely bottle feed.

Fortunately we had good feeding therapists, and they helped a lot. I would HIGHLY recommend that families with babies with cleft palate find a feeding specialist who has worked with kids with cleft lips/palates before. Some don't have the experience and so aren't very helpful. We had already gotten an assortment of bottles to try from Simon's craniofacial team prior to his birth. That is the added benefit of the team approach—they have the specialists with experience, and they give you the bottles for free.

The specialized cleft lip and palate bottles are the Haberman, which has a longer nipple and soft reservoir to squeeze, and the Mead Johnson, which is a soft bottle that you squeeze to assist the baby in getting milk out. Also, people have had success with the Doc Brown's bottles from Babies R Us and other stores. Generally, you also use a cross-cut nipple with a hole that is in the shape of an X, or you can make/expand a regular nipple by flipping it inside out and cutting it with a knife. New nipples can be kind of tough when you first get them so we would wash and chew on them a little to break them down a little and make them softer and easier for Simon to squish in his mouth. Simon learned in the first few months to move the nipple over to his gum line and then clamp down on it there so that the milk would flow. That way he didn't need full suction to get milk out."

Sandy, Parent

The previous examples illustrate some of the challenges of feeding young children with cleft lip and palate. Specialized bottles and positioning strategies are often required (Edmondson & Reinbartsen, 1998; Glass & Wolf, 1999; Morris & Klein, 2000). Other anatomical defects can also affect feeding mechanisms such as moving food boluses and liquids around the mouth and swallowing. Understanding these conditions requires knowledge of causes and treatments. There are also specialized members on the feeding teams who serve this unique group of young children. Teams often include an otoloaryngologist (an ear, nose, and throat doctor) and orthodontist (a dentist who specializes in treatment of teeth, lips, and jaw through use and management of corrective appliances). Reconstructive surgery and corresponding after care may also be necessary to address feeding difficulties.

WHAT THE LITERATURE SAYS

The ability to accept liquids and eat solid foods requires coordination of many anatomical structures, primarily the lip, palate, jaw, and tongue (Morris & Klein, 2000). Clefts are the most common anatomical anomaly that affects children's feeding. This chapter discusses them at length. Later in the chapter, malformations of the jaw such as micrognathia (small jaw), with or without an accompanying recessed chin and enlarged tongue, are discussed. The unique needs of young children with tracheotomies are briefly described. All of these conditions can complicate intake of foods and liquids. Therefore, effective interventions to promote feeding and to address possible speech, hearing, and dental complications are needed.

Historical Perspective on Clefts

Berkowitz (1994) noted that cleft lip and cleft palate have been written about since the 13th century. Other authors have noted that in the 1600s, infants with cleft palate often died of malnutrition due to a dearth of effective feeding interventions (Redford-Badwal, Mabry, & Frassinelli, 2003). However, there is documented evidence of surgery to repair cleft lip in 390 B.C. in China. In addition, Perko (1986) noted soft palate surgery in the second half of the 18th century and the first documented case of hard palate surgery in the 1800s. The later start for cleft palate repair was due, in large part, to the introduction of anesthesia. Without it, cleft repair surgery would have been very painful, and the risk of infection would have been very high.

Through the years, there have also been changes in terminology to describe cleft conditions. Recent descriptions are more respectful of the individual with the condition. A notable example is the use and subsequent phasing out of the term *hare lip*. The term referred to the similarity in appearance between a cleft lip and distinctive shape of a rabbit's mouth. The term *hare lip* was and continues to be perceived as derogatory and insulting. Consequently, individuals with a cleft condition and their families advocated for the removal of the term from the lexicon.

Anatomy of Clefts and Complications

A cleft, visible as a split, hole, or indentation in the lip and/or palate can dramatically alter a young child's facial appearance as well as adversely affect the child's feeding ability. Common feeding difficulties include problems latching on or creating a seal around the breast or bottle, loss of liquid through the cleft, frequent burping, swallowing issues, nasal regurgitation, greater likelihood of gastroesophageal reflux, and prolonged feeding sessions. Therefore, specific cleft-related feeding difficulties must be fully evaluated in order to develop appropriate feeding interventions. Authors in the field, such as Redford-Badwal, Mabry, and Frassinelli (2003), Reid, Reilly, and Kilpatrick (2007), Walter (1994), and Wolf and Glass (1992) further describe problems with movement and placement of the child's tongue, quality of the lip seal, disorganized sucking patterns, and nontypical movement of the hard and soft palates. The authors also caution that many children with clefts also have low tone around the mouth, which can further compromise feeding.

The following section describes the affected structures. A cleft lip is an opening in the upper lip between the mouth and the nose. A cleft can be unilateral (one side) or bilateral (both sides) as well as complete (through the lip and base of the nose) or incomplete (through the lip but not reaching the base of the nose). Unilateral clefts of the lip are typically evident on the left side. In some cases, a cleft lip may extend into the nasal cavity.

The palate is the roof of the mouth. It separates the nasal and oral cavities. The hard palate is the anterior (front) bony section, while the soft palate is farther back and fleshy. A cleft palate is a gap in the roof of the mouth affecting the hard and/or soft palate. Cleft palate may also occur on both sides of the center of the palate. A cleft of the lip or palate can range from so small that it is difficult to detect to a cleft encompassing both sides of the lip and the soft and hard sections of the palate.

A young child with cleft palate may also have an alveolar ridge defect. The alveolar ridge is the bony upper gum that contains the teeth. Defects of the alveolar ridge can displace or rotate permanent teeth, prevent permanent teeth from appearing, and prevent the alveolar ridge from forming (see Saal, 2002 for additional information).

The most common feeding difficulty produced by a cleft of the lip and/or palate relates to suction. Typically, positive pressure is created by the compression of an infant's lips and gums on the nipple (breast or bottle) creating a seal; then negative pressure draws liquid from the breast or bottle into the mouth. Effectiveness of the negative pressure suction depends on the location and severity of the cleft. A larger hole or indentation limits the infant's ability to fully close and seal the mouth. In addition, the cleft may cause intake of air into the nasal cavity and liquid flowing into the lungs resulting in coughing, gagging, choking, and possible aspiration (Arosarena, 2002; Morris & Klein, 2000; Reid, Kilpatrick & Reilly, 2006; Reid, Reilly, & Kilpatrick, 2007). Likewise, Masarei, Sell et al. (2007) described altered sucking patterns in infants with a cleft condition. Sucking is often not as efficient as in infants without cleft lip or palate. As a result, more energy is required to consume a smaller amount, overall intake is reduced in volume, and nutritional needs may not be fully met.

Possible Causes of Clefts

Clefts of the lip, soft palate, and hard palate are one of the most common birth defects (Arvedson & Brodsky, 2002). Clefts occur in approximately 1 in 700 live births, with males affected approximately twice as frequently as females (Berkowitz, 1994; Fraker & Walbert, 2003; Glass & Wolf, 1999; Reid, 2004; Scherer & Kaiser, 2007). Depending on the location and size of the cleft, the failure of the lip or palate to fuse together occurs between the 7th and 12th week of gestation (Morris & Klein, 2000). A history of clefting in

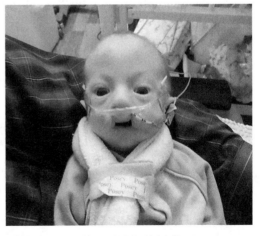

Infant with bilateral cleft lip

the child's family is considered a predisposing factor (Damiano et al., 2009). Compared with other populations, there is a higher incidence of clefts in children from Asian and Native American backgrounds (Morris & Klein, 2000).

Environmental factors contributing to clefting include the mother's use of medications such as anticonvulsants and steroids during pregnancy. Smoking and drinking alcohol during pregnancy can contribute as well (Hodgkinson et al., 2005). For example, Shaw and Lammer (1999) found higher incidence of cleft lip with and without cleft palate in a sample of mothers who drank more than 5 drinks from 1 month preconception to 3 months postconception. Hayes (2002) described a risk associated with pesticides and also noted a correlation between maternal caffeine intake and clefting. Taken together, all of these factors contribute to cleft lip and palate, but it remains unclear which agent or agents directly cause the condition.

Approximately 10% of clefts are part of genetic syndromes including Patau syndrome (trisomy 13; Jones, 2006), Treacher Collins syndrome (Posnick & Ruiz, 2000) and Turner syndrome (Starke, Wikland, & Moller, 2003). In addition, these and other genetic conditions may also produce micrognathia (small jaw), which can further affect a young child's acceptance of liquids and solid foods. Wagener, Rayatt, Tatman, Gornall, and Slator (2003) described the presence of micrognathia in a sample of children with Pierre Robin sequence. Masarei, Sell et al. (2007) and Masarei, Wade et al. (2007) also noted the potential of cleft conditions to affect tongue and jaw movements without the presence of an enlarged tongue or recessed chin. Pereira, Sacher, Ryan, and Hayward (2009) described a sample of 13 children with Alpert syndrome. Records indicated that 7 in the group were diagnosed with cleft palate (5 clefts of the hard palate; 2 clefts of the soft palate). Data further identified difficulties with the suck–swallow–breathe sequence and poor weight gain.

Parental Perceptions

Regarding children with cleft lip and/or palate, the literature indicates a range of emotional responses in parents, with some parents describing acceptance from the time of diagnosis to ambivalent feelings to emotional rejection of the infant (Nicholson, 2002). This information is critical to inform treatment options. Nackashi, Dedlow, and Dixon-Wood (2002) noted "parents of a newborn with cleft lip/palate often experience considerable anxiety due to the problems they encounter when attempting to feed their baby...these feelings can interfere with the normal interaction between parent and child" (p. 309).

Johansson and Ringsberg (2004) studied 20 families including 20 mothers and 12 fathers. The authors reported that parents adapted to their child's cleft condition and perceived it as a "flaw" rather than a disability. Furthermore, parents were most concerned about their child's speech and feeding needs over the child's appearance. Speltz, Armsden, and Clarren (1990) described greater stress for mothers with older infants and toddlers with cleft lip and palate compared with mothers with young children with only cleft palate. Results also indicated that mothers' stress was more related to perceptions of their maternal skills than their children's facial anomaly. An additional study examined needs of 12 mothers and 3 fathers with newborns with cleft lip and palate in Thailand. Their initial concerns focused on information about feeding, surgery, and care after cleft repair (Chuacharoen, Ritthagol, Hunsrisakhun, & Nilmanat, 2009). Finally, an investigation by Baker, Owens, Stern, and

Willmot (2009) reported that "those parents reporting a greater family impact resulting from their child's condition were those whose child was younger or whose child had medical problems in addition to cleft lip and palate" (p. 233).

Black, Girotto, Chapman, and Oppenheimer (2009) examined cross-cultural reactions to cleft conditions from Thai, Chinese, Uygur, Colombian, and American mothers. Thai mothers were most positive while mothers with a Chinese background were the most negative. These perceptions were hypothesized to be associated with a premium placed on physical appearance in the Chinese culture. Taken together, the findings described in this section hold import for collaboration with the professionals providing services to the child with a cleft condition and to the family (Johansson & Ringsberg, 2004; Knapke, Bender, Prows, Schultz, & Saal, 2010; Young, O'Riordan, Goldstein, & Robin, 2001).

Cleft Team

A child with a cleft lip and/or palate receives care from a team of professionals. This team is referred to as the craniofacial team or cleft team. Team members typically include the child's parents, pediatrician, speech-language pathologist, feeding specialist, dietitian, nurse, otoloaryngologist, audiologist, dentist, orthodontist, oral surgeon, and social worker or psychologist (Edmondson & Reinbartsen, 1998; Glass & Wolf, 1999; Morris & Klein, 2000; Wolf & Glass, 1992). The importance of a cleft team was underscored in a study by Austin et al. (2010) of mothers in Arkansas, Iowa, and New York participating in the National Birth Defects Prevention Study. Approximately 25% of the children were not followed by a cleft team ($n = 61$, total = 253) and received fewer surgeries to correct their clefts.

Cleft teams can be organized in a number of configurations (see Chapter 5 for a detailed examination of feeding team structures). The most important factor is that a member of the cleft team must assume the leadership position (Strauss, 2002). For example, a team member must be available as an "impartial facilitator" to discuss options about treatment and surgery (p. 296). Strauss also advocated face-to-face meetings, ongoing training and education, and information regarding additional resources (e.g., parent support group) for optimal functioning of the team. Knapke et al. (2010) described perspectives of 17 parents of infants with clefts. Parents were satisfied with care, but identified areas for improvement including providing more written information, encouraging contact with parents in similar situations, and sharing information about clefts with health care professionals not on their child's team. In addition, Hodgkinson et al. (2005) emphasized that cleft team members should do all they can to encourage confidence in parents' ability to feed their children.

A study of 26 families by Amstalden-Mendes, Magna, and Gil-da-Silva-Lopes (2007) examined the provision of feeding guidance shortly after their newborn's birth (50% diagnosed with cleft lip and palate). Interview data indicated that most feeding information was given by nurses or physicians, with a focus on breastfeeding and the use of items such as cups and droppers as necessary. Initial contact with their child's cleft team varied from 4 days–2 months after the child's birth. The authors recommended that all members of the child's team be knowledgeable about feeding interventions.

OTHER ANATOMICAL CONDITIONS

An additional type of anatomical anomaly is micrognathia (small jaw). This condition is most common in children with genetic conditions such as Alpert syndrome or Pierre Robin sequence. With regard to Pierre Robin sequence, the infant's tongue often falls back in the throat as well, which can cause blockage of the airway and feeding problems such as choking. Fortunately, the lower jaw often reaches age-appropriate size within the child's first few years (Tan et al., 2009). Many children with Pierre Robin sequence also require treatment for cleft palate. Spender et al. (1996) discussed the enlarged tongue in many children with Down syndrome. When an enlarged tongue is coupled with hypotonia (low muscle tone), feeding both liquids and solid foods can be a source of difficulty.

Finally, some young children with one or more of these conditions may also require a tracheotomy (or "tracheostomy") to assist with breathing because of a malformation in the child's airway or blockage of the airway. Some young children require use of a ventilator (a machine that gets oxygen to the lungs and removes carbon dioxide from the body) for a long period of time and may continue to need some form of mechanical assistance, such as a tracheotomy, to breathe. In addition, treatment for some children with severe sleep apnea (pauses of breathing during sleep) may require a tracheotomy. Most children with a tracheotomy can eat by mouth once they are medically cleared for oral feeding by their feeding team (Simmon & McGowan, 1989). It is critical to include a pediatric pulmonologist (a specialist in the treatment of respiratory conditions) on the child's feeding team to offer recommendations for the development of a feeding plan.

STRATEGIES AND SPECIALIZED INTERVENTIONS

The following sections provide strategies and specialized interventions to address feeding young children with anatomical anomalies. The majority of these techniques address cleft lip and palate, and additional sections address feeding assistance for young children with a recessed jaw, with an enlarged tongue, or who require a tracheotomy. Breastfeeding, bottle feeding, spoon feeding, introducing textured foods, appliance use, and presurgical and postsurgical recommendations specific to cleft lip and cleft palate are offered. Above all, feeding methods should be safe and assist the child to receive adequate nutrition. Parents and professionals are instructed to always consult with the child's feeding team before implementing new feeding strategies or interventions.

Breastfeeding

Many infants with a cleft condition are able to successfully breastfeed. Smedegaard, Marxen, Moes, Glassou, and Scientsan (2008) described comparable growth of 115 infants with cleft lip and palate or cleft palate only. A large part of the success was attributed to nurses working with parents to increase their confidence in breastfeeding. Another sample of infants with one or more clefts was found to breastfeed for a similar length of time as their peers without an anatomical anomaly (Garcez & Giugliani, 2005).

Among infants with cleft conditions, the most frequently mentioned difficulties with breastfeeding were weak suction, difficulty attaching to the breast, and breast milk escaping through the nostrils (Bannister, 2004; Glass & Wolf, 1999;

Morris & Klein, 2000; Swigert, 1998). The authors emphasized the health benefits of breastfeeding (e.g., breast milk's protection against infection), noted cleft-specific advantages of breastfeeding (including reduced opportunity for irritation of the infant's nose), and suggested options for positioning to encourage successful sealing, sucking, and swallowing. Strategies to address these difficulties are described in the following section.

Breastfeeding Infants with Cleft Lip   Strategies to support breastfeeding infants with cleft lips include the following:

• For breastfeeding a child with a small, unilateral cleft lip: The mother holds the infant with the cleft side to the breast to create a seal and places her thumb on the cleft or gently pushes the lip together. A "football hold" is recommended so that the infant faces the mother rather than lying across her lap. This position helps the infant remain more upright. The mother is also better able to guide and support her infant's head to latch on to the breast. Nackashi, Dedlow, and Dixon-Wood (2002) pointed out that infants with a small, unilateral cleft lip have the most success nursing as long as they are able to create the necessary negative pressure at the breast.

• For breastfeeding an infant with a large, unilateral cleft lip: The mother positions the infant with the cleft side toward her (rather than down toward breast). This assists with improved lip closure during sucking and swallowing.

• For breastfeeding an infant with a bilateral cleft lip: The mother positions the infant in a more upright position, such as straddling the mother's leg or lying on the mother's chest with the mother seated in a chair leaning slightly back.

• For breastfeeding all infants with clefts: Keep the infant's nose in line with the mother's nipple. This helps the infant orient to the breast by smelling the mother's milk. All positioning options should encourage the infant to open his or her mouth as wide as possible to locate and seal onto the nipple (Klein & Delaney, 1994; Morris & Klein, 2000).

A feeding wedge is an additional means to support an infant with a cleft lip during breastfeeding.

Breastfeeding Infants with Cleft Palate   The most critical consideration for breastfeeding infants with a cleft palate is the size and location of the cleft. If the cleft is in the hard palate, creating a seal using negative pressure will be difficult. Liquid can move through a hole in the soft palate and cause gastroesophageal reflux (GER) or aspiration. Positioning is critical to successful nursing at the breast along with frequent checks to determine that breast milk is not pooling (i.e., leaking from an incomplete seal or aspirated into the lungs; Garcez & Giugliani, 2005; Glass & Wolf, 1999). The authors also point out that infants with clefts may not be able to completely empty their mother's breast, which can limit milk production and adversely affect the infant's overall nutritional intake and growth.

Many infants have difficulty acquiring or simply cannot acquire sufficient calories at the breast. Supplemental nursing systems can be used to assist these infants. For example, Medela offers a supplemental nursing system to provide breast milk from an adjustable flow bottle while the infant nurses at the breast. Benefits include better monitoring of intake and positioning.

According to Glass and Wolf (1999), many infants with cleft palates will accept expressed breast milk in a specialized bottle (see next section) with milk directly from the breast as a secondary source. The authors further recommend that mothers provide pumped breast milk as long as possible to meet their infant's nutritional needs. The feeding team can provide information and assistance to develop a pumping program to maintain the mother's supply of breast milk.

Bottle Feeding Infants with Clefts

Literature indicates that most infants with both cleft lip and cleft palate cannot breast-feed due to the cleft condition, additional medical concerns (e.g., when the cleft is part of a genetic syndrome), and/or compromised respiratory status (Smedegaard et al., 2008). In these cases, pumping and providing breast milk is recommended because of its health benefits and parent–infant bonding (Gartner et al., 2005). Formula can be used as the primary source of nourishment or as a supplement.

For infants who require use of a bottle and nipple system, a number of considerations guide selection (see Table 13.1). To encourage greater intake with reduced gagging and coughing, Morris and Klein (2000) recommended taking frequent breaks for burping and offering a larger number of smaller feedings throughout the day (instead of fewer, larger feedings). Information about selecting a bottle and nipple system is provided in the following section.

Safety in bottle feeding infants with cleft conditions is essential because these infants tend to experience difficulty keeping breast milk or formula in their mouth. Bannister (2004), Morris and Klein (2000) and Swigert (1998) offered recommendations for nipples and bottles for infants with cleft conditions as well as recommendations regarding general feeding considerations. The individual providing bottle feeding must be attentive to positioning and frequency of swallows. Cradling the child is optimal and can reduce pooling of liquid in an infant's mouth. Offering concentrated or thickened formula is an additional strategy to facilitate bottle feeding. The use of flexible bottles, rather than rigid plastic or glass bottles is also recommended. Consider the following additional recommendations for bottle feeding infants with cleft lip.

Positioning Infants with Cleft Lip   If needed, adaptations can be made to feeding positions for infants with cleft lip. For example, an infant can be propped on a pillow to approximate a sitting position. The parent or caregiver feeding the child can see the child's face and help provide lip closure. Input from the feeding team guides this type of feeding support. In addition, positioning is critical to maintain the infant's airway and to reduce the swallowing of air and the aspiration of liquids, and the amount of lip support can be adjusted as the infant learns to compensate for the cleft.

Table 13.1.   Considerations When Selecting a Bottle and Nipple System

1. Can initial and replacement bottles and nipples be purchased at a local retailer, or must they be specially ordered from the manufacturer?
2. Does positioning encourage parent–infant interaction (e.g., eye contact) during bottle feeding?
3. Does positioning encourage parent's ability to read infant cues during bottle feeding?
4. Can flow rate be modified dependent on the child's needs?
5. Can different nipples be used to match changes in the child's bottle feeding skills?
6. Does the selected nipple compress to the degree needed by the infant?
7. Is the bottle easy to clean?

Bottle and Nipple Systems for Infants with Cleft Lip   Infants with cleft lip can often use commercially available bottles and nipples, and most of the nipples and bottles described in this section are available at larger retail stores. Otherwise, the manufacturer should be contacted to order the items or to find out the location of the nearest supplier. A member of the cleft team such as an SLP can also provide assistance.

Avent and Dr. Brown's Natural Flow Wide Neck bottles have a slower flow-rate compared with other commercially available bottles. The slower rate helps an infant with cleft lip to better coordinate the suck–swallow–breath sequence. In contrast, the nipple may need to have an enlarged hole or be cross-cut. NUK Orthodontic or cross-cut, premature infant nipples and Playtex nipples are commonly used with infants with cleft lip. There are also nipple systems that provide several nipples to reflect the infant's developing skills (see image of Pigeon system).

Positioning Infants with Cleft Palate or with Cleft Lip and Palate   For an infant with cleft palate, or cleft lip and palate, appropriate positioning is a primary concern. The use of a pillow or wedge to prop the infant to a more upright position is often effective (Morris & Klein, 2000). An occupational or physical therapist can also provide positioning recommendations. It is also necessary to have feeders who are attentive to the infant's satiation and fatigue cues.

Bottle and Nipple Systems for Infants with Cleft Palate or with Cleft Lip and Palate   The bottles and nipples listed in the previous section may be used with infants with cleft palate or with cleft conditions. The most important consideration is the infant's ability to coordinate the suck–swallow–breath sequence. The infant's cleft team can also provide suggestions that take into account the position and severity of the cleft(s).

Infants with cleft palate often use a Special Needs or Haberman feeder or Mead Johnson Cleft Palate Nurser and nipple for bottle feeding. With these systems, flow-rate can be adjusted to match the child's suck–swallow–breath sequence. It is best to squeeze the bottle in pulses to assist the flow-rate (squeeze after approximately every 2–3 sucks). An additional advantage of these systems is the one-way valve, which reduces or eliminates backflow and pooling of breast milk or formula in the child's mouth.

An additional option is to use Playtex Drop-Ins liners. The liners are soft plastic sleeves that can be squeezed to facilitate bottle feedings. In addition, the Soft Plas bottle assists the flow from the bottle when an infant is unable to or has a weak suck. A nipple or spout-shaped top can be used with this bottle.

The Pigeon nipple is also recommended. It can be used with most varieties of bottles and has a faster flow-rate compared with the Haberman feeder. This type of nipple has a firm side that makes contact with the roof of the infant's mouth. The other side is softer and rests on the tongue. An additional distinctive feature is inclusion of a small notch at the base of the nipple which serves as an air vent. Finally, similar to the Haberman feeder, there is a plastic one-way valve that fits into the Pigeon nipple. The feeder does not need to squeeze the bottle because the valve enables the infant to control the flow of breast milk or formula. Frequent opportunities to burp are also helpful.

Depending on the manufacturer, the bottles described in the previous two sections are available in 4-ounce, 6-ounce, 8-ounce and 9-ounce sizes. Bannister

(2004) advised caregivers to provide "two to three teaspoons of cooled boiled water after formula feeds to reduce the likelihood of infection" (p. 65). A soft cloth or gauze soaked in warm water can also be used to clean the area. Some infants with cleft lip and palate may require tube feeding due to the size of the clefts or other conditions that affect feeding and respiration (Bannister, 2004; Berkowitz, 1994; Morris & Klein, 2000). Refer to Chapter 14 for an in-depth discussion of types of tube-feeding and strategies for oral stimulation and transition to oral feeding.

Introducing Solid Foods

The following section provides a brief overview of strategies for spoon feeding and introducing textured foods to infants and toddlers with a cleft condition. The emphasis for the use of utensils and introduction of various types of solid foods is to "move slowly to feeding success" (Morris & Klein, 2000, p. 658). Information about use of a palatal obturator to assist with feeding and preparing for cleft surgery follows.

Spoon Feeding   Strategies to address spoon feeding in infants and toddlers with cleft conditions are usually similar to those for young children without anatomical anomalies (Masarei et al., 2007a; Morris & Klein, 2000). The transition to puréed, then to mashed, and then to textured foods is generally similar, especially after surgery to correct the lip and/or palate. It is best to use a soft spoon to introduce puréed foods (e.g., coated spoon, Maroon spoon). The main caution is to provide spoon feeding at a slow pace to reduce the possibility of gagging, choking, or nasal discharge of food items. It is best to let the infant or toddler set the pace for spoon feeding (Edmondson & Reinbartsen, 1998; Reid, 2004). This also encourages positive interactions during feedings (see Chapter 3). If the child has an unrepaired cleft palate, he or she must also learn to move the bolus of food around the cleft. To assist with bolus consistency, gravy or commercial thickener can be used to bind looser consistency foods together and assist with swallowing. The cleft team can assist with techniques for bolus management.

Introducing Finger Foods   The introduction of finger foods is an important milestone for young children. Children with a repaired cleft lip do not have any restrictions, but the feeder should always observe the child for gagging and choking and provide appropriately sized pieces of the food. Choking occurs in many young children during initial presentations of various finger foods. Suggested first foods include banana slices, soft crackers, cookies, pieces of cheese, and cut up cooked pasta such as macaroni or small shells. Some foods—for example cereal such as Cheerios and pieces of whole grain bread or grilled cheese sandwiches— should only be offered after the first group of foods are accepted and eaten without choking or nasal discharge. If solid food remains in the cleft after eating, the feeder should use a finger or cotton swab to clean the area. The child's cleft team should be consulted for strategies in these feeding areas (Bannister, 2004; Glass & Wolf, 1999; Nackashi et al., 2002; Reid et al., 2006).

Use of a Palatal Obturator

Infants with cleft palate may use a palatal obturator—a plastic insert made to fit a cleft in the hard palate. It is meant to familiarize the infant with the sensation of a repaired palate. It is usually taken out during feeding activities and, as a result, does not remove the need for the strategies described previously. The current literature is divided on its utility (see Masarei et al., 2007b; Murphy & Caretto, 1999; Nackashi et al., 2002; Oktay, Baydas, & Ersoz, 2006; Suzuki, Yamazaki, Sezaki, & Nakakita, 2006). Some infants do not tolerate insertion and removal of the appliance. It also must be closely monitored as the infant grows, and efforts must be made to keep it clean so infection is not introduced to the palate and the surrounding areas. In outcome after surgical repair of palate clefts at 12 months of age Murphy and Caretto (1999) found no difference between children who had and children who had not used a palatal obturator. Conversely, Oktay et al. (2006) describe successful outcomes when palatal obturators were used in place of cleft palate surgery with young children with Pierre Robin sequence. (Surgical intervention is described next.)

A palatal obturator is made from an impression of infant's upper jaw. It acts as an artificial palate to separate the nasal cavity from the mouth and helps to bring the tongue forward (Morris & Klein, 2000). When left in the mouth during feeding, the appliance can aid the suck–swallow–breath sequence for infants and can aid chewing in toddlers and preschool-age children (Berkowitz, 1994; Suzuki et al., 2006). It is important to note that a palatal obturator does not affect the negative pressure difficulties experienced by infants and young children with a cleft palate. A study by Masarei et al., 2007b confirms this. The authors found that use of palatal obturators did not improve tongue placement and overall feeding. Breastfeeding support, adaptive bottles, frequent burping, and positioning techniques were also employed to address arrhythmic tongue and jaw movements, altered rate of sucking, and difficulties coordinating the suck–swallow–breathe sequence.

For the proper fit and use of a palatal obturator, a young child's cleft team must include a professional with knowledge of its design and use. A cleft team's inability to meet this requirement is often the reason for not recommending the use of this appliance (Morris & Klein, 2000). Referrals to a teaching hospital may address this need. An additional alternative is to look for a larger feeding clinic or specialized feeding program whose staff includes more professionals with feeding expertise.

Surgical Cleft Repair

The goal for the majority of infants and young children with a cleft condition (lip and/or palate) is surgical correction. This section describes pre- and postsurgery recommendations for oral care and feeding.

Preoperative Recommendations   The primary consideration prior to surgery is for the child to meet specific weight and health guidelines. To repair a cleft lip, an infant must be at least 3 months old and weigh approximately 10 pounds. Cleft palate repair is generally not completed until after the child's first birthday (Damiano et al., 2009; Redford-Badawal et al., 2003; Reid, 2004; Skinner, Arvedson, Jones, Spinner, & Rockwood, 1997). In a study by Amstalden-Mendes et al. (2007), problems related to weight gain were the primary reason for delayed cleft surgery for a Brazilian sample. For both types of surgery, the child also must demonstrate stable respiratory status, including no episodes of pneumonia or similar illnesses in the weeks prior to surgical treatment. General anesthesia is used, which is an additional reason that respiratory health is a requirement. It should also be noted that two surgeries are needed to correct bilateral cleft lip; they are scheduled approximately 1 month apart.

Postoperative Recommendations   Following cleft repair, additional surgeries may be necessary depending upon the extent of the cleft or to assist speech development and feeding skills. These surgeries can also improve the appearance of the lip and nose and aid in stabilizing and realigning the jaw (Skinner et al., 1997). Surgeries are scheduled at least 6 months apart to allow healing and to reduce the chances of scarring.

Healing and Oral Care   Following palatal repair, the site of the repair may swell, and following cleft-lip repair there is often bruising, swelling, and/or bleeding around the affected area. In addition, both types of cleft repair may cause nasal congestion for several days, and stitches will take approximately 1 week to dissolve. All of these conditions may adversely affect appetite and overall interest in feeding. Feeders must observe the child for signs of discomfort and respond to the child's cues by alleviating the irritation.

There is also the ongoing need to keep the repaired area clean to reduce the risk of infection. Martin (2004) recommends a soft diet and rinsing the mouth after every meal and snack for approximately 2 weeks after surgery. It is important to avoid spicy and acidic foods (e.g., citrus) because they can irritate the lip and palate and slow the healing process. An additional consideration is to provide positive feeding experiences after cleft repair so that the child forms positive associations with eating rather than developing, for example, food refusal.

Postoperative Feeding   Feeding after cleft surgery focuses on offering fluids in adapted bottles and soft foods from a spoon in order to encourage healing (Martin, 2004). The main considerations are positioning, bottle and nipple type, and liquid flow-rate. An otolaryngologist, oral surgeon, and plastic surgeon are part of the surgical team and often have recommendations for postoperative feeding. An SLP also consults on the child's oral care to assist with new oral skill development and to ensure that nutritional needs are met. Coordinated follow-up care is essential.

The bottles described in the previous sections are used postoperatively, as are several additional types. For example, the Soft-Sipp bottle is often recommended postsurgery. This bottle includes multiple-size tubing to adjust for faster flow-rate and to offer thicker fluids. It is made of soft plastic, which helps reduce pain that may be associated with post-surgery feeding. VentAire, a product of Playtex, is an angled bottle that reduces air intake. VentAire Stage 2 nipples have a Y-cut tip to encourage feeding. There is also a wide nipple that approximates the shape of a breast nipple for infants who also have breastfed or who will breastfeed. Finally, the Mead Johnson Cleft Palate Nurser may be used with a variety of nipples to encourage sucking and can also be squeezed by the feeder. A bottle that approximates cup feeding is available from Medela. The SoftFeeder is a specialty device with a reservoir that controls the flow of fluid. As with the bottles described in previous sections, a squeezable design assists with the acquisition of feeding skills that were not possible or that were demonstrated in a limited way prior to surgery.

Spoon feeding can begin after surgery based on the cleft team's recommendation. Presentation of textured foods must proceed with caution depending on the child's developmental age, familiarity with textures, and extent of palatal repair. Martin (2004) pointed out that after cleft surgery, children are more likely to eat than drink, so positive experiences with spoon feeding and finger foods are critical.

Again, it is critical to work with the child's cleft team for ongoing assessment of the child's feeding skills and consistent implementation of her feeding plan. It is best to work with the child's cleft team to determine the most appropriate feeding method to use postsurgery. Sometimes syringes are used, but they require longer feeding sessions for the same amount of intake compared with bottle feeding. Arvedson and Brodsky (2002) recommended that breastfeeding begin only after using a small, open cup to offer thickened, preferred liquids. Skinner et al. (1997) also caution not to begin breastfeeding until the post-

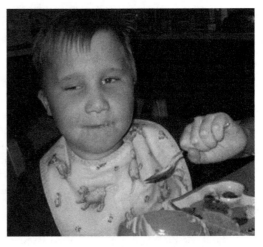

Devon (Vinny) 2 years postrepair

operative healing process is nearly complete. High calorie oral supplements such as Pediasure may be used for toddlers. Numerous resources are suggested at the end of this chapter for parents, caregivers, and professionals who have additional questions about cleft conditions and feeding.

YOUNG CHILDREN WITH RECESSED OR SMALL JAW (MICROGNATHIA)

Strategies to facilitate feeding young children with micrognathia focus on positioning, adapted bottles and nipples, and monitoring airway status. The position usually recommended is to have the child sitting upright and leaning slightly forward.

Nassar, Marques, Trindade, and Bettiol (2006) studied the effects of massage and adapted nipples on bottle fed 2-month-old infants with Pierre Robin sequence. Infants were given massage to the facial area prior to feeding, and a bottle nipple with an enlarged hole was used. When these interventions were used, the infants were able to ingest more formula in less time. Singer and Sidoti (1992) confirmed the need for modifying holes in bottle nipples and the need for determining the most appropriate positioning for feeding.

Breastfeeding children with micrognathia is often difficult, but can be attempted with advice from the child's medical team (see Nassar, Marques, Trindade, & Bettiol, 2006). If breastfeeding is unsuccessful, mothers are encouraged to pump breast milk for bottle feeding. Several authors stress the need to monitor the child's breathing pattern (Lidsky, Lander, & Sidman, 2008; Miller & Wilging, 2007; Wagener et al., 2003). Spoon feeding can proceed with similar cautions.

A mandibular distraction may be used to address micrognathia, just as it is used to address cleft palate. Mandibular distraction is a surgical procedure in which a special appliance is inserted to assist with growth of the lower jawbone. Some appliances also have an external portion with a key-type mechanism. When it is turned, the appliance stretches and so does the bone and soft tissue of the jaw. This helps accelerate jaw growth, which assists the child's respiration and facilitates feeding (Glass & Wolf, 1999).

YOUNG CHILDREN WITH AN ENLARGED TONGUE

An additional feeding complication is an enlarged tongue. This condition, combined with upper airway obstruction, is a common feature of children with Down syndrome. These conditions often interfere with feeding. Infants with an enlarged tongue and/or upper airway obstruction may be very challenging to breastfeed due to low muscle tone; in this case, expressing breast milk is recommended. The use of bottles with disposable liners (e.g., Playtex Drop-Ins) is advised because the liners can be manually squeezed to assist the infant with the suck–swallow–breath sequence. Positioning to encourage chin tuck is also helpful. When the infant is older, feeding at the breast can be attempted as long as care is taken to support the infant's head, neck, and jaw (Spender et al., 1996). Propping the infant with a pillow is also helpful for both the child and feeder because the elevation assists with more aligned positioning of the head and torso.

Spoon feeding may be difficult for this group of children. An enlarged tongue often produces tongue-thrusting or resting of the tongue outside the mouth. It also affects lip closure. It is important to establish the type of spoon the young child is able to successfully use. A Maroon spoon provides a shallow bowl and is used to address a number of oral feeding difficulties while a Lip Closure spoon offers a raised surface at the end of the bowl. For the latter type of spoon, the surface provides tactile feedback to the upper lip as the bolus is cleared from the bowl.

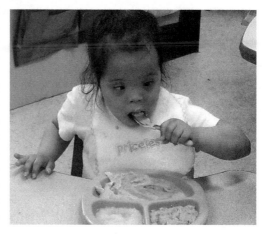

Spoon in mouth

YOUNG CHILDREN WITH TRACHEOTOMIES

A tracheotomy is a surgical procedure that places a hollow tube into the windpipe to correct a malformation or blockage in a child's airway. The trach is the resulting hole or stoma in the front of the neck. Some young children with a cleft condition or enlarged tongue require a tracheotomy (Miller & Wilging, 2007; Roger et al., 1999). In addition, there is a high incidence of young children with micrognathia requiring placement of a tracheotomy (Lidsky et al., 2008). The tracheotomy may be for the short or long term, depending on the underlying cause for placement. Furthermore, a tracheotomy may necessitate limiting or stopping oral feeding. See Bath and Bull (1997) and Lidsky et al. (2008) for examples discussing young children with Pierre Robin sequence. Smith and Sender (2006) reported on a sample of young children with Pierre Robin sequence who were successfully decannulated (progressive removal of tracheotomy resulting in return to typical breathing patterns). Over 90% of the children were able to receive a fully oral diet.

In cases when the child's medical team decides that oral feeding can continue, a number of considerations must be factored into determining the types and quantity of the child's food and liquid intake. If a child has previous negative or unpleasant feeding experiences, he or she may be hypersensitive around the mouth and hesitant to allow bottles, cups, and so forth near the face. Conversely, a child who has had enjoyable experiences may require assistance to adjust to the tracheotomy and related equipment such as a suctioning machine. With these points in mind, the list of questions in Table 13.2 provides a starting point for feeding activities.

Preparation for Oral Feeding

If a child has received primarily tube feedings and if oral intake is being introduced, it is best to provide activities to elicit sucking such as offering a pacifier. This type of oral stimulation prepares the child to tolerate tactile stimulation and begin the process of accepting liquids and solids foods. It is important to provide playful interactions so the child associates these activities with enjoyment (Morris & Klein, 2000; Wolf & Glass, 1992). Licking, mouthing, and chewing edible items and safe, nonedible objects (e.g., teethers, chewy tubes) should also be encouraged. In addition to oral stimulation, these actions promote choice-making and lets the child explore textures. The child's feeding team can provide suggestions as well.

Mealtime Strategies

A number of strategies can support feeding a child with a tracheotomy. Primary among them is the health and safety of the child. For example, protect the tracheotomy site with a bib or similar covering so that food or liquid cannot enter the tubing. Do not use bibs or coverings with a plastic liner because the liners can adhere to the tracheotomy. If a child requires suctioning, it is important to suction the child prior to a feeding because eating produces additional saliva that a child with a tracheotomy may need assistance managing (Fraker & Walbert, 2003; Klein & Delany, 1994; Oberwaldner & Eber, 2006). Additional strategies include the following:

• Always place the child in an upright position with chin tuck to assist swallowing during breastfeeding, bottle feeding, and for helping the child manage a bolus. The liquid or food item can then pass into the esophagus rather than into the lungs causing aspiration.

• Do not prop bottles. Always hold the bottle, and always monitor the infant.

• Burp an infant frequently during a feeding. Keep the infant in an upright position or on his or her right side after feeding is completed.

Table 13.2. Questions to Ask Prior to Introducing / Re-introducing Oral Feeding

1. If appropriate, did the child demonstrate age-appropriate suck–swallow–breath sequence before tracheotomy placement? If so, has the child been provided nonnutritive sucking opportunities?
2. If appropriate, was the child able to accept food items from a spoon prior to tracheotomy placement?
3. If appropriate, was the child able to finger-feed prior to tracheotomy placement?
4. What additional types of oral stimulation activities have been attempted with child? How did the child respond to these activities?
5. Does the child have necessary lung function for oral feeding?
6. Does the child have the endurance to accept a feeding without fatigue?
7. Does the child require supplemental oxygen during oral stimulation or feeding?
8. Has the child been evaluated for risk of aspiration during oral feeding?
9. Have members of the child's feeding team, including the pediatrician, approved oral intake?
10. Have parents and caregivers received training in feeding a child with a tracheotomy?

- Monitor the child's facial expressions and respiration for indications of distress (e.g., grunting, nasal flaring) and respond accordingly.
- Provide ample fluids to keep secretions thin and easy to clear.
- Keep finger foods and spoon-fed items moist because crumbs can enter the tracheotomy and cause respiratory difficulties.
- Help the child cough by modeling as well as directly teaching this skill so that the need for suctioning during mealtimes can be reduced or eliminated.
- It is best to wait a minimum of 30–40 minutes after a feeding before providing any necessary suctioning. Suctioning sooner can induce gagging and vomiting.
- If food or liquid is seen in the tracheotomy, suction immediately and call the child's primary doctor for further instructions.

SUMMARY

Taken together, the specialized interventions presented in this chapter address a variety of feeding difficulties related to anatomical anomalies. Ultimately, positioning and use of appropriate feeding items (e.g., nipples) is paramount, and specific changes to fluids and food items are important. It is also imperative to work closely with the team of professionals providing feeding-related recommendations and services.

▇ ▇ ▇ TABLE TALK ▇ ▇ ▇

Desiree is a 7-month-old infant with unilateral cleft lip and palate (the soft portion of the palate). She also has an alveolar ridge defect. Her lip was successfully repaired 2 months ago. Desiree accepts fluids from the Mead Johnson Cleft Palate Nurser and has had success with the Haberman feeder. Teresa, her maternal grandmother and primary care-giver, wants her granddaughter to use Playtex Drop-Ins in "regular" bottles. Teresa says she is more comfortable with that type of system. However, this change would conflict with the advice of Desiree's cleft team. Ms. Woods, Desiree's SLP, is firm in the use of a specialized system, especially because Desiree will undergo the first of two operations to correct her palate in approximately 5 months.

The cleft team has begun discussing the use of a palatal obturator prior to Desiree's palate repair. Teresa has not brought Desiree to two appointments set up for the purpose of preparing the mold for the palatal obturator. Teresa has also mentioned that she wants to offer her granddaughter more baby foods. Currently, Desiree eats all types of fruit but has refused most vegetables.

Desiree still experiences some episodes of gagging and choking during feeds. Teresa has been observed to use Playtex Drop-Ins and squeeze the plastic sleeves and providing an amount of fluid that Desiree's mouth cannot manage. The SLP and occupational therapist have spoken with Teresa about the need to closely monitor the flow-rate in order to provide Desiree with opportunities to better coordinate her suck–swallow–breath sequence as well as to reduce the likelihood of negative feeding experiences.

The cleft team is also concerned that Desiree has several teeth coming in at the same time. Teresa is offering her teethers and more frequent feedings. She is worried about how teething will affect Desiree's surgery. Ms. Woods has reassured Teresa that teething in infants with cleft palate is typically no different than in young children without a cleft condition. She also encouraged Teresa to return to Desiree's feeding schedule and to understand that they can work together to introduce a greater variety of puréed foods into her diet as well as soft finger foods.

Discussion Questions

▪ Do you agree with Ms. Woods's recommendations?

▪ What is your recommendation about the palatal obturator?

▪ How would you approach the issues surrounding bottle feedings and solid foods?

FEEDING NUGGETS

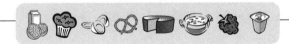

Books

Your Cleft-Affected Child: The Complete Book of Information, Resources, and Hope by Carrie T. Gruman-Trinkner and Blaise Winter, (2001)
http://www.hunterhouse.com

A Parent's Guide to Cleft Lip and Palate by Karlind T. Moller, Clark D. Starr, and Sylvia A. Johnson, (1990)
http://www.upress.umn.edu

Management of Cleft Lip and Palate by A.C.H. Watson, Debbie A. Sell, and Pamela Grunwell, (2001)
http://www.wiley.com

Web Sites

FACES: The National Craniofacial Association
faces@faces-cranio.org
http://www.faces-cranio.org

For more information regarding cleft care and feeding:
http://www.cleftline.org/

14

Young Children Who Require Tube Feeding

What You'll Learn in This Chapter

This chapter provides

- Information regarding reasons for placement of a feeding tube
- An overview of feeding procedures for nasogastric, gastrostomy, jejunostomy, and gastro-jejunostomy tubes
- A discussion of the benefits and challenges of tube feeding
- Strategies used to assist young children to transition from supplemental or full tube feeding to partial or total oral feeding

■ ■ ■ **FOOD FOR THOUGHT** ■ ■ ■

"Kiki, who has full trisomy 18, started off drinking about an ounce of formula every 3 hours. The remainder of her formula would be put through the nasogastric tube (NG-tube). She came home from the hospital when she was 1 month old, with the NG-tube still inserted. We had instructions to feed her every 3 hours. It took at least an hour to get 1.5 ounces into her, so that meant we would wake her up, feed her for an hour or more, let her sleep a bit, and then do it all again. I do not miss those days!"

Loretta, Parent

"Nick, who is 3½ years old, has the spastic quadriplegia form of cerebral palsy. He is a twin who was born at 28 weeks gestation. Nick got his gastrostomy tube (G-tube) last March. Most of his feedings (5 per day) are by the tube. He still does some bottle feeding, but it's Pediasure only. If he is congested, the Pediasure is too thick, so his mom gives him Pedialite. Nick's mother wishes she could have spoken with the parent of a child who has the same condition or someone who knows more about it. She feels like the G-tube should have been introduced earlier because Nick wasn't even on the growth charts, and now he is gaining weight more quickly than before the G-tube."

Lise, ECSE Graduate Student

WHAT THE LITERATURE SAYS

Chernoff (2006) described the evolution of tube feeding from ancient times to the present. The author emphasized the changes in enteral feeding (tube feeding) technology and changes in the children and adults who received this type of feeding intervention. Tube feeding during the late 1800s and early 1900s emphasized the provision of medications and use of infused solution containing food items such as milk, barley broth, and eggs (p. 408). Today, specialized formulas exist (e.g., Kindercal TF, Pediasure , Peptamen Jr.), and tube feedings can be received through the mouth, nose, stomach, and jejunum (middle section of small intestine; Campbell, 2006). Young children with severe feeding challenges often receive one or more types of tube feeding, whether for a short time or for long-term nourishment.

Some young children are unable to meet their caloric or nutritional requirements by oral intake alone. Others have difficulty eating due to a neurological condition (e.g. cerebral palsy) or an anatomical condition (e.g., cleft palate). Still other children experience problems with their digestive system such as esophageal problems or frequent aspiration (see Chapter 11), or they experience problems with the overall feeding process. Regardless of the underlying cause, tube feeding addresses intake and general health and development (Isaacs, 2004; Sleigh & Brocklehurst, 2004; White, Mhango-Mkandawire, & Rosenthal, 1995). Positive outcomes of tube feeding, including improved general health and weight gain, have been discussed by Cook, Hooper, Nasser, and Larsen (2005) and Craig, Scambler, and Spitz (2003).

Parents, caregivers, clinicians, and other professionals often have mixed viewpoints on the initiation and continuation of tube feeding. For example, Craig, Scambler, and Spitz (2003) interviewed parents with children with neurological disabilities who received tube feeding. The parents expressed a need for greater levels of emotional support to assist them in the daily care of their children. Greer, Gulotta, Masler, and Laud (2008) identified a similar theme in their study of families with a tube-dependent child who participated in an intensive feeding program. Many mothers commented on how feeding was one of the few "normal" things their child was able to do and said they worried that without that ability their children would be perceived as more disabled. In addition, mothers desired the positive social interactions that feeding provides (see Chapter 3). Hunt (2007) reiterated this finding and advocated for clinicians and other professionals to work closely with families to make informed decisions that match family preferences and that address family concerns.

For young children who have had very little or no exposure to eating by mouth and for whom tube feeding meets nutritional needs, skills for typical feeding (e.g., independent bottle feeding and chewing textured foods) may not be acquired when expected, may be reached later, or may never be developed (see Kerwin, 1999; Mason, Harris, & Bissett, 2005; Sullivan et al., 2005). Oral feeding is emphasized when a young child's medical problems are stabilized or resolved, anatomic conditions are corrected, or other underlying digestive system causes are managed. Infants and young toddlers should be given opportunities to suck on a pacifier to stimulate movement of lips, gums, and tongue. This type of nonnutritive sucking provides oral stimulation that can ease the transition to oral intake. Older toddlers and preschool-age children should be given a variety of foods to suck, taste, and chew. Whatever the type of oral stimulation, these occasions encourage growth and development related to feeding abilities (McKirdy, Sheppard, Osborne, & Payne, 2008). These activities can also serve to advance fine motor skills and social interaction with parents and caregivers.

TYPES OF FEEDING TUBES

This chapter considers four types of tube feeding for young children: nasogastric tubes (NG-tube; through the nose), gastrostomy tubes (G-tube; through the stomach), jejunostomy tubes (J-tube; through the small intestine) and gastro-jejunostomy tubes (GJ-tube; through stomach and small intestine). Gavage feeding (a process in which a thin, plastic tube is placed through the mouth into the stomach) is used for a different purpose compared with the feeding tubes discussed in this chapter. Gavage is commonly used with premature infants in neonatal intensive care units and is discussed in Chapter 9. An additional type of feeding is partial or total parenteral nutrition, which involves intravenous feeding that bypasses the need for eating and digestion. Parenteral feeding can be used with infants, toddlers, or preschool-age children, but it is beyond the scope of this chapter.

Nasogastric Tubes

The two main reasons for placement of a nasogastric tube (NG-tube) are to assist young children with nutritional intake and to reduce the risk of aspiration. An NG-tube is used for short periods of time until the problem is resolved (e.g., Kiki's story at the beginning of this chapter) or as a temporary measure until the child receives a long-term or permanent feeding tube such as a gastrostomy tube (G-tube). An infant with respiratory difficulties may be unable to safely accept breast milk or formula and thus may require an NG-tube until her respiratory status improves. Or a young child with Down syndrome may require supplemental NG-tube feedings as she recovers from cardiac surgery.

The NG-tube is inserted through the child's nose directly into the stomach cavity. A stethoscope should be used to ensure that the tube is inserted correctly. Otherwise, the tube may be positioned in the lung, which can cause discomfort and aspiration. It is necessary for parents, caregivers, clinicians, and other professionals to receive training before performing this procedure. Placement and removal of the

NG-tube can trigger gagging or vomiting. Suctioning may also be necessary if the child has a large amount of oral or nasal secretions. Sterile tape is typically used to secure the NG-tube to the child's face. The site must be closely monitored because the tape may cause skin abrasions and discomfort. Cleaning the area at least once daily is recommended.

Some infants receiving NG-tube feedings may require special formula. Premature infants as well as newborns with digestive system difficulties will need formula with the appropriate combinations of calories and nutrients. Similac Neosure, Enfamil Enfacare and Nutren Junior are examples of high-calorie formulas frequently prescribed for premature infants. Similac Alimentum and Enfamil Nutramigen address the needs of infants with protein allergies. Breast milk as well as commercial formulas can be passed through the NG-tube. Regardless of the type of formula, the amount and rate is determined by the child's feeding team. Decisions are made with consideration given to the child's health and daily needs. The members of the team, including the child's parents, meet to discuss the child's caloric and nutrient needs. Chapter 5 fully describes possible feeding-team members, overall team structure, and strategies to promote and maintain ongoing collaboration and communication among team members.

Surgically or Endoscopically Placed Tubes for Long-Term Feeding

While an NG-tube is inserted and removed daily or several times a week and primarily used for a short period of time, G-tubes and J-tubes are placed surgically or endoscopically and used over an extended period of time, which can be weeks, months, or throughout the child's life. Endoscopic placement refers to placing a tube into the stomach through the abdominal wall (percutaneous) or directly into the jejunum portion of the small intestine. Surgical placement entails a more invasive procedure and a hospital stay that may last several days for observation of the tube site for infection and tolerance of enteral feeds (e.g., no vomiting) prior to discharge.

G-tubes and J-tubes are commonly used for young children with significant neurological issues (e.g., as a result of bacterial meningitis) that, if untreated, can affect the oral-motor skills necessary to eat and drink safely. There are also infants, toddlers, and preschoolers with motor impairments (e.g., cerebral palsy; see Nick's story at the beginning of this chapter) and health issues (e.g., dysphagia) that cause feeding difficulties that may require tube feeding.

Gastrostomy Tube

Young children requiring a G-tube often have long-standing feeding concerns such as frequent aspiration episodes, a history of poor weight gain, and associated health concerns and anatomical anomalies such as cleft palate or a fistula. Some young children may continue to eat and drink by mouth after insertion of a G-tube, while others receive nutrition exclusively through the G-tube.

There are two types of G-tubes, and they can be placed using an endoscope at a hospital or outpatient surgery center. With the first type, a narrow, lighted tube is threaded through the esophagus to locate the abdominal wall. An opening suitable for a G-tube can then be made. A tube or porthole-like device or a "button," placed at or within approximately one inch of skin level is placed for access to the G-tube. The second type of G-tube is referred to as a percutaneous endoscopic gastrostomy tube (PEG-tube), and also requires an internal balloon catheter. The outer portion or button is known commercially as a Bard, MIC-KEY or Applied Medical Technology (AMT) MINI Classic Balloon. Both G-tube types are for long-term use. A child's recovery after a PEG-tube placement may require 1 day to several days in the hospital to monitor healing and the child's tolerance of feedings.

Daily button care is essential to reduce the risk of infection and discomfort to the child from soreness or leakage at the opening in the skin (stoma site). A 2" x 2" split gauze should be used on the skin around the button or exterior tubing. The stoma site must be cleaned at least twice a day with mild soap and warm water. Aa drawback for use of exterior tubing is that it can be pulled out by the child, can be caught on furniture, and can be more difficult to keep dry during a bath or other water activities.

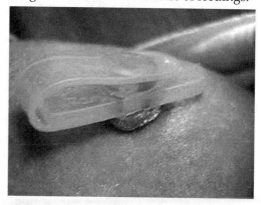

Bard button

Infant formula, breast milk, specialized formula such as Pediasure and Compleat, milk, and water can be given through a G-tube. Klein, Duperret, and Trautlein (2006) and Klein and Morris (2007) provided suggestions for homemade blended formulas (HBF). These blends include table foods prepared to a puréed consistency and thinned as necessary to pass through the G-tube. An HBF should be offered at least once a day for a 3–5 day period to encourage acceptance and to observe for adverse reactions (e.g., vomiting, diarrhea, constipation). Klein, Duperret, and Trautlein (2006) recommended offering HBF during mealtimes through a syringe; this type of feeding is referred to as a bolus feed. HBF facilitates a more active role in meal preparation and interaction for the child, the parents, and the caregivers. It also provides learning opportunities. The child can help blenderize the food, for example, while the parent labels and describes the foods' individual tastes. A final benefit is improved health because HBF can provide a more complete diet than manufactured formula. Klein and Morris (2007) developed a handbook focusing on HBF, which can serve as an important resource.

All types of enteral nutrition can be provided in one of two ways: bolus feeds or gravity feeds. Bolus feeds are given through a tube connected to the stoma site. A syringe is used to provide formula at a rapid rate. Feedings are brief, typically around 10 minutes long. If tolerated, bolus feeds are used during the child's daytime activities at a child care center or ECSE classroom, for example, and in community settings. A child's parent is typically taught how to bolus feed by a dietitian or medical professional such as a nurse or gastroenterologist (a physician who specializes in the diagnosis and treatment of disorders of the gastrointestinal tract, including the esophagus, stomach, and small intestine). In turn, the child's parent (or a program or agency nurse if available) trains the

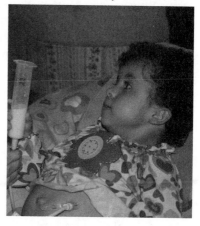

Annabel fed via Bolus feed

caregiver or classroom professional how to measure and perform bolus feeds. The parent would also advise of any change in the amount of a bolus feed. Instances of child discomfort or vomiting must be reported to the parent because the schedule or volume of feeds may need to be adjusted.

In contrast, gravity feeds are given by connecting the external section of the G-tube (i.e., the button) to a feeding pump such as the EnteraLite Infinity, Kangaroo Pet, or UltraPak Enteral Closed System. Gravity feeds provide formula at a much slower rate than a bolus feed, often taking an hour or more for a daytime feeding or running throughout the overnight hours. Some feeding pumps can be placed in a backpack or similar bag, rather than attached to an intravenous (IV) pole to improve mobility for the child and to enable caregivers and professionals to provide a gravity feed in a variety of settings. In terms of measuring the formula and relaying instances of discomfort, training is similar that provided for bolus feed. However, for gravity feeds, caregivers must also learn how to attach and remove the tubing and how to program and operate the feeding pump.

Liquid medications or crushed and diluted pills can also pass through a G-tube. It is important to always flush a G-tube with warm water following a feeding or medication. Parents report that an effective option is the use of approximately 1 ounce of Coca-Cola to flush build-up inside a G-tube. They say that the acidity helps dissolve whatever is blocking the tube.

The most important consideration for both types of G-tubes is maintaining a seal on the internal

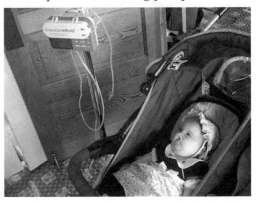

Feeding Pump

and external components. Medical attention is often necessary if the G-tube site becomes irritated or infected. Ointment should be placed on the skin after cleaning the stoma site. If there is a mechanism malfunction such as the balloon catheter deflating, medical attention is necessary. Tightness or observed discomfort around the site can also indicate the need for a larger button or tube extension due to the child's growth. Finally, if the button or tubing is pulled out, bleeding and/or leaking of stomach contents may occur. The G-tube must be replaced rapidly or the stoma will attempt to close. Parents and caregivers can be trained to replace a button, but in some cases, replacing the G-tube may require surgery.

Jejunostomy Tube

A jejunostomy tube (J-tube) is a feeding tube inserted through the abdomen and into the jejunum (part of the small intestine) to assist with feeding. Liquid nutrition bypasses the stomach and is fed directly into the intestinal tract. This is important for young children with digestive system issues resulting in an inability to properly digest food in their stomach or with difficulties emptying stomach contents into the intestine.

A J-tube is always surgically inserted. Young children must stay in the hospital for several days for care of the stoma site and to introduce J-tube feeds. Tubing or a button can be placed depending on the surgeon's and the family's preference. After discharge, use of a feeding pump is recommended, along with flushing the J-tube with water after each feeding. J-tubes have a number of possible complications including discomfort, intolerance of feedings, skin irritation or infection, and bowel obstruction. The stoma of a J-tube, similar to that of a G-tube, should be cleaned with mild soap and warm water.

Gastro-Jejunostomy Tubes

A gastro-jejunostomy tube (GJ-tube) has openings to the stomach *and* the small intestine. Medications are provided through the G-tube and formula is provided through the J-tube. Daily care is similar to that described previously, with attention to both stoma sites. Similar formulas, pumps, and flushing procedures are used with G-tubes, J-tubes, and GJ-tubes. Bolus feeds can be used with GJ-tubes if tolerated. Some young children require continuous feeds at a slow rate throughout the day and/or nighttime hours to avoid gagging or vomiting. All caregivers, clinicians, and other professionals working with a young child with any type of feeding tube should be knowledgeable regarding its use and care.

The recommendations for feeding procedures and care of the stoma site can be applied in any setting. Caregivers, clinicians, and professionals who are responsible for tube-feeding a child must work with the other members of the feeding team to ensure consistency and safety in all the aforementioned areas. Consideration must also be given to the availability of training in the use of tube-feeding materials. It is also necessary to work closely with the young child's parents for training and provision of necessary supplies.

The Tube Feeding Process

Regardless of the type of tube feeding, young children must be safe and comfortable when receiving enteral feeds. During the feeding and for approximately an hour afterward, children must be in an upright or semireclined position in an appropriate seating system (e.g., infant seat, highchair, Corner Floor Sitter). This positioning is especially critical for gravity feeds. A young child who is bolus-fed can be held or positioned in a chair or specialized seating system. The feeding team provides recommendations for optimal positioning and equipment. All adults involved in feeding the infant, toddler, or preschooler must receive training to properly position the child and properly use the feeding equipment (which can include a bottle or cup to measure formula, syringes for bolus feeds, a pump or feeding/flow bag, and extension tubing to access the Bard or MIC-KEY button). For gravity feeds, the pump must be correctly set to deliver the feed per the feeding team's specifications such as 50 ml per hour for 3 hours (i.e., 150 ml over 180 minutes).

Table 14.1 provides an overview of the four types of tube feeding, including method of placement, primary feeding methods, benefits, and challenges.

STRATEGIES AND SPECIALIZED INTERVENTIONS

Tube feeding may be a young child's sole nutrition source, or it may be supplemental. The transition from oral intake to tube feeding can be gradual or immediate. As indicated previously, young children receive tube feedings to address a number of feeding challenges. Some young children receive tube feedings to supplement what

Table 14.1. Types of tube feeding

	Placement method	Feeding method*	Benefits	Challenges
Nasogastric (NG-tube)	Intubation	Bolus gravity feed	Bypass mouth Short term use	Gagging Discomfort Not tolerating feedings Skin irritation
Gastrostomy (G-tube)	Endoscopically surgically	Bolus gravity feed	Bypass mouth Long term use Reduce risk of aspiration Offer oral stimulation and feeds as tolerated	Discomfort Not tolerating feedings Skin irritation or infection
Jejunostomy (J-tube)	Endoscopically surgically	Bolus gravity feed	Bypass stomach Long term use Reduce risk of aspiration	Discomfort Not tolerating feedings Skin irritation or infection Bowel obstruction
Gastrostomy-Jejunostomy (GJ-tube)	Endoscopically surgically	Bolus gravity feed	Access for formula and medication Long term use Reduce risk of aspiration	Discomfort Not tolerating feedings Skin irritation or infection Bowel obstruction

* Child should be positioned in as upright a position as tolerated for all types of enteral feedings

they eat by mouth. This may entail providing remaining amounts of meals in liquid form, giving a supplemental tube feeding at a specific time during the day, or providing a specified number of ounces or continuous feed overnight to ensure adequate calories. There are also infants, toddlers, and preschoolers with adequate oral intake who require tube feedings during an illness or to receive medications. Finally, as described earlier in the chapter, there are young children with anatomical, medical, and neurological conditions that necessitate long-term tube feeding (Sullivan et al., 2005).

Transitioning to Oral Feeding

Parents, caregivers, clinicians, and other professionals must be mindful of readiness indicators for oral feeding, whether or not the child has a previous history with oral feeding. Primary among these are the child's health and medical status, the child's oral-motor abilities, and parental input, which will be interpreted by the feeding team who may make recommendations for oral intake. Second, is the young child's interest in eating orally and enjoyment in the activity, whether feeding is a new experience or was preexisting prior to tube feeding (Burklow, McGrath, Allred, & Rudolph, 2002). Finally, the child must be able to tolerate at least a minimal amount of oral stimulation and participation in daily mealtime activities (Klein, 2007a; Morris & Klein, 2000). For example, during a cooking lesson, a preschool-aged child with a G-tube can smell and touch the ingredients and help prepare the food item or meal. In the home setting, the child should join the family at the table for meals and be engaged in mealtime conversation and interactions. If the child's feeding team agrees, small tastes can be offered on the child's finger, mouth, or eating utensil.

Regardless of the specific oral activity, facial and oral massage is helpful to prepare a child for the introduction or reintroduction of oral feeding (Morris & Klein, 2000). Initial oral activities must also be tailored to how well the child's digestive system can tolerate and digest the offered tastes and liquids, and the child's overall comfort with oral experiences. Some toddlers and preschoolers will be willing to participate in tastings, while others may clench their mouths shut when they see the approach of a spoon (Schauster & Dwyer, 1996). Furthermore, the child's developmental age must be considered. For example, a 4-year-old with developmental delays or a complex neurological condition may function in all developmental areas at an 18-month level. Instead of being offered tastes of only solid foods, the child should be presented with opportunities to explore mashed and soft chewable foods.

Research has established that the longer tube feeding lasts, the lower the likelihood of eating by mouth, even at a supplemental level (Mason et al., 2005). To preserve the possibility of eating by mouth, infants who are tube fed should be offered pacifiers with and without tastes, such as breast milk and puréed fruit, and they should be introduced to puréed foods using a Baby Safe Feeder or spoon. If the feeding team approves, bite-size cereal and similar finger foods should also be

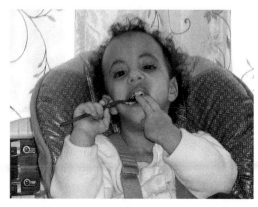

Madison

given. In addition to sampling the options for infants, toddlers can also taste items with more texture (e.g., oatmeal and blended foods) from a spoon, try more finger foods (e.g., different types of crackers), and use a cup for liquids. Self-feeding should be encouraged. Finally, oral experiences for preschoolers should be expanded to include self-feeding with a spoon and fork, finger foods from all food groups, and straws for liquids. A list of oral experiences is provided in Table 14.2.

Table 14.2.   Oral experiences for tube-dependent young children*

Infants	• Facial and oral massage as tolerated
	• Use of a Nuk® toothbrush or similar item
	• Suck on finger
	• Suck on pacifier
	• Suck on pacifier with taste provided on the tip, including breast milk, formula, puréed fruit or vegetable
	• Offer Baby Safe Feeder with fruit or vegetable (room temperature or frozen)
	• Offer biter biscuit or cracker (Gerber Graduates, Beech Nut Let's Grow, Earth's Best, Zwieback or similar)
	• Offer finger foods such as bite-size cereal and fruit chunks
Toddler	• Facial and oral massage as tolerated
	• Use of Chewy Tubes
	• Offer Baby Safe Feeder with fruit or vegetable (room temperature or frozen)
	• Offer textured foods by spoon
	• Offer finger foods such as bite-size cereal and fruit chunks
	• Encourage self-feeding of preferred foods by spoon
	• Provide cup with spout and handle(s)
Preschoolers	• Facial and oral massage as tolerated
	• Encourage self-feeding of preferred foods by spoon and fork
	• Offer variety of textured foods
	• Offer finger foods from all food groups
	• Provide cup without spout or lid as appropriate
	• Provide cup with straw

*Always consult with the child's feeding team before implementing any oral experiences and to determine appropriate amount, texture, and presentation

There are additional considerations in supporting a young child to accept foods and liquids orally. A feeding plan should be developed, including type of foods and liquids offered, weight gain, and general health must be monitored. In addition, the feeding environment should be addressed, along with positioning, appetite and satiation regulation, and family and caregiver participation and satisfaction (Burklow et al., 2002; Morris & Klein, 2000; Schauster & Dwyer, 1996). It is important to link tube feedings with opportunities for social interaction and participation in age-appropriate activities to support a successful transition to oral feeding. Some tube fed children do not associate feeding with interaction, such as passing meal items around the table and engaging in dinner table conversation. In addition to increasing oral intake, experiences should also help build the feeding relationship between the child and the parent, caregiver, and professionals on the feeding team (Mason et al., 2005; Schauster & Dwyer, 1996). Introduction of oral feeding to a young child with limited to total dependence on a feeding tube also requires the proper functioning of the mouth, tongue, esophagus, stomach, and intestines, along with the ability to swallow without aspirating and the ability to ingest adequate solids and liquids to meet nutritional needs. Whether the weaning process is partial or total, a variety of strategies and interventions exist to facilitate oral feeding.

STRATEGIES AND INTERVENTIONS TO FACILITATE ORAL FEEDING

A number of strategies exist to facilitate the introduction or reintroduction of oral feeding for a child who has been receiving tube feedings. The following sections describe ways to address each skill area described.

Development of a Feeding Plan

The young child's feeding team must collaborate to determine the type of oral stimulation, foods, and liquids to offer as well as procedures to monitor weight gain and general health. Each member of the team should share expertise and coordinate interventions so that the child receives oral feeds that are developmentally and functionally appropriate, and that can be implemented in all settings (Morris & Klein, 2000). For example, a specialized feeding chair can be used in the home, but may not be transportable to a child care center or restaurant. A portable booster seat with lateral supports (see next section on positioning aids) can be an alternative. Alternatives such as these for seating and the use of other specialized items such as a Maroon spoon or Sippy cup with handles must be addressed in the child's feeding plan.

Oral stimulation must be incorporated to prepare the child for oral feeding opportunities (McKirdy et al., 2008). Input to the hands, arms, cheeks, jaw, and mouth activate the parts of the body and face necessary for intake of solid foods and liquids. Items such as Nuk toothbrushes and Chewy Tubes, as appropriate, also offer a means for an infant, toddler, or preschooler to practice facial muscle movements in order to be better organized for the presentation of food items (Bryon, 2000; Morris & Klein, 2000). Especially for a young child with little experience with oral feeding, oral stimulation from a parent, caregiver, clinician, or other feeding-team member offers critical practice opportunities that can facilitate increased oral intake and, for some young children, assist with the discontinuation of enteral feeding.

The feeding plan must include feeding objectives describing what the child will demonstrate, needed materials, and specific criteria to determine when the objectives have been reached. This information facilitates consistency in presentation, including the specific food items and liquids, amounts, and textures that will be offered. The type of larger document that the feeding plan fits into (an Individualized Family Support Plan or an Individualized Education Plan) determines the format and types of objectives (see Chapter 7 for more information).

In addition, the feeding plan should include a description of feeding utensils and the amount of assistance the child requires for their use. This information is beneficial to parents, caregivers, clinicians, and other professionals because it provides consistency in implementation (for example when every member of the feeding team offers the same type of spoon or cup). A feeding plan must also specify how members of the feeding team can encourage greater independent feeding. A 4-year-old who has been tube-dependent since birth may require a great deal of physical assistance to bring a spoon to the mouth to taste puréed foods, while a young toddler with more oral feeding experiences may only need verbal reminders to spoon feed.

Positioning should also be specified for the child's safety. Most children with physical limitations need adaptive seating to facilitate head and trunk control for feeding experiences. Known allergies or restrictions must also be included in the feeding plan and explained for individuals who feed the child only infrequently (e.g., grandparent, babysitter) or who are not as familiar with the child, but are part of the feeding team (e.g., substitute early childhood special education teacher).

A feeding plan also assists with collecting data about the effectiveness of food presentation and the amount and types of food items and liquids the child accepts during feeding opportunities. These types of data can identify when circumstances have reached the point at which tube feeding can be discontinued. Before enteral feeding can be discontinued, oral intake must reach a point wherein the child's nutritional needs are met and sustained. For example, the feeding plan might indicate that oral feedings are sufficient (without supplemental tube feeding) when 75% of all meals over a period of 2 weeks are taken orally (Mason et al., 2005). It is important to note that some young children are able to be successfully weaned from tube feeding to 100% oral intake, but do not have their G-tube, J-tube, or GJ-tube removed because the tube ensures a means of entry for enteral nutrition and/or medication if necessary (e.g., during illness or some other event that negatively affects oral intake).

Steps must also be taken to guarantee that feeding experiences promote positive parent–child and caregiver–child interaction. These steps include creating a comfortable feeding environment for the parent and child, offering preferred tastes, food items, and liquids (as appropriate), and providing praise for all of the child's attempts. Interactions between the dyad must be positive and mutually enjoyable. The adult should be encouraged to talk with the child, sing songs, and/or describe the child's actions during feeding interactions. If interventions are difficult or unpleasant to implement, the likelihood of success in oral feeding is reduced (Burklow et al., 2002; Craig et al., 2006). Parents and caregivers must provide young children with these essential feeding experiences. Without their agreement with the feeding plan, it can be challenging to provide the interventions and adaptations necessary to wean a child partially or fully from tube feedings. Team members must work in concert with these individuals throughout development and implementation of the feeding plan. (Refer to Chapters 3 and 5 for tips on promoting parent and caregiver participation on the feeding team and in the implementation of the feeding plan.)

As briefly mentioned in a previous section of this chapter, monitoring must also be a component of the feeding plan. Data must be collected to ascertain whether feeding interventions are effective. Data collection methods can include anecdotal records, frequency charts, and food diaries. Data collection is especially critical when offering oral feedings to a tube-dependent child. The transition to eating by mouth can be a lengthy process. Sometimes the transition to complete oral feeding takes years to accomplish, especially if the child experiences setbacks (e.g., illness, medical complications; Klein & Delaney, 1994; Morris & Klein, 2000). The feeding team must engage in ongoing communication to share information and make adjustments based on child progress and potential weaning-related difficulties. This ensures a feeding plan that moves toward little to no reliance on tube feeding. (See Chapter 6 for more information on assessment and data collection.)

THE FEEDING ENVIRONMENT

Whether offering feeding experiences in the child's home, child care center, or classroom setting, a number of physical and social factors must be considered. Especially for a child who has been dependent on tube feedings, the feeding environment must meet all of the child's needs. Lighting, temperature, and related environmental factors must be thoroughly examined. For example, if the environment is too warm, a child may feel uncomfortable and eat or drink less. This condition could also negatively affect a child's swallowing and other eating-related physiological functions. Schauster and Dwyer (1996) discussed how tube-dependent children may receive feedings in areas other than a classroom or cafeteria in a school setting or a dining room at home. Some children may need to become accustomed to mealtime sounds, sights, and smells through a gradual desensitization process.

The feeding environment will also need to encourage independent feeding to the greatest extent possible. Methods such as provision of preferred food items, assistive devices such as adapted spoons and bowls, and other individualized interventions to address child-specific feeding needs can help encourage independent feeding. An additional consideration is that the child will ultimately need to accept food items from all caregivers, clinicians, and other professionals (Mason et al., 2005). Collaboration, coordination, and necessary training are required to attain this outcome. Training can occur through formal or informal methods of communication including meetings, demonstrations, and e-mail.

For the social component, the feeding environment must be familiar and calming. The social aspect of the feeding environment encourages the child's comfort through provision of feeding experiences with trusted individuals in a relaxed, comfortable setting (Bryon, 2000). Especially in a child care or classroom setting, the child needs to feel comfortable. Adults must interact with the child in a positive and age-appropriate manner. (This means, for example, no baby talk with a 4-year-old.) Infants, toddlers, and preschoolers also need consistent access to at least one preferred adult. Whenever possible, a favored child care provider or teacher should offer oral stimulation and related activities. If the child is fearful or anxious, feeding experiences will likely be negatively affected. Young children with a history of enteral feeding, especially with an NG-tube, are often wary of all types of oral stimulation. The parent or caregiver initiating oral stimulation must offer praise and encouragement for all feeding attempts. In the author's experience, holding an infant or young toddler and maintaining eye contact is helpful during these activities. In addition, assisting the child into a relaxed body position assists with lip closure and tongue movement.

The feeding team must be aware of who the child prefers as his primary feeding partner (the individual providing the feeding experiences). This may be the child's parent, other primary caregiver, or a professional on the feeding team who has frequent feeding interactions with the child. This individual plays a critical role in facilitating the child's oral intake and also in sharing information with other individuals involved in feeding experiences with the child. The collective result should be successful establishment of oral feeding skills as specified in the child's feeding plan.

Positioning

Appropriate positioning is critical to all feeding experiences (Snyder, Breath, & DeMauro, 1999). Before a child who has been relying on tube-feedings begins oral feeding, he or she must be evaluated for motor abilities including head control, shoulder and trunk stability, and hip alignment. Parents and caregivers should also be involved in the selection of a seating system that meets their child's needs, while matching space availability, allowing for use in multiple settings, and accommodating family budget constraints. All of this information is then used to select a seating system to meet the child's abilities and needs. Examples of commercially available options are the Bumbo baby seat, a highchair with or without adaptations to specialized seating, and systems manufactured by Rifton or Tumbleform. Commonly utilized adaptations to store bought items include shoulder straps, nonslip seat material such as contact paper or Dycem, and lateral supports. Some young children may also require specialized equipment such as hand, arm, leg, or foot orthotics (Snyder, Breath & DeMauro, 1999). (Further information on positioning is available in Chapter 12.)

Regulation of Appetite and Satiation

Introducing solid foods and liquids to a young child unfamiliar with eating by mouth must include a focus on satiation regulation. When a child receives continuous or scheduled tube feedings throughout a 24 hour period, he or she will not feel hunger as a child who is an oral feeder does (e.g., asking for a snack after a nap; Bryon, 2000). With input from the child's feeding team, a schedule must be developed that balances opportunities for meeting nutritional needs and encourages increasing amounts of oral intake during waking hours. This assumes that the young child is motivated to eat insofar as oral intake is a pleasant and reinforcing experience. Feelings of hunger and fullness can be developed by offering food prior to tube feeding and making corresponding alterations to the child's tube-feeding amounts and schedule (Benoit, Wang, & Zlotkin, 2000; Byars et al., 2003; Klein, 2007b).

Klein (2007a) also discusses attending to the child's verbal and nonverbal communication, including facial expressions and body language, during oral feeding experiences. When the child requests oral stimulation or a food item in sounds, words, or gestures (e.g., smiles at approach of spoon), the experience should continue. When a child says "no" or indicates "no" by shaking his or her head, or when the caregiver observes an increase in muscle tone in the child's hands or neck or clenching of the mouth, the feeding experiences should be stopped. When implementing these strategies with a young child with limited expressive language, it is important to observe the child's response to novel tastes and textures. For example, typically developing young children often grimace when a new taste or texture is introduced, and children with various disabilities can be observed to grimace in these situations as well. After additional presentations and encouragement, the child will often accept the novel item. When introducing feeding experiences to a child who has received short- or long-term tube feeding, the experiences must be individually appropriate. Consider Emme's example in the following paragraph.

Emme was a 20-month-old little girl who received primarily tube feedings since birth due to a variety of respiratory conditions. Because she had done well with oral stimulation experiences during the previous 3 months, the feeding team felt she was stable enough to try tastes of puréed fruits and other sweet flavors. Using a Maroon spoon, the speech-language pathologist (SLP) first introduced bananas and apple sauce, which Emme accepted. Emme gagged during the first three presentations of puréed peaches. The SLP and Emme's child care provider gave her opportunities to touch the puréed peaches and encouraged her to bring her fingers to her mouth. They also used Thick-it to increase the consistency of the peaches. After three additional presentations, Emme tasted the puréed peaches and, on the next presentation, accepted two tastes from the Maroon spoon. It is necessary to monitor the child for gagging, coughing, and choking; intake will not increase if the child associates oral intake with discomfort.

Family and Caregiver Participation

The feeding relationship helps form the basis of a young child's successful transition from tube to oral feedings. The interplay between the child and the feeding partner is a critical element in facilitating feeding experiences that are positive and that encourage increasing amounts of oral intake.

The child's feeding partners must fully participate during feeding interactions. For example, Klein (2007a) explained that it is imperative to have mealtime conversations that include the child, but that do not solely focus on eating. The author emphasized modeling of appropriate mealtime behaviors such as utensil use and stated that children "do not have to eat to be a participant" (p. 26). For young children who have been tube-dependent for an extended period of time, oral feeding experiences need to be planned, brief, playful, and free from pressure to eat (Bryon, 2000; McKirdy et al., 2008). There is also the potential for the child missing critical periods of feeding development, which can further interfere with increasing oral intake. Care must be taken to ensure that the feeding partner provides feeding experiences that are responsive and reinforcing for the young child.

Family and caregiver adherence to the feeding plan can be appraised through monitoring changes in the child's oral intake. The expectation is that implementation of the feeding plan will result in the child's eating more by mouth and requiring fewer tube feedings. This outcome can further encourage family and caregiver involvement in oral feeding experiences and provide mealtime interactions in the child's home, child care, and community settings.

SUMMARY

Tube feeding, whether supplemental or total, warrants input from a child's feeding team and ongoing observation of bolus and gravity feeds, tube integrity, and opportunities for presentation of oral intake. Some infants, toddlers, and preschoolers thrive solely on enteral feeding, while others can tolerate varying amounts of table foods and liquids. As indicated here, tube feedings provide support to address medical or developmental issues and require adherence to procedures and a schedule developed by the child's feeding team. The strategies and specialized interventions discussed in this chapter are intended as ways to promote nutrition and growth, as well as positive outcomes for young children requiring this type of feeding support.

▩ ▩ ▩ TABLE TALK ▩ ▩ ▩

Lawrence is 2½ years old and weighs 20 pounds. He is diagnosed with spastic cerebral palsy and asthma. Lawrence's mother, M'laya, does her best to feed her son semipuréed foods, but Lawrence's tongue thrust makes it difficult for him to strip the spoon and swallow. He is able to take several ounces of thickened liquids with each meal and generally accepts either a high-calorie pudding or a blended fruit smoothie for a morning snack.

Lawrence has had several episodes of aspiration pneumonia in the past year as well as three upper respiratory infections. His last asthma attack required a 2-day hospital stay. Lawrence has not shown any significant weight gain in the past 9 months. M'laya is very concerned about her son's feeding and general health. Lawrence's early intervention (EI) team, especially Lisa Becker, his child development specialist, and Nancy Villamayor, his speech language pathologist, share this concern.

M'laya was unprepared for the pediatrician's recommendation for placement of a G-tube. Dr. Greene acknowledged her efforts to feed her son, but pointed out that Lawrence was not on the growth chart for his age. His frequent illnesses were another cause for worry. M'laya agreed to supplemental tube feeding but wanted Lawrence to continue eating by mouth while he received additional calories needed for general health and growth.

The first 2 weeks were difficult for Lawrence as the stoma site healed and his body adjusted to the continuous overnight feedings. Dr. Greene was happy with the results until Lawrence had another aspiration episode after eating blueberry yogurt. The pediatrician informed M'laya that she should not offer Lawrence any thickened liquids or semipuréed foods and only provide tube feedings every 4 hours during the day and continuously overnight.

M'laya countered that she took great care feeding Lawrence and enjoyed feeding interactions with her son. It was a source of pride for her that she was able to feed him. She also explained that Lawrence was the most interactive during and after mealtimes. She did not feel that it was fair that Lawrence could not participate in an activity that was enjoyable to him and to her. M'laya said she would take greater care when feeding him as would Lisa and Nancy during therapy sessions.

Discussion Questions

▩ Do you agree with Dr. Greene's recommendations? Why or why not?

▩ If you were working with this family, how would you respond to M'laya's arguments?

▩ Would you provide Lawrence with supplemental oral feeding experiences? Why or why not?

FEEDING NUGGETS

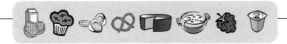

Books

Tube Feeding by Marcia Silkrocki, and Peggi Guenter (2001)

Feeding and Nutrition in Children with Neurodevelopmental Disability by Peter B. Sullivan (2009)

Web Sites

Feeding Tube Awareness
supertubimomm@gmail.com
http://www.feedingtubeawareness.com/

Kids with Tubes
info@kidswithtubes.org
www.kidswithtubes.org

Recommendations and Conclusions

INTRODUCTION

"All members of the child's team need to understand and participate in the intentional and individualized instruction deemed necessary…Thus, caregivers, therapists, and other interventionists need to work together in designing, implementing, and evaluating the effects of intervention."

(Pretti-Frontczak & Bricker, 2004, p. 181)

Section IV describes future directions and recommendations for development and implementation of feeding strategies and specialized interventions. With regard to recommendations, this book has emphasized context and strategies for feeding young children, positive feeding interactions (including the role of caregivers and the role of the child in feeding), social aspects of feeding (stressing the environment and preparation), and specialized interventions for young children with feeding difficulties. Chapter 15 further describes methods to achieve positive feeding interactions and development of feeding skills. Additional information is provided regarding the implementation of the transdisciplinary team model to work with young children with feeding difficulties. The need for integrating feeding strategies and specialized interventions throughout a child's daily activities and routines is further explored. This section provides recommendations for transdisciplinary feeding teams as well as a variety of naturalistic feeding interventions for use in home, classroom and community settings.

15

Feeding Outcomes and Future Directions

"I have boy/girl fraternal twins. They were exposed to the same flavor experiences in utero and through my breast milk, and when they were 1 year old, they pretty much ate the same foods without much encouragement. However, when they were 3, my son was eating a food in order to get dessert and threw up. Now, at 5 years old, he rarely tries new foods, gagging when encouraged to try something new, while his sister will try pretty much everything. She sometimes resists, and there are foods she dislikes. But, for the most part, she eats lots of vegetables and fruits.

My son eats fruits but only a few vegetables, and the vegetables he will eat are not the best ones (canned carrots, corn). I think he is very sensitive to bitter flavors, while his sister does not seem to be. We offer many healthy foods and have changed the techniques we use to get them to eat. For example, dessert is served infrequently and never as a reward for eating dinner. We offer fruits instead of sweets. We provide new foods to try on a weekly basis, along with foods they enjoy. We still wonder if our son will ever be a healthy eater, but we have hope."

Sally, Parent

"We were eating supper at the table the other night. Emma, who is 29 months old wanted to eat with her hands instead of her fork. She knows how to use utensils, especially when she eats pudding or applesauce. I asked her numerous times to use her fork instead of her hands. She didn't do as I asked, but ate with her left hand and just held her fork in her right hand. I guess it is much easier to use hands instead of a utensil."

Linda, Parent

"Recently Aubrey, who is 9 months old, has not wanted to eat baby food. She used to eat her food very well. Her parents told me they have been feeding her table food at mealtimes. However, at the child care we are not allowed to feed the children anything but baby food until they are a year old. I feed Aubrey turkey and rice baby food, which is warmed up before she eats it, and peaches. When I give her a bite she makes a bad face. She has a few bites of each food and then begins to cry. Eventually, she will not open her mouth for me anymore. I gave her some puffs and yogurt bites; she stopped crying and ate them. She will not open her mouth to eat anymore baby food."

Margaret, Child Care Provider

"Noel, who is 11 months old, has a cleft palate. He's due for surgery sometime soon after his first birthday, so we can't put a nipple or a bottle in his mouth anymore. When giving him something to drink (either juice or his special 'spit-up' formula), I hold the cup to his mouth and let him take little sips, then wipe whatever spills on his chin. If he grabs the cup, he usually just tips it over and spills everything out. That's why I hold it for him. For food, he usually eats a mixture of a mixed grain cereal/oatmeal with formula and two stage-1 vegetables or fruits. These these foods are thick enough to stick to the spoon, but not thick enough for it to be hard for him to swallow."

Anna, Child Care Provider

Feeding is a process. Meals are about much more than just nutrition; they are provided within a context of family and cultural rituals, as Satter (1987) so nicely elucidated. During meals, young children gain a sense of belonging to a group as well as the sense of security that a family ritual, like mealtime, provides.

Positive mealtime experiences are an important part of a child's development and predictive of positive outcomes (Fiese & Schwartz, 2008). For example, compared with children who do not share family mealtimes, children who do are better adjusted (Eisenberg, Olson, Neumark-Sztainer, Story, & Bearinger, 2004), have better communication skills (Lyttle & Baugh, 2008), and make healthier eating choices (Fiese & Schwartz, 2008). Adolescents who had family meals with their parents as young children are less likely to smoke, drink, or take illicit drugs (National Center on Addiction and Substance Abuse at Columbia University, 2007). It is critical, then, to promote positive mealtime experiences for all children in their earliest years and to equip families and other professionals with the tools they need to improve feeding outcomes for every child.

This book has explored theoretical frameworks related to feeding, examined feeding development and risk factors for feeding challenges, described specific feeding difficulties, and shared strategies and specialized interventions to improve outcomes for a range of young children. This final chapter synthesizes key points and discusses next steps for those individuals working with young children with feeding difficulties by exploring the social aspects of feeding as well as considerations related to teaming and naturalistic interventions.

CONTEXT OF FEEDING

A positive feeding context is critical for children's development. There are several theories that professionals can keep in mind when working with families to ensure that there is a positive feeding context.

Attachment Theory

The first is attachment theory. The intimate relationship that an infant forms with a caregiver is enduring and has lifelong significance for positive relationships. When a parent consistently meets the infant's needs in a caring and sensitive manner, the infant feels comforted and learns to trust others. An infant feels good when he or she is fed until full, gently burped, and allowed to fall asleep in a caregiver's arms. Providing this environment ensures that the infant is getting everything he or she needs to develop in a positive manner. One of the most basic ways that parents and caregivers feel closer to infants is by feeding them. There is little that can compare to the feeling of contentment at meeting the feeding needs of a newborn or young child.

Conversely, consider an environment where the parent does not consistently meet the infant's needs or meets them in a less than optimal way. For example, a hungry infant may be handed a cold bottle, or a bottle of curdled milk. She may not be held or talked to during feedings. This child develops no expectations for a positive feeding experience. Feeding will not be enjoyable or rewarding, only a means of gaining minimal sustenance, if that. Infants with a nonorganic failure to thrive diagnosis may receive enough to eat but do not utilize the calories and, therefore, do not gain weight. When moved to a nurturing environment, these infants start to put on weight. Young children with disabilities may also present challenges to the feeding relationship such as difficulties with intake (Cooper-Brown et al., 2008; see Chapters 11 and 13) and/or the need for tube feeding (Sleigh, 2005; see Chapter 14). Feeding-related interactions for these children may be limited in number or stressful and can have significant impact on the attachment relationship with their caregiver.

Family Systems Theory

Family systems theory is another important framework to consider in the context of feeding development. This theory describes four different types of families (chaotic, rigid, flexible, and structured). Feeding-related challenges may arise as a result of an ineffective family structure. In a chaotic family, for example, as described in Chapter 2, the family lacks leadership. The parents may provide little guidance for the child and let the child eat whatever he wants to eat rather than what he should eat. The parents may punish the child for playing with his food at one time and laugh at him the next time. This may cause a great deal of confusion for the child and potentially lead to disordered eating. A rigid family, on the other hand, expects the child to adjust to the demands and rules of the family. The child may be punished for his eating habits and behavior without fully understanding why and become stressed during mealtimes.

Children living in flexible and structured family systems (more balanced families) are less likely to have issues that occur during feeding due to the more balanced interactions. It is important for professionals working with young children to fully understand parents' perceptions of their infant's eating behaviors in order to provide the best care for families and to improve feeding outcomes for children. For example, Black (1999) notes that in families who feed infants solids before they are developmentally ready, parents may misinterpret their spitting out the foods as rejection. This can interfere with the parent–infant relationship and later feeding interactions, creating stressful feeding times for both parent and child.

Bioecological Systems Theory

Bronfenbrenner's bioecological systems theory (1993) offers another important framework for exploring feeding issues. This theory is based on the concept that development reflects the influence of several environmental factors that are woven into the child's developmental context. A child born to vegetarian parents, for example, receives some of the flavors of the mother's vegetarian diet via amniotic fluid and breastfeeding. When the child later begins receiving solid foods, the family prepares vegetarian meals consistent with the prior experiences of the infant. Later, the young child is exposed to commercials advertising sugary cereals and other treats and asks for them while shopping with her mother. There are many influences on this child's feeding preferences and habits and they will continue to evolve as the child grows, demonstrating how multiple systems affect feeding and eating patterns of young children.

Each of these theories can guide our understanding of an infant's feeding relationship, particularly if there are problems. The context, along with the interactions of important caregivers, should be explored when considering feeding challenges. With greater understanding of the child and the feeding context, key changes can be made to provide a more positive and improved feeding environment.

DEVELOPMENTALLY APPROPRIATE FEEDING AND RELATED STRATEGIES

Feeding seems like a simple process but, as has been shared throughout this book, there are many factors and potential difficulties related to feeding young children. In this next section we provide additional suggestions for enhancing young children's feeding experiences.

Breastfeed and/or Bottle Feed During the First Year

As discussed in Chapter 1, breast milk and/or formula should be the only food an infant receives until he or she is 4–6 months old. Breastfeeding is beneficial to the infant in many ways. It is important that parents-to-be receive early information about breastfeeding and that they receive support during breastfeeding. It can be difficult to help mothers make a decision as to whether to breastfeed because of the delicate nature of some of the related issues. Some women may be uncomfortable discussing breastfeeding, whereas others may be pressured by a partner or other family member to make a particular choice and reluctant to discuss options with a professional. The process of breastfeeding is influenced by many factors including sexuality, culture, society, and employment (Van Esterik, 2002). It's crucial for professionals working with families to be sensitive to unique situations and needs.

Offer Solid Foods No Earlier than 4 Months

Developmentally, infants are not ready for solid foods until they are 4–6 months old. Offering solid foods before 3 months of age can lead to an increased risk of diabetes (Norris et al., 2003) and obesity (Huh, Rifas-Shiman, Taveras, Oken, & Gillman, 2011). When infants are fed solids early, they may receive less milk because of the sensation of fullness that solids may provide. Furthermore, introducing solids before an infant is ready can lead to choking because young infants are not prepared to handle them (see Chapter 1).

Keep In Mind the Child's Development and Skills

As indicated previously, solid foods should not be offered before an infant is 4 months old. Similar attention needs to be given to other developmental considerations, such as the child's ability to bite and chew various textures (e.g., oatmeal, raw vegetables, cottage cheese). Understanding how feeding development relates to other areas of typical development is crucial (Crist & Napier-Phillips, 2001), especially when providing care for young children displaying delayed or disordered feeding, such as young children who exhibit food selectivity (Johnson, Handen, Mayer-Costa, & Sacco, 2008; Lockner, Crowe, & Skipper, 2011; see Chapter 1 and Appendix A for additional resources.)

Encourage Self-Feeding Skills   Providing activities that involve children's gross and fine motor skills can help them learn the skills necessary for self-feeding. Imitation and play activities can help a young child learn the skills needed to feed himself. Activities could be as simple as pretending to feed a baby doll with a spoon; having imaginary tea parties, picnics, or meals; using scoops and shovels in the sandbox; putting small objects through holes in containers; and scooping, stabbing, cutting, and pinching pieces of Play-Doh.

Offer Only Safe Foods   Children under the age of 1 year should not be offered cow's milk or foods that may be a choking hazard, such as nuts, round cuts of hot dogs, grapes, carrot chunks, or nuggets. Also, children under 1 year should not eat honey because of the risk of food poisoning. Attention to food allergies is also necessary (Sicherer, 2002). Food preparation in home and community settings must follow hygienic practices. Adults must wash hands before handling raw food, food preparation areas must be kept clean, and expiration dates for dairy products and other perishable foods must be monitored. Together, these practices ensure that all of the foods a child is offered are age-appropriate, developmentally appropriate, and free of germs and contaminants.

Introducing New Foods

Once it is determined that a new food is safe for an individual child and appropriate for his or her level of development, caregivers may not know when to go ahead and introduce the food. Sometimes a child is only fed a food one time before a caregiver assumes he or she does not like it. Other times, children are "bribed" into eating new foods or punished for not doing so. When possible, professionals can offer advice that supports positive new food experiences.

Offer New Foods Consistently and Repeatedly   First, new foods should be offered to a child eight or nine times before considering whether the child will accept the food. This helps an infant to develop a taste for the food (Forestell & Mennella, 2007). Young children are more likely to accept a food if it is offered more frequently over a longer period of time rather than introduced only for a few days before moving on to the next food.

In other words, parents and caregivers should repeatedly offer foods that have been previously rejected. Some foods must be repeatedly offered as many as 20 times before they are accepted. Periodic food rejection is typical for young children. This behavior may be inherited from our evolutionary predecessors for whom food neophobia served a biological function that protected omnivores against harmful foods (Cowart, 1981).

Don't Offer Incentives for Eating   Children are more likely to make better choices when they are not trying to eat enough adult-specified foods in order to get preferred foods such as desserts. In addition, desserts don't have to be unhealthy. For example, yogurt, fruits, and pudding with bananas are nutrient-rich desserts that do not provide a lot of calories. Desserts such as ice cream and cake can be offered occasionally, but they should not be a reward for cleaning a plate.

POSITIVE FEEDING INTERACTIONS

Creating a positive mealtime environment for children is important for a child's early development, and there are many ways professionals can help families achieve positive feeding experiences for children. The final aspect of healthy feeding interactions is the social context; feeding should be a warm and emotionally rewarding experience for both child and caregiver.

Social Aspects of Feeding

Mealtime conversation is important to a successful meal. Conversations should be fun and light-hearted. Child care providers, for example, can have children take turns talking so one person does not dominate the conversation during the snack or meal. A calm, warm, and accepting environment makes for better eating for all involved, and children who feel appreciated and respected at the table will feel better about what they are eating as well.

Realistic, Consistent Expectations

It's also important to help children understand what to expect at mealtime. For instance, children need to be taught where and when to come to eat, how to behave during a meal, when they can leave the meal, and how to eat each type of food. This can be done by taking pictures of the process of a meal and keeping them available for viewing in the dining room or kitchen at home or in a classroom or lunchroom. Pictures can demonstrate preparing a meal, setting out the utensils and serving dishes, eating the meal, and clearing the meal. Because children are learning appropriate eating skills and table manners between 3 and 6 years of age, they should be given opportunities to practice using serving spoons, scoops, tongs, and so forth with guidance along the way. Adults should model and teach appropriate mealtime behaviors. When children make a mistake, adults can correct them gently and demonstrate what is expected.

Children often need to shift gears from playing before they can focus on eating, so giving them time to transition is important. A premeal routine can help. Planning a quiet, calming activity before meals makes this transition easier. When young children have a consistent daily schedule with a consistent mealtime routine, they understand what is going to happen next and are more likely to have positive mealtime interactions.

Create a Calm and Pleasant Environment

First, eliminate distractions. The environment in which children eat should be calm, quiet, and welcoming. It is important to check the lighting and noise level as well as the temperature in the in the dining area. For some children these factors do not have an impact, but for others they may determine whether the child will participate in a meal or snack (Johnson et al., 2008).

Meals can be fun experiences for children and provide opportunities for humor and positive interactions with peers and family. Meals should also be texturally and visually interesting with lots of variety available for children. Lundy et al. (1998) found that offering infants different textures such as mashed or chopped and chewy foods encourages later preference for a variety of textures. Involving children in meal preparation may increase interest in the meal and increase interest in eating the foods that are offered. By allowing children to help make part of a meal, children are more excited to eat the meal. Some other ideas related to this are mentioned in Chapter 8.

HEALTHY NUTRITION

The Role of the Caregiver

Caregivers are the ultimate decision-makers when it comes to children's diets. They shop for, prepare, and serve the foods that children consume, and their decisions affect children's care and development. People who work with young children and their families should include in discussions about food and food choices, especially in terms of developmentally appropriate feeding, offering healthy choices, and making meals fun. Children often eat better in settings where the environment is different from home. Professionals, child care providers, and service providers are in a unique position to share feeding ideas about types of foods and their presentation and can model behaviors that help parents feed their children. Chapter 8 provides recommendations that can be used or adapted for the home setting.

Healthy Foods and a Healthy Weight

Nutritious eating habits developed early in life provide health benefits for a lifetime. A number of recommendations will help children maintain a healthy weight. Nutrients necessary for optimal health should be found in the food we consume daily. Yet, no one food provides all of the nutrients the body needs. Therefore, the first recommendation for parents, caregivers, and professionals is to offer a variety of foods to young children. Serving a combination of foods, both novel and familiar, will not only provide optimal nutrition for a child but will also be fun and interesting. Another suggestion is to serve meals and snacks that will help maintain a healthy body weight. Specific caloric needs differ for infants, toddlers and preschoolers due to their body size, growth spurts, and physical activity level. Menus should always include plenty of fruits, vegetables, and grain products with few fatty foods. Sugars and sweets should be offered only in moderation.

Published research shows that young children regulate their intake to match their caloric needs (Rolls, Engell, & Birch, 2000). Today, foods made of simple carbohydrates and high in fats are widely available, leading to higher rates of obesity. The Feeding Infants and Toddlers Study (FITS) revealed that toddlers are taking in over 30% more calories than they expend (Devaney & Fox, 2008). Moreover, 21% of children ages 2–5 years are overweight (Briefel, 2010). Foods provided to children should be low in fat, especially saturated fat. "The Dietary Guidelines for Americans suggest goals of 30% or less of total calories from fat and less than 10% of calories from saturated fat for everyone over two years of age" (LSU AgCenter, 2010, p. 2). Higher levels of fat have been linked to obesity, diabetes, hypertension, and cancers of the gall bladder, colon, breast, and endometrium (U.S. Department of Health and Human Services, 2001).

According to the Centers for Disease Control and Prevention, children should engage in regular physical activity and should participate in approximately 1 hour of physical activity daily to burn calories, help with weight control and prevent chronic diseases (2011). Benefits of being active include the following: increased energy, improved self esteem, a healthy heart, and a healthy weight. Bluford, Sherry, and Scanlon (2007) discussed the need for improved diet, physical activity, parent participation, and behavioral strategies to prevent obesity. Most programs in their review were multifaceted. This finding draws attention to the importance of establishing healthy eating habits early and maintaining them using a number of interrelated strategies.

Children make sound decisions when they are provided with healthy food choices. It is important to share information about healthy choices with adults who care for children because many adults are not aware of proper nutrition. The following feeding practices can lead to more positive feeding interactions, better feeding outcomes, and long-term health benefits for all young children.

Offer a Colorful Variety of Fruits and Vegetables

Today's diets frequently lack fruits and vegetables (especially vegetables). A great deal of research has been done about the introduction of vegetables and their acceptance and intake by infants and toddlers (e.g., Cooke, Wardle, Gibson, Sapochnik, Sheiham, & Lawson, 2004; Knai, Pomerleau, Lock, & McKee, 2006; Spill, Birch, Roe, & Rolls, 2010). One study found that when children were offered carrots before a meal and a double the portion size of carrots during the meal, children consumed more carrots (Spill et al., 2010). Healthy choices should be introduced early to ensure the establishment of lifelong patterns of nutritious eating (Devaney & Fox, 2008).

Limit Salt and Sugar

Foods and drinks with extra salt and sugar should be offered in limited quantities, because these foods generally have little nutritional value and add unnecessary calories to a young child's diet. Children naturally prefer sweets and salty foods at a young age. This preference likely evolved out of a need for energy-dense foods during periods of rapid growth (Mennella, 2008).

Limit Fatty Foods   Foods that get more than 35% of their calories from fat should be limited for children ages 2–3 years of age. For children 4 years and older, the fat content should not exceed 30%. Compared with children in past generations, children today are heavier, at higher risk for developing type 2 diabetes (Stevens, 2001) and more likely to have high blood pressure (Ludwig, 2007).

Limit Portion Size   Portion size should be appropriate for a child's age. Infants, toddlers, and preschoolers have different calorie needs for growth. Also, young children should learn to respond to their internal cues of hunger and satiety (Birch & Deysher, 1986). Children should generally be allowed to decide how much to eat. They may be served a second portion, but only if they decide they want more after eating an appropriately sized portion. They should be allowed to regulate the amount of food they take in because their intake is related to their energy expenditure. Children can select the foods they want to eat from healthy and balanced choices that are provided for them. If healthy choices are provided, monitoring a child's intake becomes less necessary; self-regulation develops, and caloric needs are met (Birch & Fisher, 1998; Birch, Johnson, & Fisher, 1995).

WORKING TOGETHER: THE TRANSDISCIPLINARY APPROACH

The following sections address the transdisciplinary approach used by feeding teams and the use of naturalistic interventions in home and community settings with young children with feeding difficulties. The transdisciplinary team model holistically addresses feeding difficulties within a context of communication, collaboration, and coordination (McGonigel, Woodruff, & Roszmann-Millican, 1994; Stayton & Bruder, 1999). Feeding progress is more likely to occur and be maintained through supportive interactions among team members (Bruns & Thompson, 2010).

The transdisciplinary model emphasizes communication, collaboration, and coordination among members of the feeding team in order to obtain desired feeding outcomes. Feeding teams must work very closely with families and caregivers to ensure safety and overall health and to aid feeding progress (Nijhuiset al., 2007). This is especially critical given the large number of young children with feeding difficulties such as failure to thrive and aspiration. Additional benefits offered by the transdisciplinary approach are that it addresses the need for professionals to engage in role exchange to bolster their skills and to provide the most comprehensive strategies and specialized interventions to meet each child's unique feeding needs. Role exchange emphasizes cross-discipline information sharing and implementation.

Increased Emphasis on Communication and Collaboration

The transdisciplinary approach cannot be implemented without team members' concerted efforts to communicate and collaborate about a child's feeding strengths and needs. Wooster, Brady, Mitchell, Grizzle, and Barnes (1998) pointed out the need for a team approach to provide services and supports to children with varied feeding difficulties. This approach necessitates information sharing and a willingness to learn from team members. Ongoing, frequent, and respectful communication must be observed. Team members may differ on the need for a specialized intervention. For example, in such situations, discussion and joint problem solving must occur. Without negotiation and cooperation, desired outcomes will not be attained.

Technology offers new communication options such as e-mail correspondence, text messaging, and Google Documents. Professional development may be needed so that all feeding team members gain the requisite knowledge to utilize these electronic systems. Decisions can then be made regarding the most appropriate means of communication for all team members as well as among individual professionals. Whatever the means of communication, the emphasis is directed toward provision of evidence-based practices to support feeding development (Buysse & Wesley, 2006). This interdependence and the resulting interrelationships promote collaboration (Briggs, 1997). Teamwork requires group effort and continuous information sharing, and the resulting relationships are an additional benefit offered by the transdisciplinary approach.

In order to sustain ongoing communication and collaboration, administrative support is necessary (Kaczmarek, Pennington, & Goldstein, 2000; Simonsmeier & Rodríguez, 2007). For example, time for meetings as well as the availability of technology is provided through the request of agency, program, and school supervisors. Opportunities for face-to-face and other modes of communication must be viewed as vital to the feeding team's success. Additionally, administrators can create partnerships with personnel at other community agencies and programs that offer feeding-related supports and services.

Role Exchange

One of the tenets of the transdisciplinary model and underlying the approach is sharing knowledge and specialized skills across disciplines. Team members work collectively toward achieving feeding plan goals, and they depend on each other for the implementation of discipline-specific responsibilities. Team members must also meet regularly, either face-to-face or via electronic means, to share expertise and consult with each other (Wooster et al., 1998).

Individual accountability also plays a major part in the transdisciplinary approach. Discipline-specific regulations and responsibilities influence which strategies and specialized interventions can be implemented. Team members also must be comfortable employing strategies outside their own areas of expertise. Rapport, McWilliam, and Smith (2004) reported "Although leaders in early intervention are strongly in favor of the transdisciplinary approach...it is viewed with caution among some practitioners from specialized disciplines" (p. 38). O'Donoghue and Dean-Claytor (2008) described how their sample of speech-language pathologists (SLP) did not feel confident in addressing dysphagia-related treatment needs because of an expressed lack in prerequisite knowledge. It is important to realize that not all SLPs specialize in feeding, just as not all occupational therapists (OT) have background in sensory processing and its relation to oral intake. Some professionals might be unwilling to share their expertise or have ethical constraints based on their professional organization or state oversight agency (e.g., Department of Human Services, Board of Education).

A study by Utley and Rapport (2000) examined willingness on the part of special education teachers, occupational therapists (OTs), and physical therapists (PTs) to share knowledge and implement strategies across disciplines. The therapists agreed to share information about postural alignment but felt it was inappropriate for special education teachers to provide "appropriate positioning for eating and feeding as well as how to implement feeding techniques" (p. 111). The

PTs agreed to impart information about range of motion exercises, but would only allow special education teachers to implement the exercises if they were present. The authors also noted "these team members had interacted with one another for *extended* periods of time...yet had not fully acquired one another's skills" (p. 115).

In the transdisciplinary approach, role release is the end point of a process wherein professionals learn about each other's professional responsibilities and implement new skill sets. However, as indicated previously, professionals may not feel comfortable relinquishing skills and/or knowledge that they feel is only for individuals trained in their own field. In such situations, role release may not be reached. The alternative takes place earlier in the process when role exchange is achieved (King et al., 2009).

Three stages precede role exchange. The first is role extension. This stage is exemplified by increasing expertise in one's own discipline, by staying current with field-specific literature, attending professional meetings and conferences, and participating in other types of professional development activities. Second, is role enrichment. The focus during role enrichment is sharing foundational knowledge and terminology across disciplines. Third, is role expansion. Following role enrichment, feeding team members are able to move into role expansion. This stage goes beyond information exchange. In role enrichment, professionals observe one another and share opinions and recommendations in order to learn about discipline-specific perspectives. Throughout these stages, role support should be offered via "ongoing interaction among team members" (King et al., 2009, p. 216). These interactions are characterized as opportunities for consultation and further cross-discipline training.

Role exchange is embodied by cross-discipline implementation of practices with supervision from the discipline-specific professional. In terms of feeding strategies and specialized interventions, role exchange can involve a parent implementing oral-motor exercises after an OT models them, or it can involve a PT observing an SLP positioning a child in a feeding chair. Role expansion would need to take place concurrently to promote professional development for all feeding team members.

Working with Family and Caregivers

Working together entails viewing all feeding team members as equals and respecting individual contributions. Qualifications must extend beyond professional degrees and years of experience in the field. Drobynk and Rocco (2011) described a team consisting of a parent, a personal care attendant, classroom teachers, and occupational therapy coaches working together to reintroduce fluid acceptance in a 10 year old. The child was fed orally until a negative surgery experience. The authors noted, "As mealtime routines are most often carried out by the child's parent/s, children are best served by empowering their parents to develop their own strategies and solutions" (p. 11). Furthermore, interventions to facilitate chin tuck to taste, and later, accept fluids was "developed and carried out by the mother who needed only a little 'tweaking' by the 'experts'—an approach much more likely to succeed and to be continually followed since it was one that came about naturally" (p. 11).

It is imperative that parents and caregivers work with their child's feeding team during the implementation of strategies and specialized interventions. What may not be as readily apparent is their participation in the development of the feeding plan and the evaluation of its success. Insights based on parents' intimate knowledge of their child benefit the transdisciplinary feeding team in several ways. Primary among these benefits are the recognition of family priorities (Brotherson, Sharp, Bruns, & Summers, 2008; McWilliam, 2005) and the varied contexts for provision of feeding support. Martin, Southall, Shea, and Marr (2008) also commented on the necessity of including families in all aspects of the feeding process. Treating a feeding disorder must include *all* individuals involved in meal preparation and feeding activities with the child.

There is a concomitant need to expand the possible range of feeders who work with a young child with feeding difficulties. Most often, parents provide meals, but with changing demographics and lifestyles, the "circle of feeders" can expand to include siblings, neighbors, babysitters, community program staff, and family friends. This links with provision of services in natural environments for infants and toddlers with disabilities and greater access to community-based offerings for preschoolers receiving special education services. Therefore, it becomes imperative that strategies and specialized interventions be shared with all possible caregivers (Bruns & Thompson, 2010; Scherer & Kaiser, 2007; Wooster et al., 1998). Ongoing supervision and feedback from feeding team members are necessary to ensure child safety and progress.

Respecting Culture and Diversity

As discussed in Chapter 4, views on foods and feeding practices are informed by an individual's family, culture, socioeconomic status, education, and personal beliefs. It is important to inform professionals and caregivers about appropriate feeding practices that will enhance the child's health and development without treading on beliefs and values. Some beliefs may interfere with appropriate feeding practices, and professionals must be sensitive to the underlying reasons that inform those beliefs. For example, while working in a skilled nursing facility with medically fragile young children, one of the authors of this text, Deborah A. Bruns, encountered several immigrant parents who disagreed with the recommendation to offer pureed and slightly textured foods to their infants and toddlers because they had grown up observing young babies eating solid foods in several countries in Asia. Similarly, some parents of children with cerebral palsy did not agree with recommendations for tube feeding even with medical documentation of aspiration because "feeding by a machine" was not always regarded in a positive way in some African American subcultures. (See Chapter 4 for more information on how to address feeding challenges in culturally diverse populations.)

Professionals are often called on to translate their understanding, informed by education and professional practice, of the needs of children to parents with whom they are working. Decisions about feeding are very personal and based on a rich generational and cultural history, and professionals must treat families and their traditions with dignity and respect. Respect is an integral part of a professional's work with young children and their families, especially when the family's beliefs differ from those held by the professional. As discussed in the following sections, ensuring beneficial feeding outcomes for young children requires ongoing communication and collaboration between families and professionals. Respectful interactions are a first step toward a successful partnership.

Providing Naturalistic Interventions

Another technique (in addition to the transdisciplinary approach) that is useful in order to facilitate increased intake and overall feeding development, is the use of naturalistic techniques. The following sections provide ideas for building upon naturally occurring opportunities to work on feeding skills throughout a young child's daily activities and routines. These interventions are implemented in the child's everyday settings and with the child's caregivers and peers (Grisham-Brown, Pretti-Frontczak, Hemmeter, & Ridgley, 2002; Kashinath, Woods, & Goldstein, 2006; McWilliam & Casey, 2007; Meadan, Ostrosky, Zaghlawan, & Yu, 2009; Pretti-Frontczak & Bricker, 2004; Sandall & Schwartz, 2008).

Provide Interventions in Children's Everyday Settings   Because there is a variety of feeding team members, feeding support can and should be provided in a variety of settings. For example, Chiarello and Effgen (2006) discussed the changes in service provision for PTs. Clinical settings were the norm until changes in the Individuals with Disabilities Education Improvement Act (IDEA) of 2004 (PL 108-446) encouraged professionals to offer their services in settings where young children would participate if they did not require special services. Early intervention professionals, such as developmental specialists, receive training to work in home and community environments. However, this may not be commonplace in other fields (Campbell, Chiarello, Wilcox & Milbourne, 2009; Pilkington & Malinowski, 2002). Furthermore, when working with preschool-age children, public schools and related center-based settings are the norm. The adjustment then becomes offering services in the classroom with the child's peers rather than in the context of one-to-one or small-group therapy. Professional development activities may be necessary to impart information about classroom structure and related management procedures to OTs, PTs, and SLPs. This allows training to align feeding strategies and specialized interventions with the context of small- and large-group activities and instruction.

An additional setting described in the literature is the neonatal intensive care unit (NICU). Supporting intake is critical with newborns, especially for those with an anatomical anomaly or those who are premature. In addition to medical personnel, dietitians (Olsen, Richardson, Schmid, Ausman & Dwyer, 2005; Sneve, Kattelmann, Ren & Stevens, 2008) and OTs (Caretto, Topolski, Linkous, Lowman & Murphy, 2000; Tanta & Langton, 2010) may work with newborns and help parents learn and implement specialized feeding interventions in the NICU (e.g., specialized formula) and after discharge (e.g., positioning equipment). In addition, the NICU-based feeding team must work with community-based professionals to coordinate overall care as well as feeding needs. Again, the concept of a circle of feeders is apt because a potentially large number of adults are involved in coordinating feeding activities, strategies, and specialized interventions within the NICU, at home, and in community settings such as center-based child care.

Community settings offer many opportunities for the acquisition and use of feeding skills. Many community activities, such as block parties and religious ceremonies, include participation in meal preparation and/or eating. In addition, independence is a critical outcome for all young children and should also be addressed in feeding development (Segal, 2004). It is of limited utility if a preschooler feeds himself at home and is unable to eat independently in a restaurant or at a peer's birthday party. This, again, calls for coordination so that progress is maintained and strategies to promote new skills are shared and monitored across settings.

Embedding Interventions into Daily Routines
Feeding should be addressed within an array of daily activities and routines, especially because early development is integrated rather than isolated. Gains in language, for example, affect and interact with fine and gross motor advances. Woods and Kashinath (2007) also discussed opportunities for skill development during play activities and daily routines. The authors focused on increasing social communication through naturalistic strategies, such as environmental arrangement and modeling. Results indicated that mealtimes offered many opportunities for their sample of 14 young children (ages 12–65 months). The authors noted, "this study illustrates how similar caregiving routines offer similar, and for some families, more opportunities for practice on targeted communication and social outcomes" (p. 148). The same can be said of feeding development within the context of daily routines. For example, using a toothbrush is similar to using a spoon. Working with a young child to transfer positions (e.g., standing to sitting) can also assist with midline orientation at mealtimes.

Pretti-Frontczak and Bricker (2004) and Sandall and Schwartz (2008) described the benefits of embedding for young children with disabilities. Other authors have examined the efficacy of embedding (Grisham-Brown, Pretti-Frontczak, Hemmeter, & Ridgley, 2002; Jung, 2007; Rosenkoetter & Squires, 2000). In addition, Wolery and McWiliam (1998) specifically discuss the importance of embedding opportunities to work on feeding with preschoolers with disabilities. From birth to age 5, embedding provides varied opportunities for skill acquisition and availability of natural consequences. Working with a young child to prepare and eat his snack at child care or Head Start, for example, provides many ways to address developmental skills such as eye-hand coordination, problem solving, and self-feeding. Embedding also promotes greater participation in age-appropriate activities.

Embedding holds much promise for addressing feeding difficulties. There is little reason to work on feeding skills, such as accepting textured foods and drinking from an open-mouth cup, outside of mealtimes. Working on feeding outcomes during daily activities and routines bolsters feeding development and related skills such as reaching and grasping and turn-taking. Sensory-based feeding difficulties are also best addressed through embedding because it allows the problems to be addressed within existing mealtime routines and allows for a reduction in environmental input that may adversely affect the child's intake. Furthermore, young children with a behavioral component to their feeding difficulties can make significant gains when feeders embed strategies and are responsive to the child's existing skills and preferences (Woods, 2003).

A final consideration is that embedding feeding strategies and specialized interventions does not preclude one-on-one sessions (with an SLP, for example). Some young children—such as a child who receives primarily enteral feeds but who is beginning to accept tastes of pureed foods—may require focused practice on feeding skills or require highly supervised interventions (McKirdy, Sheppard, Osborne & Payne, 2008). The feeding team will determine the appropriate menu of strategies and specialized interventions to meet an individual child's needs.

SUMMARY

As evidenced throughout this book, feeding is complex and requires the use of many interrelated skills and behaviors. There are many factors that can influence the development of age-appropriate feeding. Individualized assistance is necessary to provide needed adaptations and equipment. Young children who exhibit "red flags" and those with diagnosed feeding conditions require a team of parents, caregivers, and professionals to offer eating experiences that are supportive and enjoyable and that work toward desired feeding outcomes.

References

Adams, L., & Conn, S. (1997). Nutrition and its relationship to autism. *Focus on Autism and Other Developmental Disabilities, 12*(1), 53–58.

Addessi, E., Galloway, A.T., Visalberghi, E., & Birch, L.L. (2005). Specific social influences on the acceptance of novel foods in 2–5 year old children. *Appetite, 45*, 264–271. doi: 10.1016/j.appet.2005.07.007

Ahearn, W.H. (2003). Using simultaneous presentation to increase vegetable consumption in a mildly selective child with autism. *Journal of Applied Behavior Analysis, 36*(3), 361–365.

Ainsworth, M.D.S. (1979). Infant-mother attachment. *American Psychologist, 34*, 932–937.

Alder, E., Williams, F., Anderson, A., Forsyth, S., Florey, C., & van der Velde, P. (2004). What influences the timing of the introduction of solid food to infants? *British Journal of Nutrition, 92*, 527–531. doi:10.1079/BJN20041212

Alexander, R. (1987). Oral-motor treatment for infants and young children with cerebral palsy. *Seminars in Speech and Language, 8*(1), 87–100.

Alper, B.S., & Manno, C.J. (1996). Dysphagia in infants and children with oral-motor deficits: Assessment and management. *Seminars in Speech and Language, 17*, 283–309.

American Academy of Pediatrics. (1997). Policy statement: Breastfeeding and the use of human milk. *Pediatrics, 100*(6), 1035–1039.

American Academy of Pediatrics. (2005). Breastfeeding and the use of human milk. *Pediatrics, 115*(2), 496–506.

American Academy of Pediatrics: Bright Futures Steering Committee and Medical Home Initiatives for Children with Special Needs Project Advisory Committee. (2006). Identifying infants and young children with developmental disorders in the medical home: An algorithm for developmental surveillance and screening. *Pediatrics, 118*(1), 405–420.

American Academy of Pediatrics Committee on Nutrition. (1998). *Pediatric nutrition handbook.* Elk Grove Village, IL: American Academy of Pediatrics.

American Academy of Pediatrics Committee on Nutrition. (2008). *Pediatric nutrition handbook* (6th ed.). Elk Grove Village, IL: American Academy of Pediatrics.

American Psychiatric Association. (2000). *Diagnostic and statistical manual of mental disorders* (4th ed.). Washington, DC: American Psychiatric Association.

Amminger, G.P., Berger, G.E., Schafer, M.R., Klier, C., Fredrich, M.H., & Feucht, M. (2007). Omega-3 fatty acids supplementation in children with autism: A double-blind, randomized, placebo-controlled pilot study. *Biological Psychiatry, 61*(4), 551–553.

Amstalden-Mendes, L.G., Magna, L.A., & Gil-da-Silva-Lopes, V.L. (2007). Neonatal care of infants with cleft lip and/or palate: Feeding orientation and evolution of weight gain in a nonspecialized Brazilian hospital. *Cleft Palate-Craniofacial Journal, 44*(3), 329–334.

Anderson, A.K., Damio, G., Chapman, D.J., & Perez-Excamilla, R. (2007). Differential response to an exclusive breastfeeding peer counseling intervention: The role of ethnicity. *Journal of Human Lactation, 23*(1), 16–23.

Anderson, J.W., Johnstone, B.M., & Remley, D.T. (1999). Breastfeeding and cognitive development: A meta-analysis. American *Journal of Clinical Nutrition, 70*, 525–535.

Anderson, K.E., Nicklas, J.C., Spence, M., & Kavanagh, K. (2009). Roles, perceptions and control of infant feeding among low-income fathers. *Public Health and Nutrition, 13*(4), 522–530. doi:10.1017/S1368980009991972

Anderson, S. (1998). Daily care. In E. Geralis (Ed.), *Children with cerebral palsy: A parent's guide* (2nd ed., pp. 101–145). Bethesda, MD: Woodbine.

Aneja, S. (2004). Evaluation of a child with cerebral palsy. *Indian Journal of Pediatrics, 71*(7), 627–634.

Antunovic, E. (2009). The best place after the womb. NAP. Retrieved from: http://www.bobafamily.com/

Archer, L., Rosenbaum, P.L., & Streiner, D.L. (1991). The Children's Eating Behavior Inventory: Reliability and validity results. *Journal of Pediatric Psychology, 16*(5), 629–642.

Arenz, S., Ruckerl, R., Koletzko, B., & Von Kries, R. (2004). Breastfeeding and childhood obesity: A systematic review. International *Journal of Obesity and Related Metabolic Disorders, 28,* 1247–1256.

Armstrong, J., Reilly, J.J., & Child Health Information Team. (2002). Breastfeeding and lowering the risk of childhood obesity. *Lancet, 359,* 2003–2004.

Arosarena, O.A. (2002). Update on cleft care. *Current Opinion in Otolaryngology and Head and Neck Surgery, 10*(4), 303–308.

Arvedson, J.C. (1997). Behavioral issues and implications with pediatric feeding disorders. *Seminars in Speech and Language, 18*(1), 51–70.

Arvedson, J.C. (2000). Evaluation of children with feeding and swallowing problems. *Language, Speech, and Hearing Services in Schools, 31,* 28–41.

Arvedson, J.C. (2008). Assessment of pediatric dysphagia and feeding disorders: Clinical and instrumental approaches. *Developmental Disabilities Research Reviews, 14*(2), 118–127.

Arvedson, J.C., & Brodsky, L. (Eds.). (2002). *Pediatric swallowing and feeding: Assessment and management* (2nd ed.). San Diego, CA: Singular.

Arvedson, J., Rogers, B., Buck, G., Smart, P., & Msall, M. (1994). Silent aspiration prominent in children with dysphagia. *International Journal of Pediatric Otorhinolaryngology, 28,* 173–181.

Ashwal, S., Russman, B.S., Blasco, P.A., Miller, G., Sandler, A., Shevell, M., et al. (2004). Diagnostic assessment of the child with cerebral palsy: Report of the Quality Standards Subcommittee of the American Academy of Neurology and the Practice Committee of the Child Neurology Society. *Neurology, 62,* 851–863.

Austin, A.A., Druschel, C.M., Tyler, M.C., Romitti, P.A., West, I.I., Damiano, P.C., et al. (2010). Interdisciplinary craniofacial teams compared with individual providers: Is orofacial cleft care more comprehensive and do parents perceive better outcomes? *Cleft Palate-Craniofacial Journal, 47*(1), 1–8.

Ayres, A.J. (1979). *Sensory Integration and the Child.* Los Angeles, CA: Western Psychological Services.

Babbitt, R.L., Hoch, T.A., & Coe, D.A. (1994). Behavioral feeding disorders. In D.N. Tuchman & R.S. Walter (Eds.), *Disorders of feeding and swallowing in infants and children: Pathophysiology, diagnosis, and treatment* (pp. 77–95). San Diego, CA: Singular.

Bachrach, V.R., Schwarz, E., & Bachrach, L.R. (2003). Breastfeeding and the risk of hospitalization for respiratory disease in infancy: A meta-analysis. Archives of *Pediatric and Adolescent Medicine, 157,* 237–243.

Backstrom, C.A., Wahn, E.I.H., & Ekstrom, A.C. (2010). Two sides of breastfeeding support: experiences of women and midwives. *International Breastfeeding Journal, 5,* 1–8. doi:10.1186/1746-4358-5-20

Baikie, G., South, M.J., Reddihough, D.S., Cook, D.J., Cameron, D.J., Olinsky, A., & Ferguson, C. (2005). Assessment of aspiration tests using barium videofluoroscopy, salivagram, and milk scan in children with cerebral palsy. *Developmental Medicine & Child Neurology, 47,* 86–93.

Bailey, D.B., Hebbeler, K., Scarborough, A., Spiker, D., & Mallik, S. (2004). First experiences with early intervention: A national perspective. *Pediatrics, 113*(4), 887–896.

Baker, E.A., Schootman, M., Barnridge, E., & Kelly, C. (2006). The role of race and poverty in access to foods that enable individuals to adhere to dietary guidelines. *Preventing Chronic Disease: Public Health Research, Practice, and Policy, 3*(3), 1–11.

Baker, S.R., Owens, J., Stern, M., & Willmot, D. (2009). Coping strategies and social support in the family impact of cleft lip and palate and parents' adjustment and psychological distress. *Cleft Palate-Craniofacial Journal, 46*(3), 229–236.

Bandini, L.G., Anderson, S.E., Curtin, C., & Cermak, S. (2010). Food selectivity in children with autism spectrum disorders and typically developing children. *Journal of Pediatrics, 157*(2), 259–264.

Bandura, A. (1965). Influence of models' reinforcement contingencies on the acquisition of imitative responses. *Journal of Personality and Social Psychology, 1,* 589–595.

Bandura, A. (2001). Social cognitive theory. *Annual Review of Psychology* (Vol. 52). Palo Alto, CA: Annual Reviews.

Banks, J.W. (2003). Ka'nistenhsera: A native community rekindles the tradition of breastfeeding teiakotihshies. *AWHONN Lifelines, 17*(4), 341–347.

Bannister, P. (2004). Feeding a baby with cleft lip and palate. In V. Martin & P. Bannister (Eds.), *Cleft care: A practical guide for health professionals on cleft lip and/or palate* (pp. 45–68). Wiltshire, England: APS.

Baroni, M., & Sondel, S. (1995). A collaborative model for identifying feeding and nutrition needs in early intervention. *Infants & Young Children, 8*(2), 15–25.

Batchelor, J. (2008). Failure to thrive revisited. *Child Abuse Review, 17,* 147–159.

Bath, A.P., & Bull, P.D. (1997). Management of upper airway obstruction in Pierre Robin sequence. *The Journal of Laryngology & Otology, 111,* 1155–1156.

Baumrind, D. (1971). Current patterns of parental authority. *Developmental Psychology Monograph, 4,* 1–103.

Beckman, D. (2003). Oral-motor therapy: A protocol for speech and feeding. *Advance, 13*(36), 6–8.

Bell, H.R., & Alper, B.S. (2007). Assessment and intervention for dysphagia in infants and children: Beyond the neonatal intensive care unit. *Seminars in Speech & Language, 28*(3), 213–222.

Bell, K.E., & Stein, D.M. (1992). Behavioral treatments for pica: A review of empirical studies. *International Journal of Eating Disorders, 11*(4), 377–389.

Belsky, J. (1984). The determinants of parenting: A process model. *Child Development, 55,* 83–96.

Bener, A., Denic, S., & Galadari, S. (2001). Longer breastfeeding and protection against childhood leukemia and lymphomas. *European Journal of Cancer, 37,* 234–238.

Benoit, D. (2005). Feeding disorders, failure to thrive, and obesity. In C. H. Zeanah (Ed.), *Handbook of infant mental health* (2nd ed., pp. 339–352). New York, NY: Guilford Press.

Benoit, D., Wang, E.E.L., & Zlotkin, S.H. (2000). Discontinuation of enterostomy tube feeding by behavioral treatment in early childhood: A randomized controlled trial. *The Journal of Pediatrics, 137*(4), 498–503.

Benson, J.E., & Lefton-Greif, M.A. (1994). Videofluoroscopy of swallowing in pediatric patients: A component of the total feeding evaluation. In D.N. Tuchman & R.S. Walter (Eds.), *Disorders of feeding and swallowing in infants and children: Pathophysiology, diagnosis, and treatment* (pp. 187–200). San Diego, CA: Singular.

Bentley, M., Gavin, L., Black, M.M., & Teti, L. (1999). Infant feeding practices of low-income, African-American, adolescent mothers: An ecological, multigenerational perspective. *Social Science & Medicine, 49,* 1085–1100.

Berger, I., Weintraub, V., Dollberg, S., Kopolovitz, R., & Mandel, D. (2009). Energy expenditure for breastfeeding and bottle-feeding preterm infants. *Pediatrics, 124*(6), e1149–52.

Berkowitz, D. (1994). *The cleft palate story.* Carol Stream, IL: Quintessence.

Berlin, C.M., Jr., Paul, I.M., & Vesell, E.S. (2009). Safety issues of maternal drug therapy during breast-feeding. *Clinical Pharmacology Therapy, 85*(1), 31–35.

Bernard-Bonnin, A. (2006). Feeding problems of infants and toddlers. *Canadian Family Physician, 52,* 1247–1251.

Bernbaum, J.C., Pereira, G.R., Watkins, J.B., & Peckham, G.J. (1983). Nonnutritive sucking during gavage feeding enhances growth and maturation in premature infants. *Pediatrics, 71*(1), 41.

Baby Friendly Hospital Initiative. (2010). About the BFHI. Retrieved from http://www.babyfriendlyusa.org/eng/01.html

Birch, L.L. (1999). Development of food preferences. *American Review of Nutrition, 19,* 41–62.

Birch, L.L. (2008). Preface. In L. Birch & W. Dietz (Eds.), *Eating behaviors of the young child: Prenatal and postnatal influences on healthy eating* (pp. ix–x). Elk Grove Village, IL: American Academy of Pediatrics.

Birch, L.L., Birch, D., Marlin, D., & Kramer, L. (1982). Effects of instrumental eating on children's food preferences. *Appetite, 3,* 125–134.

Birch, L.L., & Deysher, M. (1985). Conditioned and unconditioned caloric compensation: Evidence for self-regulation of food intake by young children. *Learning and Motivation, 16,* 341–355.

Birch, L.L., & Deysher, M. (1986). Caloric compensation and sensory specific satiety: Evidence for self-regulation of food intake by young children. *Appetite, 7,* 323–331.

Birch, L.L., & Dietz, W.H. (Eds.). (2008). *Eating behaviors of the young child: Prenatal and postnatal influences on healthy eating.* Elk Grove Village, IL: American Academy of Pediatrics.

Birch, L.L., & Fisher, J.O. (1995). Appetite and eating behavior in children. *Pediatric Nutrition, 42*(4), 931–953.

Birch, L.L., & Fisher, J.O. (1996). The role of experience in the development of children's eating behavior. In E.P. Capaldi (Ed.), *Why we eat what we eat: The psychology of eating* (pp. 113–141). Washington, D.C.: American Psychological Association

Birch, L.L., & Fisher, J.O. (1998). Development of eating behaviors among children and adolescents. *Pediatrics, 101*(Suppl.), 539–549.

Birch, L.L., Fisher, J.O., Gimm-Thomas, K., Markey, C.N., Sawyer, R., & Johnson, S.L. (2001). Confirmatory factor analysis of the Child Feeding Questionnaire: A measure of parental attitudes, beliefs, and practices about child feeding and obesity proneness. *Appetite, 36*(3), 201–210.

Birch, L.L., Johnson, S.L., & Fisher, J.A. (1995). Children's eating: The development of food acceptance patterns. *Young Children, 50,* 71–73.

Birch, L.L., Marlin, D.W., & Rotter, J. (1984). Eating as the "means" activity in a contingency: Effects on young children's food preference. *Child Development, 55,* 431–439.

Birch, L.L., McPhee, L., Shoba, B.C., Pirok, E., & Steinberg, L. (1987). What kind of exposure reduces children's food neophobia? Looking vs. tasting. *Appetite, 9*(3), 171–178.

Birch, L.L., McPhee, L., & Sullivan, S. (1989). Children's food intake following drinks sweetened with sucrose or aspartame: Time course effects. *Physiology and Behavior, 45,* 387–396.

Black, J.D., Girotto, J.A., Chapman, K.E., & Oppenheimer, A.J. (2009). When my child was born: Cross-cultural reactions to the birth of a child with cleft lip and/or palate. *Cleft Palate-Craniofacial Journal, 46*(5), 545–548.

Black, M.M. (1999). Commentary: Feeding problems: An ecological perspective. *Journal of Pediatric Psychology, 24*(3), 217–219.

Blacklin, J.S. (1998). Your child's development. In E. Geralis (Ed.), *Children with cerebral palsy: A parent's guide* (2nd ed., pp. 193–229). Bethesda, MD: Woodbine.

Bluford, D., Sherry, B., & Scanlon, K.S. (2007). Interventions to prevent or treat obesity in preschool children: A review of evaluated programs. *Obesity, 15,* 1356–1372.

Boesch, R.P., Daines, C., Willging, J.P., Kaul, A., Chone, A.P., Wood, R.E., & Amin, R.S. (2006). Advances in the diagnosis and management of chronic pulmonary aspiration in children. *European Respiratory Journal, 28*(4), 847–861.

Borowitz, S.M., & Borowitz, K.C. (1997). Gastroesophageal reflux in babies: Impact on growth and development. *Infants & Young Children, 10*(2), 14–26.

Bowlby, J. (1969). *Attachment and loss (Vol. 1). Attachment.* New York, NY: Basic Books.

Bowlby, J. (1973). *Attachment and loss (Vol. 2). Separation, anxiety, and anger.* New York, NY: Basic Books.

Bowlby, J. (1989). *Secure and insecure attachment.* New York, NY: Basic Books.

Bragelien, R., Rokke, W., & Markestad, T. (2007). Stimulation of sucking and swallowing to promote oral feeding in premature infants. *Acta Paediatrica, 96*(10), 1430–1432.

Branscomb, K.R., & Goble, C.B. (2008). Infants and toddlers in group care feeding practices that foster emotional health. *Young Children, 63*(6), 28–33.

Brazelton, T.B. (1956). Sucking in infancy. *Pediatrics, 17,* 400–404.

Bricker, D. *Assessment, Evaluation, and Programming System for Infants and Children* (2nd ed.). Baltimore, MD: Paul H. Brookes Publishing Co.

Briefel, R.R. (2010). New finds from the Feeding Infants and Toddlers Study: Data to inform action. *Journal of the American Dietetic Association, 110*(12), S5–S7

Briefel, R.R., Hanson, C., Fox, M.K., Novak, T., & Ziegler, P. (2006). Feeding Infants and Toddlers Study: Do vitamin and mineral supplements contribute to nutrient adequacy or excess among US infants and toddlers? *Journal of the American Dietetic Association, 106*(Supplement 1), S52–S56.

Briefel, R.R., Reidy, K., Karwe, V., Jankowski, L., & Hendricks, K. (2004). Toddlers' transition to table foods: Impact on nutrient intakes and food patterns. *Journal of the American Dietetic Association, 104* (Suppl. 1), 38–44.

Briggs, M.H. (1993). Team talk: Communication skills for early intervention teams. *Communication Disorders Quarterly, 15*(1), 33–40.

Briggs, M.H. (1997). A systems model for early intervention teams. *Infants & Young Children, 9*(3), 69–77.

Brinich, E., Drotar, D., & Brinich, P. (1989). Security of attachment and outcome of preschoolers with histories of nonorganic failure to thrive. *Journal of Clinical Psychology, 18,* 142–152.

Britten, P., Marcoe, K., Yamini, S., & Davis, C. (2006). Development of food intake patterns for the MyPyramid Food Guidance System. *Journal of Nutrition Education and Behavior, 38,* S78–S92.

Britton, J.R., Britton, H.L., & Gronwaldt, V. (2006). Breastfeeding, sensitivity, and attachment. *Pediatrics, 118*(5), e1436–e1443. doi:10.1542/peds.2005-2916

Brodwick, M., Baranowski, T., & Rassin, D.K. (1989). Patterns of infant feeding in a tri-ethnic population. *Journal of the American Dietetic Association, 89*(8), 1129–1132.

Bronfenbrenner, U. (1993). The ecology of cognitive development: Research models and fugitive finds.

In R.H. Wozniak & K.W. Fischer (Eds.). *Development in Context* (pp. 3–44). Hillsdale, NJ: Erlbaum.

Bronner, Y.L., Gross, S.M., Caulfield, L., Bentley, M.E., Kessler, L., Jensen, J., Weathers, B., & Paige, D.M. (1999). Early introduction of solid foods among urban African-American participants in WIC. *Journal of the American Dietetic Association, 99*, 457–461.

Bronte-Tinkew, J., Zaslow, M., Capps, R., Horowitz, A., & McNamara, M. (2007). Food insecurity works through depression, parenting, and infant feeding to influence overweight and health in toddlers. *Journal of Nutrition, 137*, 2160–2165.

Brotherson, M.J., Sharp, L., Bruns, D.A., & Summers, J.A. (2008). Family-centered practices: Working in partnership with families. In P.J. Winton, J.A. Mc-Collum, & C. Catlett (Eds.), *Practical approaches to early childhood professional development: Evidence, strategies, and resources* (pp. 53–80). Washington, DC: Zero To Three Press.

Bruns, D.A., & Thompson, S.D. (2010). Feeding challenges in young children: A best practices model. *Infants & Young Children, 23*(2), 93–102.

Bryon, M. (2000). Interventions for children who are tube-fed. In A. Southall & A. Schwartz (Eds.), *Feeding problems in children* (pp. 191–202). Abingdon, Oxon, England: Radcliffe Medical Press.

Buhimschi, C., & Weiner, C.P. (2009). Medications in pregnancy and lactation. *Obstetrics & Gynecology, 114*(1), 167–168. doi: 10.1097/AOG.0b013e3181a89522

Bullock, F., Woolridge, M.W., & Baum, J.D. (1990). Development of co-ordination of sucking, swallowing, and breathing: Ultrasound study of term and preterm infants. *Developmental Medicine and Child Neurology, 32*, 669–678.

Burklow, K.A., McGrath, A.M., Allred, K.E., & Rudolph, C.D. (2002). Parent perceptions of mealtime behaviors in children fed enterally. *Nutrition in Clinical Practice, 17*(5), 291–295.

Burklow, K.A., McGrath, A.M., & Kaul, A. (2002). Management and prevention of feeding problems in young children with prematurity and very low birth weight. *Infants & Young Children, 14*(4), 19–30.

Burklow, K.A., McGrath, A.M., Valerius, K.S., & Rudolph, C. (2002). Relationship between feeding difficulties, medical complexity, and gestational age. *Nutrition in Clinical Practice, 17*(6), 373–378.

Burklow, K.A., Phelps, A.N., Schultz, J.R., McConnell, K., & Rudolph, C. (1998). Classifying complex pediatric feeding disorders. *Journal of Pediatric Gastroenterology & Nutrition, 27*(2), 143–147.

Burroughs, A.K., Asonye, V.O., Anderson-Shanklin, G.C., & Vidyasagar, D. (1978). The effects of nonnutritive sucking on transcutanious oxygen tension in noncrying preterm infants. *Research in Nursing Health, 1*(2), 69–75.

Buskens, I., Jaffe, A., Mkhatshwa, H. (2007). Infant feeding practices: Realities and mindsets of mothers in southern Africa. *AIDS Care 19*(9), 1101–1109.

Buswell, C.A., Leslie, P., Embleton, N.D., & Drinnan, M.J. (2009). Oral-motor dysfunction at 10 months corrected gestational age in infants born less than 37 weeks preterm. *Dysphagia, 24*, 20–25.

Buysse, V., & Wesley, P.W. (2006). *Evidence-based practice in the early childhood field.* Washington, DC: Zero To Three Press.

Byars, K.C., Burklow, K.A., Ferguson, K., O'Flaherty, T., Santoro, K., & Kaul, A. (2003). A multicomponent behavioral program for oral aversion in children dependent on gastrostomy feedings. *Journal of Pediatric Gastroenterology and Nutrition, 37*, 473–480.

Call, J.D. (1984). Child abuse and neglect in infancy: Sources of hostility with the parent-infant dyad and disorders of attachment in infancy. *Child Abuse & Neglect, 8*, 185–202.

Camp, K.M., & Kalscheur, M.C. (1994). Nutritional approach to diagnosis and management of pediatric feeding and swallowing disorders. In D.N. Tuchman & R.S. Walter (Eds.), *Disorders of feeding and swallowing in infants and children: Pathophysiology, diagnosis, and treatment* (pp. 153–185). San Diego, CA: Singular.

Campbell, P.H., Chiarello, L., Wilcox, M.J., & Milbourne, S. (2009). Preparing therapists as effective practitioners in early intervention. *Infants & Young Children, 22*(1), 21–31.

Campbell, P.H., & Halbert, J. (2002). Between research and practice: Provider perspectives on early intervention. *Topics in Early Childhood Special Education, 22*(4), 213–226.

Campbell, S. (2006). An anthology of advances in enteral tube feeding formulations. *Nutrition in Clinical Practice, 21*(4), 411–415.

Carbajal, R., Veerapen,S., Couderc, S., Jugie, M., & Ville, Y. (2003). Analgesic effect of breast feeding in term neonates: Randomized controlled trial. *British Medical Journal, 326*, 13–17.

Caretto, V., Topolski, K.F., Linkous, C.M., Lowman, D.K., & Murphy, S.M. (2000). Current parent education on infant feeding in the neonatal intensive care unit: The role of the occupational therapist. *American Journal of Occupational Therapy, 54*(1), 59–64.

Carruth, B.R., Skinner, J., Houck, K., Moran, J., Coletta, F., & Ott, D. (1998). The phenomenon of "picky eater": A behavioral marker in eating patterns of toddlers. *Journal of the American College of Nutrition, 17*(2), 180–186.

Carruth, B.R., Ziegler, P.J., Gordon, A., & Barr, S.I. (2004). Prevalence of picky eaters among infants and toddlers and their caregivers' decision about offering a new food. [Supplemental Material 1]. *Journal of the American Dietetic Association, 104*, 57–64.

Carta, J., Greenwood, C., Walker, D., & Buzhardt, J. (2010). *Using IGDIs: Monitoring progress and improving intervention for infants and young children.* Baltimore, MD: Paul H. Brookes Publishing Co.

Carter, A.S., Briggs-Gowan M.J., & Davis, N.O. (2004). Assessment of young children's social-emotional development and psychopathology: Recent advances and recommendations for practice. *Journal of Child Psychology and Psychiatry, 45*(1), 109–134.

Cassidy, J., & Shaver, P. (Eds.). (2008). *Handbook of attachment: Theory, research, and clinical applications* (2nd ed.) New York, NY: Guilford Press.

Centers for Disease Control and Prevention (2011a). *How much physical activity do children need?* Retrieved from: http://www.cdc.gov/physicalactivity/everyone/guidelines/children.html

Centers for Disease Control and Prevention (2011b). Breastfeeding among U.S. children born 1999–2005. *CDC National immunization Survey.* Retrieved from: http://www.cdc.gov/breastfeeding/data/NIS_data/

Charney, P. (2008). Nutrition screening vs nutrition assessment: How do they differ? *Nutrition in Clinical Practice, 23*(4), 366–372.

Chatoor, I. (2009). *Diagnosis and treatment of feeding disorders in infants, toddlers, and young children.* Washington, DC: Zero To Three Press.

Chatoor, I., Ganiban, J., Colin, V., Plummer, N., & Harmon, R. (1998). Attachment and feeding problems: A reexamination of nonorganic failure to thrive and attachment insecurity. *Journal of the American Academy of Child and Adolescent Psychiatry, 37*, 1217–1224.

Chatoor, I., Getson, P., Menvielle, E., Brasseaux, C., O'Donnell, R., Rivera, Y., & Mrazek, D.A. (1997). *Infant Mental Health Journal, 18*(1), 76–91.

Chatoor, I., & Khushlani, D. (2006). Eating disorders. In J.L. Luby (Ed.), *Handbook of preschool mental health: Development, disorders, and treatment* (pp. 115–136). New York, NY: Guilford Press.

Chatoor, I., & Macaoay, M. (2008). Feeding development and disorders. In M.M. Haith & J.B. Benson (Eds.), *Encyclopedia of Infant and Early Childhood Development* (pp. 524–533). New York, NY: Academic Press.

Chen, A., & Rogan, W.J. (2004). Breastfeeding and the risk of postneonatal death in the United States. *Pediatrics, 113*(5), e435-e439.

Chernoff, R. (2006). An overview of tube feeding: From ancient times to the future. *Nutrition in Clinical Practice, 21*(4), 408–410.

Chiarello, L., & Effgen, S.K. (2006). Updated competencies for physical therapists working in early intervention. *Pediatric Physical Therapy, 18*(2), 148–158.

Chiarello, L.A., Palisano, R.J., Maggs, J.M., Orlin, M.N., Almasri, N., Kang, L., & Chang, H.J. (2010). Family priorities for activity and participation of children and youth with cerebral palsy. *Physical Therapy, 90*(9), 1254–1264.

Chua, S. Arulkumaran, S., Lim, I., Selamat, N., & Ratnam, S.S. (1994). Influence of breastfeeding and nipple stimulation on postpartum uterine activity. *British Journal of Obstetrics and Gynaecology, 101,* 804–805.

Chuacharoen, R., Ritthagol, W., Hunsrisakhun, J., & Nilmanat, K. (2009). Felt needs of parents who have a 0- to 3-month-old child with a cleft lip and palate. *Cleft Palate-Craniofacial Journal, 46*(3), 252–257.

Chulada, P.C., Arbes, Jr, S.J., Dunson, D., & Zeldin, D.C. (2003). Breastfeeding and the prevalence of asthma and wheeze in children: Analyses from the Third National Health and Nutrition Examination Survey, 1988–1994. *Journal of Allergy and Clinical Immunology, 111,* 328–336.

Clark, R.H., Wagner, C.L., Merritt, R.J., Bloom, B.T., Neu, J., Young, T.E., & Clark, D.A. (2003). Nutrition in the neonatal intensive care unit: How do we reduce the incidence of extrauterine growth restriction. *Journal of Perinatology, 23,* 337–344.

Coe, D.A., Babbitt, R.L., Williams, K.E., Hajimihalis, C., Snyder, A.M., Ballard, C., & Efron, A. (1997). Use of extinction and reinforcement to increase food consumption and reduce expulsion. *Journal of Applied Behavior Analysis, 30,* 581–583.

Collaborative Group on Hormonal Factors in Breast Cancer. (2002). Breast cancer and breastfeeding: Collaborative reanalysis of individual data from 47 epidemiological studies in 30 countries, including 50,302 women with breast cancer and 96,973 women without the disease. *Lancet, 360,* 187–195.

Committee on Nutrition. (2000). Soy protein-based formulas: Recommendations for use in infant feeding. American Academy of Pediatrics. Retrieved from http://aappolicy.aappublications.org/cgi/content/full/pediatrics%3B101/1/148#otherarticles

Conroy, M.A., & Brown, W.H. (2004). Early identification, prevention, and early intervention with young children at risk for emotional/behavioral disorders: Issues, trends, and a call for action. *Behavioral Disorders, 29*(3), 224–236.

Cook, S., Hooper, V., Nasser, R., & Larsen, D. (2005). Effects of gastrostomy on growth in children with neurodevelopmental disabilities. *Canadian Journal of Dietetic Practice and Research, 66*(1), 19–24.

Cooke, L. (2007). The importance of exposure for healthy eating: A review. *Journal of Human Nutrition and Dietetics, 20*(4), 294–301.

Cooke, L.J., Wardle, J., Gibson, E.L., Sapochnik, M., Sheiham A., & Lawson, M. (2004). Demographic, familial and trait predictors of fruit and vegetable consumption by pre-school children. *Public Health Nutrition, 7*(2), 295–302.

Cooley, W.C., and the Committee on Children with Disabilities. (2004). Providing a primary care medical home for children and youth with cerebral palsy. *Pediatrics, 114,* 1106–1113.

Cooper-Brown, L., Copeland, S., Dailey, S., Downey, D., Petersen, M.C., Stimson, C., & Van Dyke, D.C. (2008). Feeding and swallowing dysfunction in genetic syndromes. *Developmental Disabilities, 14,* 147–157.

Corbett, K.S. (2000). Explaining infant feeding style of low-income Black women. *Journal of Pediatric Nursing, 15*(2), 73–81.

Core, J. (2003). Nutrition's role in feeding children's brains. *Agricultural Research, 51*(12), 15–17.

Cornish, E. (1998). A balanced approach towards healthy eating in autism. *Journal of Human Nutrition and Dietetics, 11,* 501–509.

Cornish, E. (2002). Gluten and casein free diets in autism: A study of the effects on food choice and nutrition. *Journal of Human Nutrition and Dietetics, 15,* 261–269.

Cowart, B. (1981). Development of taste perception in humans: Sensitivity and preferences throughout the lifespan. *Psychological Bulletin, 90,* 43–73.

Cowart, B., & Beauchamp, G.K. (1986). Factors affecting acceptance of salt by human infants and children. In M.R. Kare & J.G. Brand (Eds.), *Interaction of the chemical senses and nutrition* (pp. 25–44). New York, NY: Academic Press.

Craig, G.M., Carr, L.J., Cass, H., Hastings, R.P., Lawson, M., Reilly, S.,...Spitz, L. (2006). Medical, surgical, and health outcomes of gastrostomy feeding. *Developmental Medicine & Child Neurology, 48,* 353–360.

Craig, G.M., Scambler, G., & Spitz, L. (2003). Why parents of children with neurodevelopmental disabilities requiring gastrostomy feeding need more support. *Developmental Medicine & Child Neurology, 45,* 183–188.

Crist, W., Dobbelsteyn, M., Brousseau, A.M., & Napier-Phillips, A.N. (2004). Pediatric Assessment Scale for Severe Feeding Problems: Validity and reliability of a new scale for tube-fed children. *Nutrition in Clinical Practice, 19*(4), 403–408.

Crist, W., & Napier-Phillips, A. (2001). Mealtime behaviors of young children: A comparison of normative and clinical data. *Journal of Developmental and Behavioral Pediatrics, 22*(5), 279–286.

Crockenberg, S., & Leerkes, E. (2005). Infant social and emotional development in family context. In C.H. Zeanah (Ed.), *Handbook of infant mental health* (2nd ed., pp. 60–90). New York, NY: Guilford Press.

Dailey Hall, K. (2001). *Pediatric dysphagia: Resource guide.* Clifton Park, NY: Delmar/Cengage Learning.

Daley Hall, K., & Kennedy, C.M. (2000). Meta analysis: Effects of interventions on premature infants feeding. *Journal of Perinatal and Neonatal Nursing, 14*(3), 62–77.

Damiano, P., Tyler, M., Romitti, P.A., Druschel, C., Austin, A.A., Burnett, W., ... Robbins, J.M. (2009). Demographic characteristics, care, and outcomes for children with oral clefts in three states using participants from the National Birth Defects Prevention study. *Cleft Palate-Craniofacial Journal, 46*(6), 575–582.

Daniel, M., Kleis, L., & Cemeroglu, A.P. (2008). Etiology of failure to thrive in infants and toddlers referred to a pediatric endocrinology outpatient clinic. *Clinical Pediatrics, 47*(8), 762–765.

Darrow, D.H., & Harley, C.M. (1998). Evaluation of swallowing disorders in children. *Otolaryngologic Clinics of North America, 31*(3), 405–418.

Davis, C.M. (1939). Results of the self-selection of diets by young children. *Canadian Medical Association Journal, 41,* 257–261.

Dawson, J.E., Piazza, C.C., Sevin, B.M., Gulotta, C.S., Lerman, D., & Kelley, M. (2003). Use of the high-p instructional sequence and escape extinction in a child with a feeding disorder. *Journal of Applied Behavior Analysis, 36,* 105–108.

de Vries, J.I., Visser, G.H., & Prechtl, H.F. (1982). The emergence of fetal behavior: Qualitative aspects. *Early Human Development, 7,* 301–322.

DeMatteo, C., Matovich, D., & Hjartarson, A. (2005). Comparison of clinical and videofluoroscopic evaluation of children with feeding and swallowing difficulties. *Developmental Medicine & Child Neurology, 47,* 149–157.

Denham, S.A. (2003). Relationships between family rituals, family routines, and health. *Journal of Family Nursing, 9*(3), 305–330.

Dennis, C L. (2002). Breastfeeding initiation and duration: A 1990–2000 literature review. *Journal of Obstetric, Gynecologic, and Neonatal Nursing, 31,* 12–32.

Department of Child and Family Services. (2010). *Licensing standards for daycare centers.* Retrieved from http://www.state.il.us/dcfs/docs/407.pdf

Derkay, C.S., & Schechter, G.L. (1998). Anatomy and physiology of pediatric swallowing disorders. *Otolaryngologic Clinics of North America, 31*(3), 397–404.

Dettwyler, K.A. (1989). Styles of infant feeding: Parental/caretaker control of food consumption in young children. *American Anthropologist, 91,* 696–703.

Dettwyler, K.A., & Fishman, C. (1992). Infant feeding practices and growth. *Annual Review of Anthropology, 27,* 171–204.

Devaney, B., & Fox, M.K. (2008). Dietary intakes of infants and toddlers: Problems start early. In L. Birch & W. Dietz (Eds.), *Eating behaviors of the young child: Prenatal and postnatal influences on healthy eating* (pp. 59–68). Elk Grove Village, IL: American Academy of Pediatrics.

Dewey, K.G. (2008). Breastfeeding and other infant feeding practices that may influence child obesity. In L. Birch & W. Dietz (Eds.), *Eating behaviors of the young child: prenatal and postnatal influences on healthy eating.* (pp. 69–93). Elk Grove Village, IL: American Academy of Pediatrics.

Dewey, K.G., Heinig, M.J., & Nommsen, L.A. (1993). Maternal weight-loss patterns during prolonged lactation. *American Journal of Clinical Nutrition, 58,* 162–166.

DeWitt, S.J., Sparks, J.W., Swank, P.B., Smith, K., Denson, S.E., & Landry, S.H. (1997). Physical growth of low birthweight infants in the first year of life: Impact of maternal behaviors. *Early Human Development, 47*(3), 19–34.

Dibley, M.J., Roy, S.K., Senarath, U., Patel, A., Tiwari, K., Agho, K.E., & Mihrshahi, S. (2010). Across-country comparisons of selected infant and young child feeding indicators and associated factors in four South Asian countries. *Food and Nutrition Bulletin, 31*(2), 366–374.

Dibley, M.J., Senarath, U., & Agho, K. (2010). Infant and young child feeding indicators across nine East and Southeast Asian countries: An analysis of National Data 2000–2005. *Public Health Nutrition, 13*(9), 1296–1303.

Didden, R., Seys, D., & Schouwink, D. (1999). Treatment of chronic food refusal in a young developmentally disable child. *Behavioral Interventions, 14,* 213–222.

Dietz, W.H. (2001). Breastfeeding may help prevent child overweight. *Journal of the American Medical Association, 285*(19), 2506–2507. doi: 10.1001/jama.285.19.2506

Dix, T. (1991). The affective organization of parenting: Adaptive and maladaptive processes. *Psychological Bulletin, 110*(3), 25.

Dodgson, J.E., & Struthers, R. (2003). Traditional breastfeeding practices of the Ojubwe of Northern Minnesota. *Health Care for Women International, 24,* 49–61.

Donato, J., Fox, C., Mormon, J., & Mormon, M. (2008). Feeding & motor functioning: Start at the hips to get to the lips. *Exceptional Parent, 38*(6), 64–66.

Dong, D., & Lin, B-H. (2009). *Fruit and vegetable consumption by low-income Americans: Would a price reduction make a difference?* Economic Research Report, 70. Department of Agriculture, Economic Research Service.

Douglas, J. (2000). Behavioural approaches to the assessment and management of feeding problems in young children. In A. Southall & A. Schwartz (Eds.), *Feeding problems in children* (pp. 41–57). Abingdon, UK: Radcliffe Medical Press.

Dovey, T.M., Farrow, C.V., Martin, C.I., Isherwood, E., & Halford, J.C.G. (2009). When does food refusal require professional intervention? *Current Nutrition & Food Science, 5,* 160–171.

Drobynk, W., & Rocco, K. (2011). Collaboration between school, family, and occupational therapy coaches to restore oral feeding skills in a young child. *Exceptional Parent, 41*(2), 10–11.

Dubignon, J., & Campbell, D. (1969). Sucking in the newborn during a feed. *Journal of Experimental Child Psychology, 7,* 282–298.

Duca, A.P., Dantas, R.O., Rodrigues, A.A.C., & Sawamura, R. (2008). Evaluation of swallowing in children with vomiting after feeding. *Dysphagia, 23,* 177–182.

Dunn, W. (1997a). Supporting children to participate successfully in everyday life by using sensory processing knowledge. *Infants and Young Children, 20*(2), 84-101, 23–35.

Dunn, W. (1997b). The impact of sensory processing abilities on the daily lives of young children and their families: A conceptual model. *Infants and Young Children, 9*(4), 23–35.

Dunn, W. (2001). The sensations of everyday life: Empirical, theoretical, and pragmatic considerations. *American Journal of Occupational Therapy, 55,* 608–620.

Dunn, W. (2002). *The Infant/Toddler Sensory Profile manual.* San Antonio, TX: The Psychological Corporation.

Dunn, W. (2007). Supporting children to participate successfully in everyday life by using sensory processing knowledge. *Infants & Young Children, 20*(2), 81–101.

Dunn, W., & Daniels, D. (2002). *Infant/Toddler Sensory Profile: Caregiver Questionnaire.* San Antonio, TX: Pearson.

Dunn, W., & Westman, K. (1997). The sensory profile: The performance of a national sample of children without disabilities. *American Journal of Occupational Therapy, 51*(1), 25–34.

Dunne, L., Sneddon, H., Iwaniec, D., & Stewart, M.C. (2007). Maternal mental health and faltering growth in infants. *Child Abuse Review, 16*(5), 283–295.

Dutton, G.N., & Jacobson, L.K. (2001). Cerebral visual impairment in children. *Seminars in Neonatology, 6,* 477–485.

Dykes, F., Moran, V.H., Burt, S., & Edwards, J. (2003). Adolescent mothers and breastfeeding: Experiences and support needs: An exploratory study. *Journal of Human Lactation 19,* 391–401.

Economic Research Service (ERS)/USDA. (2002). Major uses of Land in the United States Cropland. *EIP*-14, 12–21.

Edmondson, R., & Reinbartsen, D. (1998). The young child with cleft lip and palate: Intervention needs in the first three years. *Infants & Young Children, 11*(2), 12–20.

Eigenmann, P.A., & Sampson, H.A. (1998). Interpreting skin prick tests in the evaluation of food allergy in children. *Pediatric Allergy and Immunology, 9*(4), 186–191.

Einarsson-Backes, L.M., Deitz, J., Price, R., Glass, R., & Hays, R. (1993). The effect of oral support on sucking efficiency in preterm infants. *American Journal of Occupational Therapy, 48*, 490–498.

Eisenberg, M.E., Olson, R.E., Neumark-Sztainer, D., Story, M., & Bearinger, L.H. (2004). Correlations between family meals and psychosocial well-being among adolescents. *Archives of Pediatrics and Adolescent Medicine, 158*, 792–796.

Elder, J.H. v(2008). The gluten-free, casein-free diet in autism: An overview with clinical implications. *Nutrition in Clinical Practice, 23*(6), 583–588.

Elder, J.H., Shankar, M., Shuster, J., Theriaque, D., Burns, S., & Sherrill, L. (2006). The gluten-free, casein-free diet in autism: Results of a preliminary double blind clinical trial. *Journal of Autism and Developmental Disorders, 36*(3), 413–420.

Eliassen, E.K. (2011). The impact of teachers and families on young children's eating behaviors. *Young Children, 66*(2), 84–89.

Epstein, L.H., Gordy, C.C., Raynor, H.A., Beddome, M., Kilanowski, C.K., & Paluch, R. (2001). Increasing fruit and vegetable intake and decreasing fat and sugar intake in families at risk for childhood obesity. *Obesity Research, 9*(3), 171–178.

Epstein, L.H., Myers, M.D., Raynor, H.A., & Saelens, B.E. (1998). Treatment of pediatric obesity. *Pediatrics, 101*, 554–570.

Ermer, J., & Dunn, W. (1998). The Sensory Profile: The performance of a national sample of children with and without disabilities. *American Journal of Occupational Therapy, 52*(4), 283–289.

Faith M.S., Scanlon, K.S., Birch, L.L., Francis, L.A., & Sherry, B. (2004). Parent-child feeding strategies and their relationships to child eating and weight status. *Obesity Research, 12*, 1711–1722.

Faith, M.S., Storey, M., Kral, T.V., & Pietrobelli, A. (2008). The Feeding Demands Questionnaire: Assessment of parental demand cognitions concerning parent-child feeding relations. *Journal of the American Dietetic Association, 108*(4), 624–630.

Farm and Food Policy Project. (2007). Making Healthy Food more accessible for low-income people. Retrieved from www.farmandfoodproject.org/

Fazzi, E., Signorini, S.G., Bova, S.M., La Piana, R., Ondei, P., Bertone, C., ... Bianchi, P.E. (2007). Spectrum of visual disorders in children with cerebral visual impairment. *Journal of Child Neurology, 22*(3), 294–301.

Fein, S.B., Bidisha, M., & Roe, B.E. (2008). Success of strategies for combining employment and breast-feeding. *Pediatrics, 122*, S56–S62. doi:10.1542/peds.2008-1315g

Field, D., Garland, M., & Wiliams, K. (2003). Correlates of specific childhood feeding problems. *Journal of Paediatrics and Child Health, 39*(4), 299–304.

Field, T.M. (2001). Massage therapy facilitates weight gain in preterm infants. *Current Directions in Psychological Science, 10*, 51–55.

Field, T.M., Hernandez-Reif, M., & Freedman, J. (2004). Stimulation programs for preterm infants. *SRCD Social Policy Reports, XVIII (No. 1)*, 1–20.

Fiese, B.H., & Schwartz, M. (2008). Reclaiming the family table: Mealtimes and child health and wellbeing. *Society for Research in Child Development, 22*(4). 1–20.

Fiese, B.H., Foley, K.P., & Spagnola, M. (2006). Routine and ritual elements in family mealtimes: Contexts for child well-being and family identity. *New Directions for Child and Adolescent Development, 111*, 67–89. doi: 10.1002/cad

Finnbogadóttir, H., Crang Svalenius, E., & Persson, E. (2003). Expectant first-time fathers' experiences of pregnancy. *Midwifery, 19*(2), 96–105.

Fischer, E., & Silverman, A. (2007). Behavioral conceptualization, assessment, and treatment of pediatric feeding disorders. *Seminars in Speech & Language, 28*(3), 223–231.

Fisher, W.W., Piazza, C.C., Bowman, L.G., Kurtz, P.F., Sherer, M.R., & Lachman, S.R. (1994). A preliminary evaluation of empirically derived consequences for the treatment of pica. *Journal of Applied Behavior Analysis, 27*(3), 447–457.

Flammarion, S., Santos, C., Guimber, D., Jouannic, L., Thumerelle, C., Gottrand, F., & Deschildre, A. (2011). Diet and nutritional status of children with food allergies. *Pediatric Allergy and Immunology, 22*, 161–165.

Flanagan, M.A. (2008). *Improving speech and eating skills in children with autism spectrum disorders: An oral-motor program for home and school*. Shawnee Mission, KS: Autism Asperger.

Flidel-Rimon, O., & Shinwell, E. (2002). Breastfeeding multiples. *Seminars in Neonatology, 7*, 231–239. doi:10.1053/siny.2002.0110

Fomon, S.J. (1993). *Nutrition of normal infants*. St. Louis, MO: Mosby-Year.

Food and Nutrition Service. (2011). About WIC. USDA. Retrieved from http://www.fns.usda.gov/wic/aboutwic/

Ford, R.P.K., Taylor, B.J., Mitchell, E.A., Enright, S.A., Stewart, A.W., Becroft, D.M.O., & Roberts, A.P. (1993). Breastfeeding and the risk of sudden infant death syndrome. *International Journal of Epidemiology, 22*, 885–890.

Forestell, C.A., & Mennella, J.A. (2007). Food, folklore, and flavor preference development. In C. J. Lammi-Keefe, S.C. Couch, & E.H. Philipson (Eds.), *Nutrition and Health: Handbook of Nutrition and Pregnancy* (pp. 55–64). Totowa, NJ: Humana Press.

Forste, R., Weiss, J., & Lippincott, E. (2001). The decision to breastfeed in the United States: Does race matter? *Pediatrics, 108*(2), 291–296.

Forsyth, B.W., & Canny, P.F. (1991). Perceptions of vulnerability 3½ years after problems of feeding and crying behavior in early infancy. *Pediatrics, 88*, 757–763.

Fox, M.K., Pac, S., Devaney, B., & Jankowski, L. (2004). Feeding infants and toddlers study: What foods are infants and toddlers eating? *Journal of the American Dietetic Association, 104* (Suppl.1), 22–30.

Fraker, C., & Walbert, L. (2003). *From NICU to childhood: Evaluation and treatment of pediatric feeding disorders*. Austin, TX: PRO-ED.

France, L. (2007). Does baby formula have to be warmed up? *Babycenter*. Retrieved from http://www.babycenter.com/404_does-baby-formula-have-to-be-warmed-up_7260.bc

Friend, M., & Cook, L. (2009). *Interactions: Collaboration skills for school professionals*. (6th ed.). Boston, MA: Pearson.

Fucile, S., & Gisel, E.G. (2010). Sensorimotor interventions improve growth and motor function in preterm infants. *Neonatal Network, 29*(6), 359–366.

Fucile, S., Gisel, E., & Lau, C. (2002). Oral stimulation accelerates the transition from tube to oral feeding in preterm infants. *The Journal of Pediatrics, 141*(2), 230–236.

Fucile, S., Gisel, E.G., & Lau, C. (2005). Effect of an oral stimulation program on sucking skill maturation of preterm infants. *Developmental Medicine & Child Neurology, 47*(3), 158–162.

Fulton, D.R. (2000). Shaken baby syndrome. *Critical Care Nursing Quarterly, 23*(2), 43–50.

Fung, C., Khong, P., To, R., Goh, W., & Wong, V. (2004). Video-fluoroscopic study of swallowing in children with neurodevelopmental disorders. *Pediatrics International, 46*(1), 26–30.

Fung, E.B., Samson-Fung, L., Stallings, V.A., Conaway, M., Liptak, G., Henderson, R.C., ... Stevenson, R.D. (2002). Feeding dysfunction is associated with poor growth and health status in children with cerebral palsy. *Journal of the American Dietetic Association, 102,* 361–368, 373.

Furstenberg, F.F., Jr., & Brooks-Gunn, J. (1986). Teenage childbearing: Causes, consequences and remedies. In L. Aiken & D. Mechanic (Eds.), *Applications of social science to clinical medicine and health policy* (pp. 307–334). New Brunswick, NJ: Rutgers University Press.

Furuno, S., O'Reilly, K.A., Hosaka, C.M., Inatsuka, T.T., Zeisloft-Falbey, B., & Allman, T. (1988). *Hawaii Early Learning Profile.* Palo Alto, CA: VORT.

Futagi, Y. (2006). Neurodevelopmental outcome in children with intraventricular hemorrhage. *Pediatric Neurology, 34*(3), 219–224.

Gaebler, C.P., & Hanzlik, J.R. (1996). The effects of a prefeeding stimulation program on preterm infants. *American Journal of Occupational Therapy, 50,* 184–192.

Garcez, L.W., & Giugliani, E.R.J. (2005). Population-based study on the practice of breastfeeding in children born with cleft lip and palate. *Cleft Palate–Craniofacial Journal, 42*(6), 687–693.

Garcia, J.M., Chambers, E., Matta, Z., & Clark, M. (2005). Viscosity measurements of nectar- and honey-thick liquids: Product, liquid, and time comparisons. *Dysphagia, 20,* 325–335.

Gartner, L.M., Morton, J., Lawrence, R.A., Naylor, A.J., O'Hare, D., Schanler, R.J., ... American Academy of Pediatrics Section on Breastfeeding. (2005). Breastfeeding and the use of human milk. *Pediatrics, 115*(2), 496–506.

Gdalevich, M., Mimouni, D., & Mimouni, M. (2001). Breastfeeding and the risk of bronchial asthma in childhood: a systematic review with meta-analysis of prospective studies. *Journal of Pediatrics, 139,* 261–266.

Ghasia, F., Brunstrom, J., Gordon, M., & Tychsen, L. (2008). Frequency and severity of visual, sensory and motor deficits in children with cerebral palsy: Gross Motor Function Classification Scale. *Investigative Ophthalmology & Visual Science, 49*(2), 572–580.

Gilliam, J., & Laney, S. (2008). A Look at Your Child's Nutrition. *In Nutrition screening for infants and young children with special health care needs* (pp. 12–13). Spokane County, Washington, WA: Washington State Department of Health. Retrieved from http://www.doh.wa.gov/cfh/mch/documents/SpokaneScreen.pdf

Gillman, M.W., Rifas-Shiman, S.L., Camargo, C.A., Jr., Berkey, C.S., Frazier, A.L., Rockett, H.R.H., ... Colditz, G.A. (2001). Risk of overweight among adolescents who were breastfed as infants. *Journal of the American Medical Association, 285*(19), 2461–2467.

Giovannini, M., Riva, E., Banderali, G., Scaglioni, S., Beehof, S.H.E., Sala, M., ... Agostoni, C. (2004). Feeding practices of infants through the first year of life in Italy. *Acta Paediatrica, 93,* 492–497.

Girolami, P.A., & Scotti, J.R. (2001). Use of analog functional analysis in determining the function of mealtime behavior problems. *Education and Training in Mental Retardation and Developmental Disabilities, 36,* 207–223.

Gisel, E.G. (1994). Oral-motor skills following sensorimotor intervention in the moderately eating-impaired child with cerebral palsy. *Dysphagia, 9,* 180–192.

Gisel, E.G., & Alphonce, E. (1995). Classification of eating impairments based on eating efficiency in children with cerebral palsy. *Dysphagia, 10,* 268–274.

Gisel, E.G., Applegate-Ferrante, T., Benson, J., & Bosma, J.F. (1996). Oral motor skills following sensorimotor therapy in two groups of moderately dysphagic children with cerebral palsy: Aspiration vs. nonaspiration. *Dysphagia, 11,* 59–71.

Gisel, E.G., Birnbaum, R., & Schwartz, S. (1998). Feeding impairments in children: Diagnosis and effective intervention. *International Journal of Orofacial Myology, 24,* 27–33.

Gisel, E.G., Tessler, M., Lapierre, G., Seidman, E., Drouin, E., & Filion, G. (2003). Feeding management of children with severe cerebral palsy and eating impairment: An exploratory study. *Physical & Occupational Therapy in Pediatrics, 23*(2), 19–44.

Glass, R.P., & Wolf, L.S. (1999). Feeding management of infants with cleft lip and palate and micrognathia. *Infants & Young Children, 12*(1), 70–81.

Goldfarb, L. (2011). Breastfeeding, adoption, and surrogacy FAQ page. *CreatingAFamily.org.* Retrieved from: http://www.creatingafamily.org/component/search/index.php?option=com_content&view=article&id=522:breastfeeding-faq-page&catid=51:adoption-resourse

Gonzalez-Cossio, T., Rivera-Dommarco, J., Moreno-Macias, H., Monterrubio, E., & Sepulveda, J. (2006). Poor compliance with appropriate feeding practices in children under 2 years in Mexico. *The Journal of Nutrition,136,* 2928–2933.

Good, W.V., Jan, J.E., Burden, S.K., Skoczenski, A., & Candy, R. (2001). Recent advances in cortical visual impairment. *Developmental Medicine & Child Neurology, 43,* 56–60.

Gordon, H.J., Kang, M.S.Y., Cho, P., & Sucher, K.P. (2000). Dietary habits and health beliefs of Korean–Americans in the San Francisco Bay area. *Journal of the American Dietetic Association, 100*(10), 1198–1231.

Grandin, T. (1995). *Thinking in pictures and other reports from my life with autism.* New York, NY: Random House.

Grassley, J., & Eschiti, V. (2007). Two generations learning together: Facilitating grandmothers' support of breastfeeding. *International Journal of Childbirth Education, 22*(3), 23–26.

Gray, L., Miller, L.W., Phillip, B.L, & Blass, E.M. (2002). Breastfeeding is analgesic in healthy newborns. *Pediatrics, 109,* 590–593.

Greer, A.J., Gulotta, C.S., Masler, E.A., & Laud, R.B. (2008). Caregiver stress and outcomes of children with pediatric feeding disorders treated in an intensive interdisciplinary program. *Journal of Pediatric Psychology, 33*(6), 612–620.

Greer, F.R. (2001). Feeding the premature infant in the 20th century. *Journal of Nutrition, 131,* 426S–430S.

Greer, R.R., Sicherer, S., Burks, A.W., & the Committee on Nutrition and Section on Allergy and Immunology. (2008). Effects of early nutritional interventions on the development of atopic disease in infants and children: The role of maternal dietary restriction, breast feeding, timing of introduction of complementary foods, and hydrolyzed formulas. *Pediatrics, 121,* 183–191.

Grisham-Brown, J., & Pretti-Frontczak, K. (2003). Using planning time to individualize instruction for preschoolers with special needs. *Journal of Early Intervention, 26*(1), 31–46.

Grisham-Brown, J., Pretti-Frontczak, K., Hemmeter, M.L., & Ridgley, R. (2002). Teaching IEP goals and objectives in the context of classroom routines and activities. *Young Exceptional Children, 6*(1), 18–27.

Gromada, K.K., & Spangler, A.K. (1998). Breastfeeding twins and higher-order multiples. *Journal of Obstetric, Gynecologic, & Neonatal Nursing, 27*(4), 441–449.

Gross, S.J. (1983). Growth and biochemical response of preterm infants fed human milk or modified infant formula. *New England Journal of Medicine, 308,* 237–241.

Grulee, C.G. (1912). *Infant feeding.* Philadelphia, PA: Sanders.

Grummer-Strawn, L.M., & Mei, Z. (2004). Does breastfeeding protect against pediatric overweight? Analysis of longitudinal data from the Centers for Disease Control and Prevention Pediatric Nutrition Surveillance System. *Pediatrics, 113*(2), e81–e86. www.pediatrics.org/cgi/content/full/113/2/e81

Grummer-Strawn, L.M., & Shealy, K. (2009). Progress in protecting, promoting, and supporting breastfeeding: 1984–2009. *Breastfeeding Medicine, 4,* S31–S39.

Gryboski, J.D. (1969). Suck and swallow in the premature infant. *Pediatrics, 43,* 96–102.

Guenther, P.M., Dodd, K.W., Reedy, J., & Krebs-Smith, S.M. (2006). Most Americans eat much less than recommended amounts of fruits and vegetables. *Journal of American Dietetic Association, 106,* 1371–1379.

Gunderson, C., Lohman, B.J., Garasky, S., Stewart, S., & Eisenmann, J. (2008). Good security, maternal stressors, and overweight among low-income U.S. children: Results from the National Health and Nutrition Examination Survey (1999–2002). *Pediatrics, 122,* e529–e540.

Guralnick, M. J., & Conlon, C. (2007). Early intervention. In M. Batshaw, L. Pelligrino, & N. Roizen (Eds.), *Children with disabilities* (6th ed., pp. 511–521). Baltimore, MD: Paul H. Brookes Publishing Co.

Gutentag, S., & Hammer, D. (2000). Shaping oral feeding in a gastronomy tube–dependent child in natural settings. *Behavior Modification, 24*(3), 395–410.

Gutierrez, F.L., Clements, P.T., & Averill, J. (2004). Shaken baby syndrome: Assessment, intervention and prevention. *Journal of Psychosocial Nursing, 42*(12), 22–29.

Guyer, B., Hoyert, D.L., Martin, J.A., Ventura, S.J., MacDorman, M.F., & Strobino, D.M. (1999). Annual summary of vital statistics – 1998. *Pediatrics, 104,* 1229–1246.

Haddad, J., & Prestigiacomo, C. (1995). Otolaryngology considerations. In S.R. Rosenthal, J.J. Sheppard, & M. Lotz (Eds.), *Dysphagia and the child with developmental disabilities* (pp. 209–225). San Diego, CA: Singular.

Hane, A.A., Fox, N.A., Polak-Toste, C., Ghera, M.M., & Guner, B.M. (2006). Ordinary variations in maternal caregiving influence human infants' stress reactivity. *Developmental Psychology, 42,* 1077–1088.

Hannon, P.R., Willis, S.K., Bishop-Townsend, V., Martinez, I.M., & Scrimshaw, S.C. (2000). African-American and Latina adolescent mothers' infant feeding decisions and breastfeeding practices: A qualitative study. *Journal of Adolescent Health, 26,* 399–407.

Harry, B. (2008a). Collaboration with culturally and linguistically diverse families: Ideal versus reality. *Exceptional Children, 74*(3), 372–388.

Harry, B. (2008b). *Melanie: Bird with a broken wing: A mother's story.* Baltimore, MD: Paul H. Brookes Publishing Co.

Hayes, C. (2002). Environmental risk factors and oral clefts. In D.F. Wysznski (Ed.), *Cleft lip and palate: From origin to treatment* (pp. 159–169). New York, NY: Oxford University Press.

Heinig, M.J. (2001). Host defense benefits of breastfeeding for the infant. Effect of breastfeeding duration and exclusivity. *Pediatric Clinics of North American, 48,* 105–123.

Heise, D. (2002). Hispanic American Influence on the U. S. Food Industry. USDA, Agricultural Research Service. Retrieved from http://www.nal.usda.gov/outreach/HFood.html

Hendy, H.M. (1999). Comparison of five teacher actions to encourage children's new food acceptance. *Annals of Behavioral Medicine, 21*(1), 20–26.

Hill, A.S., Kurkowski, T.B., & Garcia, J. (2000). Oral support measures used in feeding the preterm infant. *Nursing Research, 49,* 2–10.

Hoch, T.A., Babbitt, R.L., Coe, D.A., Krell, D.M., & Hackbert, L. (1994). Contingency contacting: Combining positive reinforcement and escape extinction procedures to treat persistent food refusal. *Behavior Modification, 18,* 106–128.

Hodges, E.A., Houck, G.M., & Kindermann, T. (2009). Validity of the Nursing Child Assessment Feeding Scale during toddlerhood. *Western Journal of Nursing Research, 31,* 662–678.

Hodgkinson, P.D., Brown, S., Duncan, D., Grant, C., McNaughton, A., Thomas, P., & Mattick, C.R. (2005). Management of children with cleft lip and palate: Describing the application of multidisciplinary team working in this condition based upon the experiences of a regional cleft lip and palate centre in the United Kingdom. *Fetal and Maternal Medicine Review, 16*(1), 1–27.

Holland, M., & Murray, P. (2004). Diet and nutrition. In B.L. Lucas, S.A. Feucht, & L.E. Grieger (Eds.), *Children with special health care needs: Nutrition care handbook* (pp. 23–57). Chicago, IL: American Dietetic Association.

Homer, E.M. (2003). An interdisciplinary team approach to providing dysphagia treatment in the schools. *Seminars in Speech and Language, 24,* 215–234.

Horne, R.S., Parslow, P.M., Ferens, D., Watts, A.M., & Adamson, T.M. (2004). Comparison of evoked arousability in breast and formula fed infants. *Archives of Disease in Childhood, 89*(1), 22–25.

Horner, E.M., Bickerton, C., Hill, S., Parham, L., & Taylor, D. (2000). Development of an interdisciplinary dysphagia team in the public schools. *Language, Speech, and Hearing Services in Schools, 31,* 62–75.

Høst, A., Andrae, S., Charkin, S., Diaz-Vazquez, C., Dreborg, S., Eigenmann, P.A., … Wickman, M. (2003). Allergy testing in children: Why, who, when and how? *Allergy, 58,* 559–569.

Houck, G.M., & Spegman, A.M. (1999). *Snack coding manual.* Unpublished manuscript. Portland, OR: Oregon Health & Science University.

Houghton, M.D., & Graybeal, T.E. (2001). Breastfeeding practices of Native American mothers participating in WIC. *Journal of the American Dietetic Association, 101*(2), 245–247.

Howie, P.W., Forsyth, J.S., Ogston, S.A, Clark, A., & Florey, C.D. (1990). Protective effect of breast feeding against infection. *British Medical Journal, 300,* 11–16.

Huber, C.J. (1991). Documenting quality of parent-child interaction: Use of the NCAST Scales. *Infants & Young Children, 4*(2), 63–75.

Hughes, D. (2006). *Building the bonds of attachment: Awakening love in deeply troubled children* (2nd ed.). Lanham, MD: Aronson.

Hughes, S.O., Power, T.G., Fisher, J.O., Mueller, S., & Nicklas, T.A. (2005). Revisiting a neglected construct: Parenting Styles in a child feeding context. *Appetite, 44,* 83–92.

Huh, S., Rifas-Shiman, S.L., Taveras, E.M., Oken, E., & Gillman, M.W. (2011). Timing of solid food introduction and risk of obesity in preschool-aged children. *Pediatrics, 127*(3), e544-e551. doi: 10.1542/peds.2010-0740

Hunt, F. (2007). Changing from oral to enteral feeding: Impact on families of children with disabilities. *Paediatric Nursing, 19*(7), 30–32.

Hyman, P.E. (1994). Gastroesophageal reflux: One reason why baby won't eat. *The Journal of Pediatrics, 125*(6), Part 2, S103–S109.

Individuals with Disabilities Education Improvement Act Amendments of 2004, Pub. L. No. 108–446, U.S.C. 20 § 1400 et seq.

Isaacs, J.S. (2004). Non-oral enteral feeding. In B.L. Lucas, S.A. Feucht, & L.E. Grieger (Eds.), *Children with special health care needs: Nutrition care handbook* (pp. 87–102). Chicago, IL: American Dietetic Association.

Jacobi, C., Agras, W.S., Bryson, S., & Hammer, L.D. (2003). Behavioral validation, precursors, and concomitants of picky eating in childhood. *Journal of the American Academy of Child and Adolescent Psychiatry, 42*(1), 76–84.

Jadcherla, S.R., & Shaker, R. (2001). Esophageal and upper esophageal sphincter motor function in babies. *American Journal of Medicine, 111*(Suppl 8A), 64S–68S.

Jana, L.A., & Shu, J. (2008). *Food fights: Winning the nutritional challenges of parenthood armed with insight, humor and a bottle of ketchup.* Elk Grove Village, IL: American Academy of Pediatrics.

Jelm, J.M. (1990). *Oral-Motor Feeding Rating Scale.* San Antonio, TX: Pearson.

Jernstrom, H., Lubinski, J., Lynch, H.T., Ghadirian, P., Neuhausen, S., Issacs, C., & Narood, S.A. (2004). Breastfeeding and the risk of breast cancer in BRCA1 and BRCA2 mutation carriers. *Journal of the National Cancer Institute, 96,* 1094–1098.

Jiang, M., Foster, E.M., Gibson-Davis, C.M. (2010). The effect of WIC on breastfeeding: A new look at an established relationship. *Children and Youth Services Review, 32,* 264–273. doi:10.1016/j.childyouth.2009.09.005

Johansson, B., & Ringsberg, K.C. (2004). Parents' experiences of having a child with cleft lip and palate. *Journal of Advanced Nursing, 47,* 165–173.

Johnson, C.R., Handen, B.L., Mayer-Costa, M., & Sacco, K. (2008). Eating habits and dietary status in young children with autism. *Journal of Developmental and Physical Disabilities, 20*(5), 437–448.

Johnson, S.L. (2000). Improving preschoolers' self-regulation of energy intake. *Pediatrics, 106,* 653–661.

Johnson, S.L. (2002). Children's food acceptance patterns: The interface of ontogeny and nutrition needs. *Nutrition Reviews, 60*(5), S91–S94.

Johnson, S.L., & Birch, L.L. (1994). Parents' and children's adiposity and eating style. *Pediatrics, 94*(5), 653–661.

Johnson, S.L., McPhee, L., & Birch, L.L. (1991). Conditioned preferences: Young children prefer flavors associated with high dietary fat. *Physiology and Behavior, 50,* 1245–1251.

Johnson, S.B., Silverstein, J., Rosenbloom, A., Carter, R., & Cunningham, W. (1986). Assessing daily management in childhood diabetes. *Health Psychology, 5,* 545–564.

Jones, K.L. (2006). *Smith's recognizable patterns of human malformation* (6th ed.). Philadelphia, PA: Elsevier/Saunders.

Jones, M.W., Morgan, E., Shelton, J.E., & Thorogood, C. (2007). Cerebral palsy: Introduction and diagnosis (Part I). *Journal of Pediatric Health Care, 21*(3), 146–152.

Jung, L.A. (2007). Writing individualized family service plan strategies that fit into the ROUTINE. *Young Exceptional Children, 10*(3), 2–9.

Jung, L.A., & Grisham-Brown, J. (2006). Moving from assessment information to IFSPs: Guidelines for a family-centered process. *Young Exceptional Children, 9*(2), 2–11.

Kaczmarek, L., Pennington, R., & Goldstein, H. (2000). Transdisciplinary consultation: A center-based team functioning model. *Education and Treatment of Children, 23,* 156–172.

Kahng, S.W., Boscoe, J.H., & Byrne, S. (2003). The use of an escape contingency and a token economy to increase food acceptance. *Applied Behavior Analysis, 36,* 349–353.

Kannan, S., Carruth, B.R., & Skinner, J. (1999). Infant feeding practices of Anglo American and Asian Indian American mothers. *Journal of the American College of Nutrition, 18*(3), 279–286.

Kanner, L. (1943). Autistic disturbances of affective contact. *Nervous Child, 2,* 217–250.

Kashinath, S., Woods, J., & Goldstein, H. (2006). Enhancing generalized teaching strategy use in daily routines by parents of children with autism. *Journal of Speech, Language, and Hearing Research, 49,* 466–485.

Kedesdy, J.H., & Budd, K.S. (1998). *Childhood feeding disorders: Biobehavioral assessment and intervention.* Baltimore, MD: Paul H. Brookes Publishing Co.

Keet, C.A., Matsui, E.C., Dhillon, G., Lenehan, P., Paterakis, M., & Wood, R.A. (2009). The natural history of wheat allergy. *Annals of Allergy, Asthma & Immunology, 102*(5), 410–415.

Kelly, J.F., & Barnard, K.E. (2000). Assessment of parent-child interaction: Implications for early intervention. In S. Meisels & J.P. Shonkoff (Eds.), *Handbook of early childhood intervention* (pp. 258–289). Cambridge, UK: Cambridge University Press.

Kennedy, K.I., Labbok, M.H., & Van Look, P.F. (1996). Lactational amenorrhea method for family planning. *International Journal of Gynaecolgoy and Obstetrics, 54,* 55–57.

Kenny, D.J., Koheil, R.M., Greenberg, J., Reid, D., Milner, M., Moran, R., & Judd, P.L. (1989). Development of a Multidisciplinary Feeding Profile for children who are dependent feeders. *Dysphagia, 4*(1), 16–28.

Kern, L., Starosta, K., & Adelman, B.E. (2006). Reducing pica by teaching children to exchange inedible items for edibles. *Behavior Modification, 30*(2), 135–158.

Kerwin, M.E. (1999). Empirically supported treatments in pediatric psychology: Severe feeding problems. *Journal of Pediatric Psychology, 24*(3), 193–214.

KidsheaIth. (2009). Formula feeding FAQs: Preparation and storage. Retrieved from: http://kidshealth.org/parent/pregnancy_newborn/formulafeed/formulafeed_storing.html

King, G., Strachan, D., Tucker, M., Duwyn, B. Desserud, S., & Shillington, M. (2009). The application of a transdisciplinary model for early intervention services. *Infants & Young Children, 22*(3), 211–223.

Kittler, P.G., & Sucher, K.P. (2008). *Food and culture* (5th ed.). Belmont, CA: Thomson Learning.

Klein, M.D. (2007a). *Tube feeding transition plateaus. Exceptional Parent, 37*(2), 22–25.

Klein, M.D. (2007b). Turn those feedings into mealtimes! *Exceptional Parent, 37*(2), 26.